Understanding Anxiety Disorders

Understanding Anxiety Disorders

Edited by **Peter Garner**

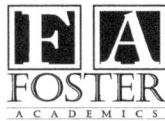

FA
FOSTER
ACADEMICS

New Jersey

Published by Foster Academics,
61 Van Reypen Street,
Jersey City, NJ 07306, USA
www.fosteracademics.com

Understanding Anxiety Disorders
Edited by Peter Garner

International Standard Book Number: 978-1-63242-469-3 (Hardback)

Printed in the United States of America.

Contents

Preface

Anxiety is the feeling of fear accompanied by nervous behavior caused by anticipation of future threat. It is generally characterized by uneasiness, worry, overreaction, somatic anxiety and rumination. Anxiety disorders can be genetic or may arise due to drug abuse. This condition might be considered appropriate if it surfaces occasionally but if it persists for a longer duration it might interfere with the mental and physical well-being of the person. The topics included in this book on anxiety disorders are of utmost significance and bound to provide incredible insights to readers. This book will also provide innovative topics for research which interested readers can take up. It will help the professionals, students and researchers in keeping pace with the rapid changes in this field.

This book unites the global concepts and researches in an organized manner for a comprehensive understanding of the subject. It is a ripe text for all researchers, students, scientists or anyone else who is interested in acquiring a better knowledge of this dynamic field.

I extend my sincere thanks to the contributors for such eloquent research chapters. Finally, I thank my family for being a source of support and help.

Editor

Evaluation of Anxiety and Depression in Caregivers of Patients Affected by Alzheimer's Disease

Anna Vespa[1]*, Maria Velia Giulietti[2], Marica Ottaviani[3], R. Spatuzzi[4], F. Merico[5], Guido Gori[6], Olimpia Claudia Rossi[3], L. Paciaroni[3], Giuseppe Pelliccioni[3], Pietro Scendoni[7], Cristina Meloni[8]

[1]Department of Neurology, INRCA-IRCCS Italian National Institute of Health and Science on Aging, Ancona, Italy
[2]Unity of Neurology, INRCA-National Institute of Health and Science on Aging, Ancona, Italy
[3]Department of Neurology, INRCA-IRCCS National Institute of Health and Science on Aging, Ancona, Italy
[4]U.O.C. Hospice/Palliative care Departments, A.O.R. San Carlo di Potenza, Italy
[5]Hospice Casa di Betania Palliative Care Center, Lecce, Italy
[6]Director Day Alzheimer Center "Le Civette", ASL-Florence, Italy
[7]Department of Rheumatology, INRCA-IRCCS National Institute of Health and Science on Aging, Fermo, Italy
[8]INRCA-IRCCS National Institute of Health and Science on Aging, Ancona, Italy
Email: *a.vespa@inrca.it, giulietti.mariavelia@libero.it, marica_O@libero.it, roberta.spatuzzi@yahoo.com, fabianamerico@yahoo.it, olimpia_rossi@hotmail.it, guigor@libero.it, g.pelliccioni@inrca.it, p.scendoni@inrca.it, melcri86@hotmail.it

Abstract

Background: Many studies have been underlined as care giving for people with Alzheimer's disease (AD) is highly stressful and has significant negative consequences, such as anxiety and depression. Objective: The specific aim of our study is to establish whether a difference exists in the prevalence of depression of family caregivers of Alzheimer's disease patients and healthy subjects not caregiver. Methods: Study group (n = 60) consists of caregivers of patients affected by Alzheimer's disease, whereas control group (n = 120) consists of healthy individuals who are not care giving (from at least 5 years). All the subjects were subdivided on the basis of the following independent variables: sex, age, marital status and educational level. The subjects of study and control groups studied have filled in the following tests: IPAT CDQ e IPAT ASQ Tests by Cattell which describe depression and anxiety. Such tests have been validated on the adult and elderly Italian population. Statistical analysis: Student t test has been applied for the comparison between experimental and control groups. Results: The caregivers show higher levels of anxiety (medium to

---

*Corresponding author.

high, P < 0.001) and depression in comparison to the group of control (medium to high, P < 0.001). This result indicates the caregiver shows serious depression. Conclusions: The high levels of depression and anxiety suggest the following considerations: interventions of social and psychological support are fundamental not only to maintain the patient in the family nucleus but also to maintain the caregiver's psychological health.

Keywords

Caregiver, Alzheimer's Disease, Anxiety, Depression

1. Introduction

The complexity of care and the constant effort make it difficult to maintain emotional balance of the caregiver and the family of a patient with Alzheimer's dementia.

The family, in fact, is still the privileged place of care for the illness of Alzheimer patient. In Italy, the caregiver is primarily a woman with a percentage up to 80% in the severe phase of illness.

The health and personal conditions of the patients and the caregivers influence the style and the quality of the care giving [1]-[4].

A progressive illness as the Alzheimer's disease leads to a profound change in the style of life of the whole family system. The changes imposed by the progression of illness set different problems in the various stadiums from a practical and organizational to the emotional point of view [3] [4]. All these can lead to the activation of new conflicts with fatigue, due to financial problems or decisions to be made. They can also reactivate ancient tensions that bring at times to definitive breakups [5]-[11].

The problematic relationship in the family system influences so much the stress of the caregiver and the quality of the daily management. The consequences invest the physical and the emotional (fatigue, scarce ability of coping) and social spheres (social isolation) [2] [5]-[17].

The deterioration of mental and physical abilities of a loved one can be for the caregiver (which has to do with behaviors related to dementia) an even bigger contributor to developing symptoms of depression. Moreover dementia- related symptoms such as wandering, agitation, hoarding and embarrassing conduct make very day challenging and make it harder for a caregiver to get rest or assistance in providing care [9] [11] [12].

In fact to assist a person with dementia can lead, therefore, to the limit the emotional resources and the caregiver can show anxious-depressive symptoms with somatic troubles that often limit the relief abilities of the caregiver [2] [5] [6] [13]-[17].

This contributes to reduce the time of permanence of the patients in the family nucleus, accelerating the appeal to live in an institution [7].

For all these reasons caregiver needs to receive psychological support [10] [12] [16]-[18].

The emotional support is a means of coping to deal with and reduce stress levels and also increases the sense of managerial competence. This promotes a caregiver emotional stability that reduces frictions and useless oppositions with positive relapses in the relationship [14] [17] [19] [20] [21].

The specific aim of our study is to establish whether a difference exists in the prevalence and depression of family caregivers of Alzheimer's disease patients and not care giving subjects. This may suggest areas of the rapeutic intervention.

2. Methods

Sampling-Choice of patients-The study groups was composed of n = 60 caregivers (male and female-age range: 40 - 75 years old; care giving from 3 to 9 years) sampled randomly from a total of 170, relatives (wife, husband, son, daughter and so on) of patients affected by Alzheimer's disease. Control group (n = 104) consists of healthy individuals who were not care giving for almost five years (**Table 1**).

The caregivers were obtained from the Alzheimer Disease Daily Center of Florence, Unity of Geriatrics in Florence Hospital the Fraticini, Florence Italy.

Table 1. Descriptive statistics of demographic variables for breast cancer patients group.

	Caregivers N = 60	Healthy Subjects N =104
Sex		
Male	34%	36%
Female	76%	74%
Age		
Range	40 - 75	40 - 75
Mean	59.96	56
Civil Status		
Single	9.30%	10.40%
Married	79.80%	77.60%
Widow	8.50%	7.50%
Divorced	2.40%	3.50%
Educational Level		
Elementary School	29.50%	28.30%
Middle School	32.90%	35.20%
High School	27.05%	26%
University	9.30%	10.30%
CDQ (mean)	6.8	3.7

All the subjects studied were subdivided on the basis of the following independent variables sex, age marital status and educational level. All the patients were affected by Dementia of Alzheimer with clinical diagnosis through Tac.

The diagnosis of Alzheimer's disease has been carried out in accordance with the criteria of the DSM-IV while its degenerative nature has been individualized following the standardized criteria NINCDS-ADRDA-Alzheimer's Criteria (specify cognitive domains) for the diagnosis of illness of Alzheimer. Particularly all the criteria have been satisfied for the diagnosis of "probable Illness of Alzheimer" (with the exception of the liquorale examination).

All the patients of this study show the level 6 of the Functional Assessment Staying Test.

The Control group was composed of n = 104 healthy subjects chosen on the basis of the same independent variables (sex, age, marital status and educational level) of the case group. There are no differences between the two study and control groups for these variables.

Inclusion criteria included age (40 - 75 yrs). Exclusion criteria included: Refusal to participate; inability to provide informed consent; previous history of depression; use of psychotropic drugs (all, included antide- pressant).

One hundred twenty threecaregivers were approached in the clinic by the physician and asked to participate in the study. All participants signed a consensus form regarding study protocol after detailed explanation by the physician at the day center for Alzheimer disease patients. Only ninety caregivers (73.17%) decided to par- ticipate and to fill out and sign the consent form. The caregiver was free to complete the questionnaire either in the center or at home. Caregivers electing to complete forms at home were given a self-addressed, stamped envelope to return the form.

Forty one patients have not responded to all the questions in the questionnaires: it was therefore decided not to consider them for the analysis. All subjects (case and control groups), were asked to complete the following psychological and psychosocial questionnaires:

1) Social schedule, which describes all demographic characteristics like sex, age, marital status, educational level and diagnosis, date of disease onset, disease severity, and so on.

2) IPAT-ASQ Test describing anxiety and IPAT-CDQ Test describing depression by Cattell [22] [23]. These

tests have been used as self report methods which describe anxiety and depression respectively. The Italian version is validated on Italian population. The range is subdivided between: 0 - 3 which indicates absence or low anxiety or depression; 4 - 7 which indicates medium and medium high level of anxiety and depression; 8 - 10 which indicates high level of depression and anxiety.

Statistical Analysis

Student's t test was employed to compare study and control group. Student's t test was used to compare the variables that measure anxiety and depression.

Statistical analyses were performed with SPSS software version 17.0. $P < 0.05$ was regarded as level of significance.

3. Results

From the comparison of Student t test between the experimental group of caregivers and the control healthy people (not care giving) a significant difference emerges for the varying anxiety ($P < 0.001$).

The caregivers of patients affected by Alzheimer disease show higher (medium high) levels of anxiety in comparison to the group of control.

From the comparison of Student t test between the experimental group of caregivers and the control healthy people not assistants of family patients a significant difference emerges for the varying depression ($P < 0.001$).

The caregivers show high level of depression instead of control group. This result means the caregiver shows serious depression (medium-high level CDQ) while the not care giving subjects show low levels of depression (CDQ).

The results show levels of anxiety and depression incaregiversmedium-high. These levels indicate the relevant issuesandaminor depression (**Table 1**).

4. Discussion

From the results it emerges that the family caregivers of Patients affected by Alzheimer disease have levels of anxiety and depression so high to indicate the presence of serious psychological problems.

Such result suggests some considerations.

To assist a person with dementia can bring the emotional resources to the limit and lead to anxious-depressive moods. So high level of depression, show that the caregiver may not be more able to assist the patients.

Implications for nursing care resulting from the results of this study consists in giving more support to caregivers in order to avoid their excessive involvement in caring and in guaranteeing educational interventions to help caregivers to manage the behavioral disturbances of the patients and to face on the depression and anxiety.

On the basis of these considerations it is fundamental to sustain caregivers adopting the following interventions to prevent the stress, the sense of uneasiness and the state of depression (de Rotrou, 2011, Ducharme, 2009; Ducharme 2011; Roth, 2005):

1) Psychological psychotherapy of support in sessions of group or individual.

The psychological support owes: a) give the possibility to elaborate the emotional reaction and integrate them; prevent or to face the levels of stress and to realize an acceptance of the illness (Roth, 2005).

In short, the purpose of the intervention of social and psychological support are as follows (Nápoles, 2010; de de Rotrou, 2011).

1) Facilitate management of the emotional conflicts and the stress connected to the degeneration of the personality of the patient (García-Alberca, 2012) and favour an emotional integration throw the elaboration and integration of the motional conflicts and the loss (Boots, 2013);

2) Give support from the social services.

These interventions are fundamental to maintain the psychological and physical health of the caregiver. In fact many studies have underlined that depression constitutes a factor of risk for the onset of various pathologies.

5. Conclusions

In conclusion this study raises a question.

The presence of high level of anxiety and depression may be markers of caregivers with a bad adaptation to the care giving conditions. Nurse practitioners can address depression through early detection and prevention (Papastavrou, 2012; Epstein-Lubo, 2012).

Further studies could highlight the importance of psychological factors and personality. These factors could be used for the planning of a psychotherapeutic intervention aimed to promote the management of stress of caregivers.

There are many studies showed that the screening for caregiver burden stress can help to identify those who are at increased risk (Mohamed, 2010).

The small sample is the limitation of the present study.

References

[1] Mohamed, S., Rosenheck, R., Lyketsos, C.G. and Schneider, L.S. (2010) Caregiver Burden in Alzheimer Disease: Cross-Sectional and Longitudinal Patient Correlates. *The American Journal of Geriatric Psychiatry*, 18, 917-927. http://dx.doi.org/10.1097/JGP.0b013e3181d5745d

[2] Schulz, R., McGinnis, K.A., Zhang, S., Martire, L.M., Hebert, R.S., Beach, Scott, R., *et al.* (2008) Dementia Patient Suffering and Caregiver Depression. *Alzheimer Disease & Associated Disorders*, 22, 170-176. http://dx.doi.org/10.1097/WAD.0b013e31816653cc

[3] Mausbach, B.T., Chattillion, E., Roepke, S.K., Ziegler, M.G., Milic, M., von Känel, R., *et al.* (2012) A Longitudinal Analysis of the Relations among Stress, Depressive Symptoms, Leisure Satisfaction, and Endothelial Function in Caregivers. *Health Psychology*, 31, 433-440. http://dx.doi.org/10.1037/a0027783

[4] García-Alberca, J.M., Cruz, B., Lara, J.P., Garrido, V., Lara, A., Gris, E. and Gonzalez-Herero, V. (2013) The Experience of Caregiving: The Influence of Coping Strategies on Behavioral and Psychological Symptoms in Patients with Alzheimer's Disease. *Aging & Mental Health*, 17, 615-622. http://dx.doi.org/10.1080/13607863.2013.765833

[5] Papastavrou, E., Charalambous, A., Tsangari, H. and Karayiannis, G. (2012) The Burdensome and Depressive Experience of Caring: What Cancer, schizopHrenia, and Alzheimer's Disease Caregivers Have in Common. *Cancer Nursing*, 35, 187-194. http://dx.doi.org/10.1097/NCC.0b013e31822cb4a0

[6] Papastavrou, E., Kalokerinou, A., Papacostas, S.S., Tsangari, H. and Sourtzi, P. (2007) Caring for a Relative with Dementia: Family Caregiver Burden. *Journal of Advanced Nursing*, 58, 446-457. http://dx.doi.org/10.1111/j.1365-2648.2007.04250.x

[7] Epstein-Lubo, G., Gaudiano, B., Darling, E., Hinckley, M., Tremont, G., Kohn, R., *et al.* (2012) Differences in Depression Severity in Family Caregivers of Hospitalized Individuals with Dementia and Family Caregivers of Outpatients with Dementia. *The American Journal of Geriatric Psychiatry*, 20, 815-819. http://dx.doi.org/10.1097/JGP.0b013e318235b62f

[8] Roth, D.L., Mittelman, M.S., Clay, O.J., Madan, A. and Haley, W.E. (2005) Changes in Social Supports as Mediators of the Impact of a Psychosocial Intervention for Spouse Caregivers of Persons with Alzheimer's Disease. *Psychology and Aging*, 20, 634- 644. http://dx.doi.org/10.1037/0882-7974.20.4.634

[9] Papastavrou, E., Tsangari, H., Karayiannis, G., Papacostas, S., Efstathiou, G. and Sourtzi, P. (2011) Caring and Coping: The Dementia Caregivers. *Aging & MentL Health*, 15, 702-711. http://dx.doi.org/10.1080/13607863.2011.562178

[10] García-Alberca, J.M., Cruz, B., Lara, J.P., Garrido, V., Gris, E., Lara, A. and Castilla, C. (2012) Disengagement Coping Partially Mediates the Relationship between Caregiver Burden and Anxiety and Depression in Caregivers of People with Alzheimer's Disease. Results from the MÁLAGA-AD Study. *Journal of Affective Disorders*, 136, 848-856. http://dx.doi.org/10.1016/j.jad.2011.09.026

[11] Watson, L.C., Lewis, C.L., Moore, C.G. and Jeste, D.V. (2011) Perceptions of Depression among Dementia Caregivers: Findings from the CATIE-AD Trial. *International Journal of Geriatric Psychiatry*, 26, 397-402. http://dx.doi.org/10.1002/gps.2539

[12] Rocca, P., Leotta, D., Liffredo, C., Mingrone, C., Sigaudo, M., Capellero, B., *et al.* (2010) Neuropsychiatric Symptoms Underlying Caregiver Stress and Insight in Alzheimer's Disease. *Dementia and Geriatric Cognitive Disorders*, 30, 57-63. http://dx.doi.org/10.1159/000315513

[13] Berger, G., Bernhardt, T., Weimer, E., Peters, J., Kratzsch, T. and Frolich, L. (2005) Longitudinal Study on the Relationship between Symptomatology of Dementia and Levels of Subjective Burden and Depression among Family Caregivers in Memory Clinic Patients. *Journal of Geriatric Psychiatry and Neurology*, 18, 119-128. http://dx.doi.org/10.1177/0891988704273375

[14] Thomas, P., Lalloué, F., Preux, P.M., Hazif-Thomas, C., Pariel, S., Inscale, P., *et al.* (2006) Dementia Patients Caregivers Quality of Life: The PIXEL Study. *International Journal of Geriatric Psychiatry*, 21, 50-56. http://dx.doi.org/10.1002/gps.1422

[15] Burgio, L., Stevens, A., Guy, D., Roth, D.L. and Haley, W.E. (2003) Impact of Two Psychosocial Interventions on White and African American Family Caregivers of Individuals with Dementia. *The Gerontologist*, **43**, 568-579. http://dx.doi.org/10.1093/geront/43.4.568

[16] Boots, L.M., de Vugt, M.E., van Knippenberg, R.J., Kempen, G.I.J.M. and Verhey, F.R.J. (2013) A Systematic Review of Internet-Based Supportive Interventions for Caregivers of Patients with Dementia. *International Journal of Geriatric Psychiatry*, **29**, 331-334. http://dx.doi.org/10.1002/gps.4016

[17] García-Alberca, J.M., Cruz, B., Lara, J.P., Garrido, V., Lara, A. and Gris, E. (2012) Anxiety and Depression Are Associated with Coping Strategies in Caregivers of Alzheimer's Disease Patients: Results from the MÁLAGA-AD Study. *International Psychogeriatrics*, **24**, 1325-1334. http://dx.doi.org/10.1017/S1041610211002948

[18] de Rotrou, J., Cantegreil, I., Faucounau, V., Wenisch, E., Chausson, C., Jegou, D., *et al.* (2011) Do Patients Diagnosed with Alzheimer's Disease Benefit from a Psycho-Educational Programme for Family Caregivers? A Randomised Controlled Study. *International Journal of Geriatric Psychiatry*, **26**, 833-842. http://dx.doi.org/10.1002/gps.2611

[19] Nápoles, A.M., Chadiha, L., Eversley, R. and Moreno-John, G. (2010) Developing Culturally Sensitive Dementia Caregiver Interventions: Are We There Yet? *American Journal of Alzheimer's Disease and Other Dementias*, **25**, 389-406. http://dx.doi.org/10.1177/1533317510370957

[20] Ducharme, F.C., Lévesque, L.L., Lachance, L.M., Kergoat, M.-J., Legault, A.J., Beaudet, L.M. and Zarit, S.H. (2011) "Learning to Become a Family Caregiver" Efficacy of an Intervention Program for Caregivers Following Diagnosis of Dementia in a Relative. *The Gerontologist*, **51**, 484- 494. http://dx.doi.org/10.1093/geront/gnr014

[21] Ducharme, F., Beaudet, L., Legault, A., Kergoat, M.-J., Lévesque, L. and Caron, C. (2009) Development of an Intervention Program for Alzheimer's Family Caregivers Following Diagnostic Disclosure. *Clinical Nursing Research*, **18**, 44-67. http://dx.doi.org/10.1177/1054773808330093

[22] Vigneau, F. and Cormier, S. (2008) The Factor Structure of the State-Trait Anxiety Inventory: An Alternative View. *Journal of Personality Assessment*, **90**, 280-285. http://dx.doi.org/10.1080/00223890701885027

[23] Ramanaiah, N.V., Franzen, M. and Schill, T. (1983) A Psychometric Study of the State-Trait Anxiety Inventory. *Journal of Personality Assessment*, **47**, 531-535. http://dx.doi.org/10.1207/s15327752jpa4705_14

Feeling Good about Teaching Mathematics: Addressing Anxiety amongst Pre-Service Teachers

Wendy Boyd[1], Alan Foster[1], Jubilee Smith[1], William Edgar Boyd[2]

[1]School of Education, Southern Cross University, Lismore, Australia
[2]School of Environment, Science & Engineering, Southern Cross University, Lismore, Australia
Email: wendy.boyd@scu.edu.au

Abstract

Research regarding pre-service teachers' attitudes towards teaching mathematics has revealed that many pre-service teachers experience high levels of mathematics anxiety about both the learning of mathematics and the teaching of the mathematics curriculum. Little is known about the particular characteristics of pre-service teachers that make them more likely to experience anxiety about mathematics in the early years. Addressing anxiety towards mathematics and the teaching of mathematics could effectively eliminate later problems in teaching. Teaching mathematics confidently is associated with teachers' beliefs about their mathematical ability, which is their mathematical self-efficacy. This paper reports on an investigation into the anxiety of first-year pre-service teachers towards their future teaching of mathematics. 223 students enrolled in a first-year mathematics unit for birth to eight years, in the Bachelor of Education of Early Childhood and Primary Education Courses attributed their beliefs about mathematics to external—their past teachers—or internal factors: that one is either good at mathematics or not. The findings highlight the need for pre-service teacher's anxiety about mathematics to be addressed within the university education classroom context so that pre-service teachers become capable and competent teachers of mathematics.

Keywords

Mathematics Anxiety; Teacher Education; Mathematical Self-Efficacy

1. Introduction

Understanding mathematics is recognised as being important in everyday life, and cuts across many professional occupations including engineering, medicine, science and education. There is a strong societal expectation that teachers themselves will be competent at mathematical skills, have a deep understanding of mathematics, and be able to teach effectively so that their students are successful in mathematics. Furthermore, it is widely accepted that having good understanding and knowledge of mathematics, and confidence in one's ability to learn mathematics, are of prime importance for teachers (Wilson, 2009). Results from the Programme for International Student Assessment, Pisa (OECD, 2010) indicate that Australia ranked significantly above the OECD average for mathematics for 65 countries, but did not score as well as Singapore, Korea, Finland and New Zealand. Mathematics is a priority area for the national curriculum in Australia and viewed as essential for providing a solid foundation in education (knowledge, skills and values) and life-long learning (ACARA, 2011). There is concern, however, that standards need to lift in mathematics education. Nobel Laureate Brian Schmidt has warned that it was important to "make sure the skill set of teachers ... is there and, if not, we need to train them up" (Schmidt, 2012).

Children need to be exposed to mathematical concepts prior to formal schooling (Lago & DiPerna, 2010), and the Early Years Learning Framework (EYLF) (DEEWR, 2009) identifies that early childhood educators need to have "a rich mathematical vocabulary to accurately describe and explain children's mathematical ideas and to support numeracy development" including "spatial sense, patterning, number, measurement, data argumentation, connections and exploring the world mathematically" (p. 38). Educators thus need to be fluent in mathematical concepts, and this should be addressed in early childhood educators' preparation in mathematics teaching needs to improve (Gülteke, Tomul, & Korur, 2013; Lee & Ginsburg, 2009).

2. Theoretical Background

Students' beliefs and attitudes to mathematics, that is their self-efficacy (Bandura, 1997), affects one's teaching of mathematics, and many people suffer from anxiety about mathematics (Goos, Smith, & Thornton, 2008). Self-efficacy influences one's personal approach to mathematics. Based on Bandura's theory (1997), Warwick (2008: pp. 31-32) asserts there are four main areas of mathematical self-efficacy comprised of:

1) Performance experience derived from the level of success in mathematics where successful achievement strengthens self-efficacy, and repeated failures weakens it.

2) Vicarious experience obtained when students compare themselves with others on maths scores which affects self-efficacy negatively or positively.

3) Verbal persuasion which relates to feedback from others on one's mathematical ability

4) Emotional arousal and anxiety about performance of doing/teaching mathematical tasks. Lower levels of anxiety are associated with increased self-efficacy and higher levels of confidence.

Much of the discussion regarding pre-service teachers and mathematics is centred on mathematics anxiety, and if not addressed in the teacher, is thought to be transferred from teacher to student with immediate and long term educational implications (Sloan, Daane, & Giesen, 2002; Vinson, 2001; Warwick, 2008). The most often used definition of mathematics anxiety is that of Richardson and Suinn's (1972), who describe mathematics anxiety as "feelings of tension ... that interfere with the manipulation of numbers and solving mathematical problems in a wide variety of ordinary life and academic situations" (p. 551). These authors devised a tool to measure mathematics anxiety, called the Mathematics Anxiety Rating Scale (MARS). Numerous studies have investigated anxiety and negative attitudes to mathematics (Bekdemir, 2010; Uusimaki & Kidman, 2004; Uusimaki & Nason, 2004; Wilson, 2009), some finding that these negative attitudes were found to affect a high proportion of students preparing to be teachers (Trujillo & Hadfield, 1999 in Townsend et al., 1999). Some studies suggest that having some anxiety, that is low level anxiety, about teaching mathematics is beneficial in that it is a motivator to engage more deeply in the course of the unit to reach an understanding of the discipline and be a better teacher than they had experienced (Young-Leveridge, 2010).

Pre-service teachers in the USA and Australia experience higher levels of mathematics anxiety than other university undergraduate students (Gresham, 2007), with the incidence of mathematics anxiety significantly higher among elementary (early years) education students (Swars, Hart, Smith, Smith, & Tolar, 2007). Research has identified reasons for pre-service teachers experiencing mathematics anxiety: past experiences of failing mathematics (Bekdemir, 2010); the pedagogical approach to the teaching of mathematics (Gresham, 2007); classroom instruction techniques (Hawera, 2004); teaching practices associated with negative attitudes towards mathematics (Swan, 2004) and students' experiences during their own primary school education (Uusimaki &

Nason, 2004). Research has also shown that females have greater anxiety compared to male counterparts (Bowd & Brady, 2003).

Anxiety associated with mathematical tasks has been observed via neuroimaging. Lyons and Beilock (2012) identified that when a person is anxious about mathematics and is confronted with a mathematics task, then more activity in the visceral threat detection area of the brain is recorded, which is associated with pain. They also found that when the person was engaged in the actual mathematics task then this activity was absent. Therefore the engagement in the task reduced the anxiety levels. The implications are that raising awareness that anxiety will subside once the task is may be beneficial for pre-service teachers and contribute to their self-efficacy in the teaching of mathematics.

The Study's Focus

Anxiety about mathematics, and the teaching of mathematics, is of concern for educators training future early years' teachers. However, feeling incompetent and anxious about teaching has often gone unacknowledged and where it is acknowledged, it has been shown to be effective in helping students start to address their anxiety (Boyd et al., 1998; Zimmerman, 1998a,b). In this study we examined students' awareness of their own individual performance at mathematics, and what reasons they give for their mathematical self-efficacy. It is argued that if students feel that anxiety towards mathematics is common amongst their student population then this will raise awareness enabling reflection on learning and motivation for addressing this anxiety.

This study was initiated by educators who teach primary school and early childhood pre-service teachers. Feedback from the 2010 student cohort after completion of the foundational mathematics course, which focused on teaching mathematics to children aged six weeks to eight years, had indicated that students experienced low levels of mathematical self-efficacy and did not feel capable with their skills in mathematics. In order to address students' self-efficacy regarding the teaching of mathematics this study investigated

1) pre-service teacher's anxiety towards mathematics at the beginning and the end of the session,
2) pre-service teacher's memories of mathematics' experiences
3) pre-service teacher's views of teaching mathematics at the beginning and end of the teaching session.

3. Method

The questionnaire and associated analysis: This study involved a questionnaire at the beginning and end of the teaching session in mathematics. The questionnaire was developed to measure students' anxiety towards the learning and teaching of mathematics, and was comprised of three parts:
- Part 1 was the demographic data of the students including age, gender, course, and educational background.
- Part 2 of the questionnaire included short answer open-ended questions about their attitudes and beliefs regarding mathematics, and to identify reasons for their beliefs. The analysis of short answer open-ended questions identified themes to understand attitudes to the learning and teaching of mathematics, and reasons students cited for attitudes towards mathematics. Participants' responses were read, and re-read as part of the analysis. This systematic analysis of the textual data, via content analysis, revealed that key themes were common across the cohort (Krippendorff, 2012). Open-ended responses to the questions were read and re-read and categories were developed. Flick, Von Kardoff and Steinke (2004) stress the importance of re-reading data so that the researchers' theoretical prior knowledge and the research questions can guide the reading of the transcript.
- Part 3 was designed to measure students' attitudes to mathematics. Eight items presented on a 5-point scale rated from 1 = strongly disagree to 5 = strongly agree. Items designed to measure the key construct of Attitudes towards Mathematics. Negatively worded items (Items 5 and 6) were reverse scored before analysis. The scale had acceptable internal reliability (Cronbach's alpha = 0.73). The items were:
1) I feel confident about teaching mathematics;
2) I expected to study mathematics in my course;
3) Studying mathematics will be useful to my training;
4) I understand mathematical concepts well;
5) I struggled with mathematics at primary school;
6) I feel anxious about teaching mathematics;
7) I am keen to learn how to teach mathematics well;

8) It is important that I teach mathematics well.

Analysis of this scale of items was conducted by the following procedure: Numeric data were entered into the SPSS statistical package to generate descriptive statistics. Scores for the 8 items were summed, and a new variable was formed: Attitude towards Mathematics. The maximum score possible was 32.

3.1. Participants

The participants were 223 pre-service teachers studying a foundation (first year) unit of mathematics in the Bachelor of Education Early Childhood Education (n = 73; 34%) and Primary Education Degrees (n = 155; 66%). The student cohort was predominately women (n = 180; 80%); the age range was 17 to 42 years old (mean $22.3 \pm 5.1\sigma$). Approximately 38% had finished school the previous year, and just over half had finished school within the past two years. Eight students held a previous degree, 88 had a Technical and Further Education (TAFE) qualification, and 35 had completed the university's Preparing for Success course.

3.2. Procedure

In this teaching unit students had a one hour weekly lecture, followed by a two hour face to face tutorial. The lecturer prepared the unit material for all tutors of the content and learning activities for each week's tutorial. The content of the mathematics unit focused on the teaching mathematics in the early years that is for children aged from six weeks to eight years old. Each week the tutorials included discussions addressing anxiety towards mathematics so that it was embedded within the unit.

Participants were recruited during the first tutorial for the session following the lecture that had introduced the topic regarding attitudes and anxiety towards mathematics. This is known in this study as Time 1. The students were informed that research indicated that attitudes and beliefs about one's ability in mathematics, and affects a teacher's own ability to teach in these areas (Sloan, Daane, & Giesen, 2002; Vinson, 2001). The topic also included a discussion of how feeling anxious in mathematics can be transferred to teachers' students. The students were invited to participate in the study and advised that there were no negative consequences for those not participating. The University's Human Research Ethics Committee approval had been obtained, and participants had the option of completing the survey, or opting out.

The students were informed that the study was investigating changes of attitude towards mathematics over the course of the teaching of the unit, and would be re-surveyed at the end of the teaching session. To ensure that analysis was of the same students each student's identity number was recorded, and matched when entering the data from the beginning of the session to the end of the session. The second questionnaire was handed out and completed at the end of the teaching session (nine weeks later) by these participants, following class discussions of anxiety regarding mathematics and strategies to approach anxiety throughout the session. This is known as Time 2 in this study. This paper reports on the results from the questionnaires from Time 1 and Time 2. Participants' response rates were 81% (n = 223) of the cohort. The questionnaire took approximately 20 minutes to complete during the tutorials.

4. Results

4.1. Pre-Service Teacher's Anxiety

There was considerable anxiety towards teaching mathematics amongst this student cohort. The mean scores for anxiety at the commencement and end of the session were compared to obtain a difference of mean scores. The range of possible scores resulting from the 8 items was 0 to 32, with the actual range for this cohort of students being from 1 - 32. The mean score for Time 1 was $23.2 \pm 4.6\sigma$, and for Time 2 was $23.4 \pm 4.6\sigma$. Mean scores were not significantly different at Time 1 to Time 2 with paired sample t tests being $t(210) = -1.1$, $p = 0.27$. This indicated that students' attitudes to mathematics did not change significantly on these eight items.

Figure 1 shows the mean scores on each item. Feeling anxious about teaching mathematics was the lowest scored item (Item 6, M = 1.9) and was identical at both time points. The data verified that 40% of students (n = 88) were anxious about teaching mathematics. The highest scored items at Time 1 were that students were keen to teach mathematics well (item 7, M = 3.7), and that it was important to teach maths well (Item 8, M = 3.7). Of interest is the change in attitude to understanding mathematical concepts which on paired sample t tests was significantly different $t(210) = -6.2$, $p = 0.000$. So while anxiety about teaching mathematics remained constant

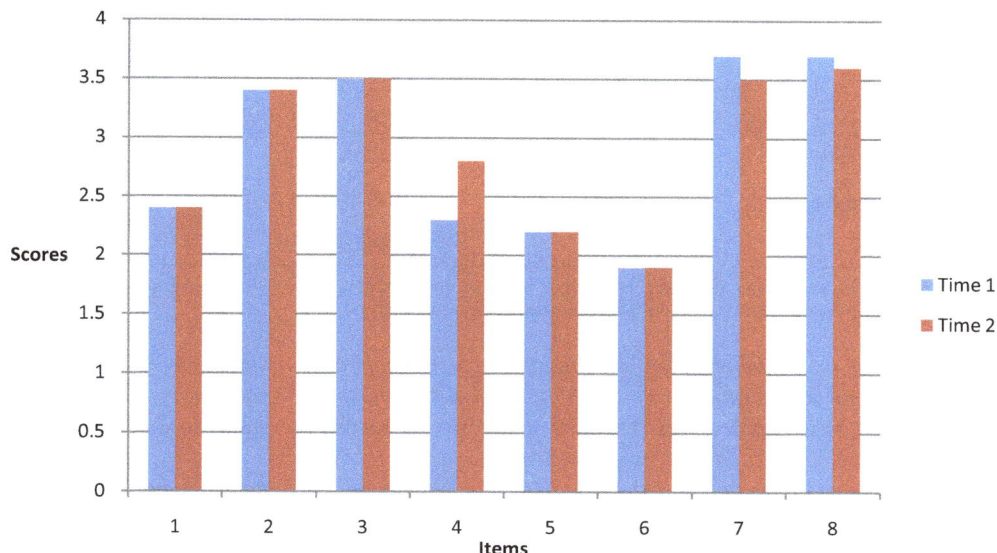

Figure 1. Mean scores for the 8 items for attitude to mathematics at time 1 and time 2 (n = 211).

throughout the session students reported that they understood mathematical concepts better at the end of the teaching session than at the commencement.

To identify the characteristics of the students who felt anxious about teaching mathematics, correlational analysis indicated a weak correlation that female students were significantly more anxious about teaching mathematics than male students ($r = 0.2$, n = 223, $p = 0.004$). Gender was the only demographic item that presented significant associations with the items in the scale.

To examine the reasons for students' anxiety a correlational analysis was conducted on the Item 5: I struggling with maths at primary school and Item 6: I feel anxious about teaching mathematics. This showed a moderate correlation ($r = 0.4$, n = 223, $p = 0.000$) at both time points indicating that students remembered finding maths at primary school difficult. The idea that they were training to be a primary school teacher may have elevated their anxiety.

4.2. Pre-Service Teacher's Memories of Mathematics' Experiences

There were 183 responses (87%) to this question: Please describe your memories of your mathematics experiences prior to this course at Time 1. Participants' memories of mathematics were either overwhelmingly positive or negative and the participants' judged their memories on the reasons why they felt that way. The analysis of memories students reported were categorised into: (1) external reasons with negative or positive attitudes to mathematics; and (2) internal reasons with their negative or positive attitudes to mathematics. These were then counted and results are reported in **Table 1**.

4.2.1. External Reasons Associated with Mathematics Ability

The main external reason given for students' attitudes to mathematics (n = 77; 47%) was the teaching approaches they had been exposed to as students in schools. The following quotes were chosen to highlight this theme from the pre-service teachers' comments. Student is identified as S.

1) Positive Attitudes

The participants identified that having a teacher who was passionate about teaching mathematics, provided hands on activities, made it fun and consequently engaged the students contributed to positive learning of mathematics. Examples of the teaching approaches that influenced students' attitudes to mathematics positively are given in the following quotes:

Thanks to my teacher who had a passion for mathematics and made it fun, enjoyable, and gave us activities to do outside which made the class interesting (S16).

My mathematics classes were always fun in primary school. The teachers made sure we had different ways of

Table 1. Students' memories of their mathematics experiences (n = 183*).

	Attitude to mathematics		
	Positive	Negative	Total
External reasons	27 (16%)	50 (30%)	77 (47%)
Internal reasons	38 (23%)	49 (30%)	87 (53%)
Total	65 (40%)	99 (60%)	164* (100%)

Note: *Note that 19 participants' responses could not be coded according to this matrix owing to insufficient information—for example: a response that said "Bad" with no explanation was omitted from analysis.

explaining situations and numbers. For example, through songs, books, pictures, etc. (S25).

Had primary school teachers who were passionate about mathematics and it rubbed off (S100).

The participants' also recalled their teachers took time to ensure the students understood the mathematics concepts:

Not great until year 11 when I had the privilege of a wonderful math teacher who loved teaching math and took the time to make sure we all understand all formulas (S115).

I enjoyed mathematics at school. If I had trouble understanding something, the teacher would take the time to explain it to me and give me extra practice, specifically for what I was finding difficult, until I understood it. I enjoyed working towards understanding of mathematics concepts (S130).

Three participants recognised that the quality of the teaching influenced their memories and subsequent learning, and intended to apply this concept in their future teaching. The following quote is an example of these three responses:

I have had some bad memories and some good memories. Throughout high school it depended on the teacher and their teaching skills. Therefore, I would like to become a success teacher so I bring a quality learning experience to all children (S3).

2) Negative attitudes

Fifty participants (27%) cited external reasons for their negative attitudes to mathematics. They recalled teaching approaches, use of resources and the teacher' classroom management style as contributing to negative attitudes to mathematics. Teaching approaches included poor explanations, teaching as too fast a pace and could not keep up, a lack of hands on experiences, and teaching directed approaches that did not support the students' learning. Examples of quotes from these participants follow:

Not very positive memories. Teachers did not provide the help I needed in high school and I would fall behind, thus losing interest in the subject (S194).

My mathematics experiences are all horrible; I've never known mathematics or how to do mathematics. Every mathematics teacher I've never had, always worked through the mathematics too fast, so I was never able to keep up, so I got left behind and I've been scared of it ever since (S68).

At school mathematics wasn't my strongest subject and the teachers just stood out the front of the class and told us how they wanted it done, they didn't really help when it was needed (S195).

Of this group of 50 participants 20 of them said that they had negative memories of mathematics because of the resources used. The use of work books, work sheets and text books were cited by 20 participants as being poor teaching practices that did not support their learning, and participants felt that these resources were often boring, as the following two quotes indicate:

I enjoyed math in Primary school, I enjoyed reasoning and questioning. When I got to high school I found it difficult to learn straight from the textbook and could not make meaning or connections with what I was learning about (S67).

I strongly disliked mathematics in primary school and high school. The teaching was boring and mostly taken from a textbook and the teachers did not take time to help individual students (S126).

Boring same old same old, worksheets—no hands on (S81).

The teacher's classroom management styles were reasons students cited for their negative attitude to mathematics. Being embarrassed by the teacher for not knowing the answer when asked was cited by four participants:

I had a mean teacher in year 6 who laughed at me because I did not know something, and now I hate offering answers in case they're wrong (S27).

Horrifying. Made to feel inadequate and like an idiot (S56).

I strongly dislike mathematics. In school I struggled with mathematics and never received any help. I was often embarrassed in front of the class due to my low knowledge of mathematics (S48).

Not very enjoyable. Mathematics teacher made me feel anxious and was not supportive, made me feel stupid for not understanding (S91).

4.2.2. Internal Reasons

Analysis of the students' memories of mathematics revealed that 87 (n = 53%) of the students believed that an ability to be good at mathematics is internally determined. You are either a mathematics person or you are not. The following examples indicate how students viewed their memories of maths and the causes of these memories.

1) Positive attitudes

Thirty-eight students (23%) recorded that mathematics was easy for them: some of their quotes include: (maths) *comes easy (S 98)*, (I am) *good at it (S41)*, (I am) *capable (S196)*, and (I am) *successful (109)*. For these students it was the nature of mathematics being logical with problems to solve with one answer that they found easy.

I loved mathematics; I was always quite good at mathematics. It's just logical which makes sense to me (S42).

I enjoyed mathematics. It is interesting and I learnt there is many ways to solve mathematics problems, and I like that there is only one answer to a question (S62).

Very positive, easy to learn, got lots of success in mathematics (S109).

I enjoyed problem solving, however disliked working out of textbooks in high school where we just did a chapter per week (S192).

The notion that mathematics comes easy to some people, and not to others, is evident in these quotes and the following quotes also support this theme. However these quotes indicate that these students believe themselves not to be a maths person.

2) Negative attitudes

Thirty percent of participants (*n* = 49) felt that their inability to do mathematics was a personal internal characteristic that could not be altered. A list of words that were used to describe their memories of their mathematics included (Maths is) *hard, it didn't gel*, (I) *couldn't understand it*, (I) *don't get it*, (maths is) *frustrating, scary, horrible, terrible, horrifying* and even (I have) *a hatred of mathematics*. The notion that people are born a mathematics person, or not, was a common theme in these comments as the following quotes indicate.

I was never an "A+" student in mathematics. I tried my hardest at primary high school but was never able to really understand the concepts of mathematics. Even today I still struggle! (S10)

Negative attitude towards mathematics in K-12 (didn't do mathematics in year 11 and 12) I was convinced that I was bad at it and not a mathematics person and I never had a teacher that reassured me (S121).

Of particular interest in this quote is that this student identified that perhaps a teacher could have changed his/her self-perception. This gives hope to those students who sense that their negative experiences that derived from internal qualities may be able to be changed by a supportive teacher, and this is valuable learning for these pre-service teachers who will be teaching mathematics to children in the classrooms. Two students who felt that they were not particularly scholarly in mathematics were motivated and willing to learn what they could to be good teachers for their future children as the following quotes indicate.

Not great, I studied mathematics throughout school and my HSC. I wasn't great at it and didn't enjoy it very much but I think that will help me now, in making me a better and more engaged teacher (S72).

Wasn't my most enjoyable subject at school. However I find learning how to teach mathematics is enjoyable (S146).

What is clear from these comments is the way maths has aroused student emotions. Students did not just like or dislike mathematics they loved it or hated it. Maths seems to have the power to rouse extreme emotions in their memory, and now they were to learn how to teach it.

4.3. Views of Teaching Mathematics

The 23 participants' responses who rated their anxiety towards teaching mathematics at 5 (the highest level) on the Likert-type scale at Time 1 to the question "Please describe your views to teaching mathematics" were chosen for analysis. This group were chosen to see first see how these student's viewed their teaching of mathematics, and then to see if these views had changed by the end of the teaching session. Only 12 of the 23 students completed this part of the questionnaire so the nine responses below demonstrate the three categories of responses. The students fell into three categories: they still felt the same about teaching mathematics; they felt slightly more confident, or they viewed teaching mathematics as a responsibility they had to conquer. T1 is at Time 1, and T2 is Time 2.

4.3.1. The Same: Still Quite Anxious

T1: *I am hoping that I can be confident in teaching maths by improving my understanding of maths. T2: I would like to teach maths in a fun way that allows children to be involved confident learners* (S2).

T1: *That I wish to become a lot more confident in my abilities to teach maths well and that my "maths anxiety" will slowly disappear. T2: Still the same as the start of this unit. Nervous, not confident, scared and very unsure about my abilities to become a great mathematics teacher* (S5).

T1: *I need to become confident in my own abilities in order to teach math well. T2: I still need to learn A LOT* (S36).

4.3.2. Slightly More Confident

T1: *I do not enjoy math as I have never understood it but children need to be taught mathematics. So I will teach it to the best of my abilities. T2: I am more confident to teach math now but I still have some anxiety. I do not fully understand all concepts though* (S5).

T1: *I don't feel that at this stage I am confident to teach maths but I understand that it is really important to teach it well. I hope that I succeed. T2: I feel slightly more confident and look forward to my future studies in maths* (S8).

T1: *At present I am very nervous about teaching maths. However I am looking forward to making maths enjoyable to making maths enjoyable for the children I teach and giving them fun, memorable learning experiences. I want to support the children and make them feel safe about giving maths a go. T2: I feel a little more confident with teaching maths, but will not feel totally ready until I am putting my knowledge into practice* (S151).

4.3.3. Taking Responsibility for Teaching and Learning

T1: *I want to give students the best possible start to maths because I know how important it is to succeed in schooling and life. Mostly, I want them to enjoy maths. T2: I am a bit nervous about teaching the later stages as the work gets more complex. However, I feel confident in that I could teach the students different techniques* (S79).

T1: *Making it fun and hands on and making children feel safe, supported and like they can have a go. Children are valued in the classroom. T2: (Maths) can be enjoyable. It is up to me as the educator to motivate students and get them excited about maths by fun, authentic, hands on experiences that children can use in real life* (S91).

T1: *I realise how important math is! Seeing children in early childhood experiment and early concepts is exciting and I want to learn how to extend this exploration and knowledge in later years!! Maths is a lifelong skill and essential to functioning in our modern world. T2: I still have some anxiety about how to make concepts clear and concise and catering for such a diversity of ability. I know how important math is and it feels like a big responsibility—this is part of my journey as I become a teacher I suppose* (S112).

5. Discussion

This study sought to understand pre-service teachers' attitudes towards teaching mathematics, the prevalence of anxiety about teaching mathematics, and pre-service teacher's understanding of the sources of their attitudes to mathematics. Students reported being anxious about teaching mathematics and this score did not change from the beginning to the end of the session. It is likely that this feeling will remain until students have the opportunity to "put my knowledge into practice", as Student 151 stated. That is their self-efficacy towards teaching mathematics will change once they have mastered the first part of self-efficacy—what Bandura terms "performance experience". They were viewed as taking responsibility for their learning how to teach mathematics, even though many of them had negative past experiences of being taught mathematics.

Overall the students were positive about studying mathematics, based on the score of Attitude to Mathematics. This result is reassuring, as past research indicates that a positive attitude to teaching mathematics influences learning, even without the knowledge about the subject (Lazarus, 1974). While a significant number of students were anxious about teaching mathematics, students viewed the teaching of mathematics to be important and were positive about learning how to teach mathematics. Indeed, students self-rated scores for understanding mathematical concepts increased significantly throughout the course of the session indicating that students felt more capable mathematically.

The results indicated that students who were positive about mathematics recalled quality teaching practices of mathematics such as engaging the students, student centred learning, supporting the students' learning by giving time, assistance and assurance about mathematics skills. This points to the power the teacher has in supporting children to learn mathematics. Choosing a teacher-centred approach, especially in the early years of learning mathematics has been found to be far more effective than a child-centred approach where children "discover" knowledge by interacting with concrete materials. Children's learning has been found to be optimised by having an effective pedagogue working alongside and supporting children's learning (Polly, Margerison, & Piel, 2014).

Unfortunately, the results also indicated that students who had struggled with mathematics identified that their teachers had used poor teaching practices, such as inadequate explanation of concepts, working from the text-book, worksheets, and poor teaching management practices. What can be learned from this is that the resources and pedagogical approaches used by teachers in classrooms need to be appropriate and respectful: teachers need to have a range of strategies to engage students in learning about mathematics in an enjoyable manner.

The cited practice of "naming and shaming" students in front of their class by asking students answers that they could not work out nor understand is likely to weaken a student's mathematical self-efficacy. Such practices constructed barriers to learning for these students, and were associated with negative attitudes to mathematics. While the study of mathematics for these students elicited strong emotional arousal, including anxiety, as a result of these practices, this study has enhanced these pre-service teacher's awareness of such practices, and the influence upon their own learning. It is hoped that by reflecting on such practices they will take this understanding with them into their own professional practices.

The results from the qualitative data identify significant issues that need to be addressed in the teaching of mathematics in undergraduate teacher education mathematics courses. Past experiences of teaching were closely linked to current perceptions, and many students had identified teaching practices that they themselves would, or would not, take into their own classroom when they taught. Even the students who identified high levels of anxiety about teaching mathematics recognised that they need to develop confidence about teaching mathematics.

6. Conclusion

The results from this study provide an insight into societal views about mathematical ability: that we are either good or bad at mathematics, and this is a result of how we were taught. That said, many of the students in this study who linked their poor mathematical ability to "I am not a maths person" labelling, recognised that they could change their ability in mathematics and wanted to learn how to teach it well. It also needs to be stated that female students were more anxious about teaching mathematics than male, and this finding supports previous research by Bowd and Brady (2003).

University teachers of mathematics can raise pre-service teacher's awareness regarding these issues identified in this study to improve student's mathematical self-efficacy. For students, to know that they are not alone in feeling like this about mathematics may enhance their self-efficacy. This second part of self-efficacy identified by Bandura (1997), that is vicarious experience, may be enhanced.

While this study focused on mathematics anxiety, this is just one part of mathematical self-efficacy. The results indicate that anxiety has the power to influence other aspects of self-efficacy—participants made strong links between their mathematics anxiety to their personal experiences of mathematics. It would be useful to survey pre-service students as they progress through their four-year teaching degree to see if anxiety towards mathematics lessens as they prepare to embark on their career as a teacher. If the anxiety did not diminish it would be recommended that pre-service teachers with low mathematical self-efficacy seek support from a mentor. In conclusion the study found that pre-service teacher's anxiety did not significantly diminish throughout the teaching session, however there was no doubt that there was heightened awareness regarding addressing one's self-efficacy about the teaching of mathematics.

Acknowledgements

The authors thank the Schools of Education, and Environment, Science & Engineering for grant assistance to publish this research.

References

ACARA (2011). Mathematics: Rationale. http://www.australiancurriculum.edu.au/Mathematics/Rationale

Bandura, A. (1997). *Self-Efficacy: The Exercise of Control.* New York: Freeman.

Bekdemir, M. (2010). The Pre-Service Teachers' Mathematics Anxiety Related to Depth of Negative Experiences in Mathematics Classroom While They Were Students. *Educational Studies in Mathematics, 75,* 311-328. http://dx.doi.org/10.1007/s10649-010-9260-7

Bowd, A. D., & Brady, P. H. (2003). Gender Differences in Mathematics Anxiety among Preservice Teachers and Perceptions of Their Elementary and Secondary School Experience with Mathematics. *Alberta Journal of Educational Research, 49,* 24-36.

DEEWR (2009). *Being, Belonging and Becoming: The Early Years Learning Framework for Australia.* Barwon, ACT: Commonwealth of Australia.

Flick, U., Von Kardoff, E., & Steinke, I. (2004). *A Companion to Qualitative Research.* London: Sage.

Goos, M., Smith, T., & Thornton, S. (2008). Research on the Pre-Service Education of Teachers of Mathematics. In H. Forgasz (Ed.), *Research in Mathematics Education in Australasia* 2004-2007. Rotterdam: The Netherlands Sense Publishers.

Gresham, G. (2007). A Study of Mathematics Anxiety in Pre-Service Teachers. *Early Childhood Education Journal, 35,* 181-188. http://dx.doi.org/10.1007/s10643-007-0174-7

Gülteke, M., Tomul, E., & Korur, F. (2013). Mathematics Special Content Competencies of Elementary School Teachers. *Creative Education, 4,* 1-10. http://dx.doi.org/10.4236/ce.2013.412A2001

Hawera, N. (2004). *Addressing the Needs of Mathematically Anxious Preservice Primary Teachers.* The Mathematics Education for the Third Millennium: Towards 2010, Townsville.

Krippendorff, K. (2012). *Content Analysis: An Introduction to Its Methodology* (3rd ed.). Thousand Oaks, CA: Sage Publications.

Lago, R., & DiPerna, J. (2010). Number Sense in Kindergarten: A Factor-Analytic Study of the Construct. *School Psychology Review, 39,* 164.

Lyons, I., & Beilock, S. (2012). When Math Hurts: Math Anxiety Predicts Pain Network Activation in Anticipation of Doing Math. *PLoS ONE, 7,* 10. http://dx.doi.org/10.1371/journal.pone.0048076

OECD (2010). OECD Programme for International Student Assessment. http://www.oecd.org/pisa/

Polly, D., Margerison, A., & Piel, J. (2014). Kindergarten Teachers' Orientations to Teacher-Centred and Student-Centred Pedagogies and Their Influence on Their Students' Understanding of Addition. *Journal of Research in Childhood Education, 28,* 1-17. http://dx.doi.org/10.1080/02568543.2013.822949

Richardson, F., & Suinn, R. M. (1972). The Mathematics Anxiety Rating Scale: Psychometric Data. *Journal of Counseling Psychology, 9,* 551-554. http://dx.doi.org/10.1037/h0033456

Schmidt, B. (2012). Speech: Brian Schmidt's Mathematical Argument. http://www.theaustralian.com.au/higher-education/speech-schmidts-argument-for-numeracy/story-e6frgcjx-1226265595923

Sloan, T., Daane, C. J., & Giesen, J. (2002). Mathematics Anxiety and Learning Styles: What Is the Relationship in Elementary Preservice Teachers? *School Science and Mathematics, 102,* 84-87. http://dx.doi.org/10.1111/j.1949-8594.2002.tb17897.x

Swan, P. (2004). I Hate Mathematics. http://www.mav.vic.edu.au/files/conferences/2004/Swan.pdf

Swars, S., Hart, L. C., Smith, S. Z., Smith, M. E., & Tolar, T. (2007). A Longitudinal Study of Elementary Pre-Service Teachers' Mathematics Beliefs and Content Knowledge. *School Science and Mathematics, 107,* 325-335. http://dx.doi.org/10.1111/j.1949-8594.2007.tb17797.x

Townsend, M., Lai, M. K., Lavery, L., Sutherland, C., & Wilton, K. (1999). Mathematics Anxiety and Self-Concept: Evaluating Change Using the "Then-Now" Procedure. Research Report, University of Auckland. http://www.aare.edu.au/99pap/tow99213.htm

Uusimake, L., & Kidman, G. (2004). Reducing Maths-Anxiety: Results from an Online Anxiety Survey.

http://eprints.qut.edu.au/974/1/kid04997.pdf

Uusimake, L., & Nason, R. (2004). Causes Underlying Pre-Service Teachers' Negative Beliefs and Anxieties about Mathematics. http://emis.matem.unam.mx/proceedings/PME28/RR/RR141_Uusimaki.pdf

Vinson, B. M. (2001). A Comparison of Pre-Service Teachers' Mathematics Anxiety before and after a Methods Class Emphasizing Manipulatives. *Early Childhood Education Journal, 29,* 89-94. http://dx.doi.org/10.1023/A:1012568711257

Warwick, J. (2008). Mathematical Self-Efficacy and Student Engagement in the Mathematics Classroom. *MSOR Connections, 8,* 31-37. http://dx.doi.org/10.11120/msor.2008.08030031

Wilson, S. (2009). "*Better You than Me*": *Mathematics Anxiety and the Bibliography in Primary Teacher Professional Learning.* Palmerston North, NZ: MERGA.

Young-Loveridge, J. (2010). *Two Decades of Mathematics Education Reform in New Zealand: What Impact on the Attitudes of Teacher Education Students?* Fremantle, WA: The Shaping the Future of Mathematics Education.

Psychosocial Moderators of Perceived Stress, Anxiety and Depression in University Students: An International Study

Aileen M. Pidgeon[1], Stephanie McGrath[2], Heidi B. Magya[3], Peta Stapleton[1], Barbara C. Y. Lo[4]

[1]PhD (Clin) Bond University, Gold Coast, Australia
[2]Bond University, Gold Coast, Australia
[3]ARNP, University of Florida, Gainesville, USA
[4]PhD University of Hong Kong, Hong Kong, China
Email: stephy.mcgrath87@gmail.com

Abstract

Extensive research shows university students experience high levels of stress, which can lead to the development of mental health problems such as anxiety and depression. Preliminary evidence supports the role of psychosocial factors such as perceived social support (PSS) and campus connectedness (CC) as protective factors in the development of mental health problems in university students. However, research conducted on the potential ameliorating effects of social support on stress applying Cohen and Wills' (1985) stress-buffering hypothesis produced weak, inconsistent, and even contradictory results. In addition, little attention has been given to examining the protective role of CC in the relationships between perceived stress, anxiety, and depression. The current study examined the applicability of CC and PSS in buffering the relationships been perceived stress, anxiety, and depression across an international sample comprised of university students (*N* = 206) from Australia, Hong Kong, and the United States. The prediction that CC and PSS would moderate the relationships between perceived stress, anxiety, and depression was partially supported. The results indicated CC moderated the relationship between perceived stress and depression but did not moderate the relationship between perceived stress and anxiety. PSS did not moderate the relationship between perceived stress and depression or the relationship between perceived stress and anxiety, thus rejecting the stress-buffering hypothesis. These findings suggest less emphasis should be placed on PSS as a protective factor, with universities focusing on enhancing CC to reduce the high prevalence of mental health problems to promote psychological wellbeing among students.

Keywords

Perceived Stress, Anxiety, Depression, Psychosocial, Perceived Social Support, Campus Connectedness, Stress-Buffering Hypothesis, Moderating, Buffering

1. Introduction

The transition into higher education is a stressful time as university students face multiple stressors such as academic overload, constant pressure to succeed, competition with peers, and in some countries financial burden as well as concerns about future career prospects [1]. While many university students adjust effectively to the university context, a large proportion of students are adversely impacted by stress and are at risk of developing mental health problems [2].

The prevalence of mental health issues in university students is of universal concern, with international studies revealing clinical levels of psychopathology, including anxiety and depression in student populations globally [2]-[5]. Thus, the mental health of university students has been the subject of increasing focus in recent years with evidence demonstrating that university students experience higher levels of psychological distress, including anxiety and depression, in comparison to non-student populations [2] [6]. Moreover, research has shown approximately 40% of university students with diagnosable mental health conditions do not seek clinical services or access university support services [7].

Research suggests psychosocial factors such as perceived social support and campus connectedness may play a protective role in the adverse consequences of perceived stress among university students. Perceived social support has been shown to be positively associated with psychological wellbeing [8]-[10]. While campus connectedness is a relatively new construct defined as a form of social connectedness and belonging that is specific to the university context and is also positively associated with psychological wellbeing and adjustment in university students [11]. Considering many university students are not seeking professional assistance for psychological issues, an investigation into the protective role that key psychosocial factors play in promoting psychological wellbeing and protecting university students from the development of mental health problems is warranted. The current study will examine the protective role of campus connectedness and perceived social support on the relationships between perceived stress, anxiety, and depression among university students.

1.1. Perceived Stress, Anxiety, and Depression

While the literature suggests various risk factors are associated with the development of anxiety and depression, the positive association between perceived stress, anxiety, and depression has been demonstrated in numerous studies [12] [13]. High levels of perceived stress increases the risk for an individual to develop anxiety and depression. However, university students worldwide are shown to be a high risk group with prevalence rates being higher than the general population [14]. Stallman [15] found a significantly higher prevalence of mental health problems in Australian university students than the general population with 83.9% of students reporting heightened levels of psychological distress including stress, anxiety, and depression. Eisenberg, Hunt, and Speer [16] assessed students across 26 United States universities and found 17.3% met the criteria for depression, 7.8% generalised anxiety disorder, 4.1% panic disorder, and a total of 6.3% reported suicidal ideation. A study conducted by Wong, Cheung, Chan, Ma, and Tang [17] in a sample of university students across 10 universities in Hong Kong revealed a prevalence of anxiety, depression, and stress with 21% of students experiencing moderate depression, 41% moderate anxiety, and 27% moderate stress. This research highlights the importance of developing an understanding of the psychosocial factors that protect students against the adverse effects of perceived stress.

1.2. Perceived Social Support

Perceived social support has been consistently shown to be positively associated with psychological wellbeing [8]-[10]. Perceived social support is defined as an individual's potential access to social support resources, that is, an individual's belief that support is available if needed [18]. Perceived social support has been repeatedly linked to positive psychological and health outcomes [18]. The breadth of research on perceived social support has led researchers to examine its role in moderating the effects of perceived stress on anxiety and depression [8] [19] [20]. A moderator is a variable that alters the strength of the relationship between a predictor variable and an outcome variable [21].

The stress-buffering hypothesis developed by Cohen and Wills [22] suggests perceived social support ameliorates the adverse effects of stressful situations. Cohen and Wills' hypothesis links with Lazarus and Folkman's [23] transactional theory of stress in that perceptions of social support may lead an individual to appraise a threatening situation as less stressful. Cohen and Wills proposed that perceived social support acts as a protective psychosocial factor for individuals experiencing high levels of perceived stress. As such, perceived social support is thought to reduce the adverse effects of perceived stress through the belief that an individual can access coping resources such as social support if needed [8]. Perceived social support may decrease the experience of stress by providing a reappraisal of the stressor, thereby reducing the affective, physiological, and cognitive reactions that make up the experience of stress [24]. Since Cohen and Wills' proposal of the stress-buffering hypothesis, many researchers have tested this process, however the literature contains inconsistent findings. Some studies have demonstrated support for a buffering model of perceived social support consistent with the stress-buffering hypothesis [25] while others have only found support for a main effect model of perceived social support [26].

1.3. Campus Connectedness

In comparison to perceived social support, social connectedness is a global construct that encompasses much more than just perceived interpersonal relations [27]. According to Lee and Robbins [28] social connectedness is a person's subjective awareness of closeness with their social world. Social connectedness has been found to be negatively associated with perceived stress, anxiety, and depression [29] [30]. Therefore, connectedness within a university context is an important psychosocial variable to examine, as many university students experience maladjustment issues in adapting to a new social environment upon transitioning into university [31]. Campus connectedness refers to social connectedness within the university context and has been defined by Lee and Robbins [28] as a student's sense of psychological belonging in a university environment. Research demonstrates that a lack of connectedness in university students has a negative impact on adjustment and psychological functioning. University students who report low connectedness also report fewer meaningful and supportive relationships with others [31]. Furthermore, university students with low levels of connectedness report higher levels of psychological distress due to their lack of meaningful connections with others [27]. Research has also demonstrated social connectedness is inversely related to perceived stress, anxiety, and depression in university students [28]-[30]. This research suggests that university students with higher levels of connectedness have lower levels of perceived stress, anxiety, and depression. Additionally, Furthermore, Rude and Burham [32] proposed connectedness should be investigated as a protective factor against depression. It is therefore essential that students feel connected on campus to ensure they adjust to university life and maintain their psychological well-being throughout their studies.

Although campus connectedness has been found to be negatively associated with perceived stress, anxiety, and depression, its moderating effect on these relationships is yet to be investigated. A paucity of research exists in examining the protective role of additional psychosocial characteristics such as campus connectedness, in moderating (buffering) the relationships between perceived stress, anxiety, and depression in university students. Further research is required to investigate the dynamic interplay among these variables. The current study will address the gap in the literature by evaluating the applicability of campus connectedness in buffering the relationship between perceived stress, anxiety, and depression.

1.4. The Current Study

The purpose of the current study was to examine psychosocial moderators of perceived stress, anxiety, and depression in an international sample of university students. The study also aimed to evaluate Cohen and Wills' [22] stress-buffering hypothesis of perceived social support, in addition to investigating the role of campus connectedness as a moderator in the relationships between perceived stress, anxiety, and depression. A series of four moderations were planned to investigate the following hypotheses:

H1. Perceived social support moderates the relationship between perceived stress and depression. Higher levels of perceived social support would buffer the effects of perceived stress on depression.

H2. Campus connectedness moderates the relationship between perceived stress and depression. Higher levels of campus connectedness would buffer the effects of perceived stress on depression.

H3. Perceived social support moderates the relationship between perceived stress and anxiety. Higher levels of perceived social support would buffer the effects of perceived stress on anxiety.

H4. Campus connectedness moderates the relationship between perceived stress and anxiety. Higher levels of campus connectedness would buffer the effects of perceived stress on anxiety.

2. Method

2.1. Participants

Participants for the current study consisted of 206 university students aged between 18 to 59 years ($M = 22.08$, $SD = 5.57$) including 160 (77.7%) females and 46 (22.3%) males. The sample included university students from Bond University, Australia, The University of Hong Kong, and The University of Florida. Inclusion criteria required participants to be aged 18 years and over.

2.2. Measures

Perceived Stress Scale (PSS). The PSS [33] is a 10-item scale designed to measure perceptions of stress. Four positively stated items require reverse scoring. To calculate a global measure of percieved stress the total number of items on the scale are summed with higher scores indicating higher levels of percieved stress.

The Depression Scale and Anxiety Scale (DASS-21). The current study used the Depression Scale and Anxiety Scale from the DASS-21, a short form version of the DASS-42 [34]. Scores for each scale are calculated through the summation of items. As the DASS-21 is a shortened version of the full DASS-42, the scores for each of the scales are to be multiplied by two. Higher scores on each scale are indicative of higher scores of depression or anxiety.

Campus Connectedness Scale (CCS). The CCS is a 14-item self report scale designed to measure university student's perception of belongingness on the university campus [28]. Eight negatively worded items require reverse scoring. The 14-items are summed with higher scores indicative of higher levels of campus connectedness.

Multidimensional Scale of Perceived Social Support (MSPSS). The MSPSS is a 12-item self-report scale designed to measure how individuals perceive their global social support system across three sources: family, friends, and significant other [9]. A global measure of perceived social support is obtained by summing the responses on the 12-items with higher values indicating higher levels of perceived social support.

3. Results

Separate moderated multiple regression analyses were conducted to determine if each of the moderators interacted to buffer the effects of perceived stress on the outcome variables of anxiety and depression. Moderation effects are assessed through the creation of a statistical interaction term comprised of the predictor variable multiplied by the moderator variable. Chaplin [35] conducted a comprehensive review of the literature and found that interaction term effect sizes generally account for between 1% and 3% of the variance in the outcome variable. Additionally, Evans [36] states moderation effects are so difficult to detect that even interaction terms accounting for 1% of the variance should be considered important. To reduce potentially problematic family wise inflation the four moderations were conducted within two separate regression models [37]. The first model investigated whether campus connectedness or perceived social support moderated the relationship between perceived stress and depression. The second model investigated whether campus connectedness or perceived social support moderated the relationship between perceived stress and anxiety. In each model, university was entered at Step 1 as a covariate to control for differences between universities on the outcome variables. At Step 2 the centered predictor and moderators were entered simultaneously, at Step 3 the interaction of the first moderator and predictor were entered, and at Step 4 the interaction of the second moderator and predictor were entered.

Model 1. At Step 1 of the analysis, university was added to the regression equation and the overall model was significant, $F(1, 194) = 7.59$, $p = 0.006$. University explained a significant 4% of the variance in depression scores. Thus, university was significantly predictive of depression scores, $\beta = .19$, $p = 0.006$, such that university students from Hong Kong had higher depression scores than university students from Australia and the United States. At Step 2, after controlling for the effects of university, perceived stress, perceived social support, and campus connectedness were added to the regression equation and the overall model was significant, $F(4, 191) = 42.74$, $p < 0.001$. Perceived stress, perceived social support, and campus connectedness accounted for 44% of the variance in depression, $\Delta F (3, 191) = 52.44$, $p < 0.001$. At this step, perceived stress was a significant positive predictor of depression, $\beta = 0.55$, $p < 0.001$, indicating that a 1 SD increase in perceived stress resulted in a 0.55 SD increase in depression. Perceived social support at this step was a non-significant predictor of depression, $\beta = -0.10$, $p = 0.124$. Campus connectedness at this step was a significant negative predictor of depression, $\beta = -0.15$ p = 0.031, indicating that a 1 SD increase in campus connectedness results in a 0.15 SD decrease in depression. At Step 3 of the analysis, the perceived stress ^{X} campus connectedness interaction term was added to the regression equation and the overall model was significant, $F(5, 190) = 36.33$, $p < 0.001$. Consistent with hypotheses, the perceived stress ^{X} campus connectedness interaction term was significantly predictive of depression, explaining an additional 2% of the variance in scores on depression, $\Delta F(1, 190) = 6.13$, $p = 0.01$. Therefore, the predictive relationship between perceived stress and depression varied according to campus connectedness. At Step 4, the perceived stress ^{X} perceived social support interaction term was added to the regression equation and the overall model was significant, $F(6, 189) = 30.30$, $p < 0.001$. Inconsistent with hypotheses, the perceived stress ^{X} perceived social support interaction term was non-significantly predictive of depression, explaining no further variance in scores on depression, $\Delta F(1, 189) = 0.56$, $p = 0.457$. Therefore the predictive relationship between perceived stress and depression did not vary according to perceived social support (**Table 1**).

To follow up the significant interaction effect of perceived stress ^{X} campus connectedness Dawson's [38] simple slope analyses were conducted to assess the nature of the interaction through a comparison of high campus connectedness scores (+ 1 SD) with low campus connectedness scores (−1 SD). The findings revealed, when campus connectedness was low, perceived stress was significantly predictive of depression, $\beta = 0.68$, $p < 0.001$. At high levels of campus connectedness, perceived stress was significantly predictive of depression, $\beta = 0.45$, $p < 0.001$. As such, the nature of the interaction appeared to be that campus connectedness at high levels had a buffering effect on the relationship between perceived stress and depression as represented by the decrease in the strength of the positive slope. Therefore, an increase in levels of campus connectedness results in a decrease in the magnitude of the effect of perceived stress on depression. A graphical representation of the interaction is displayed in **Figure 1**.

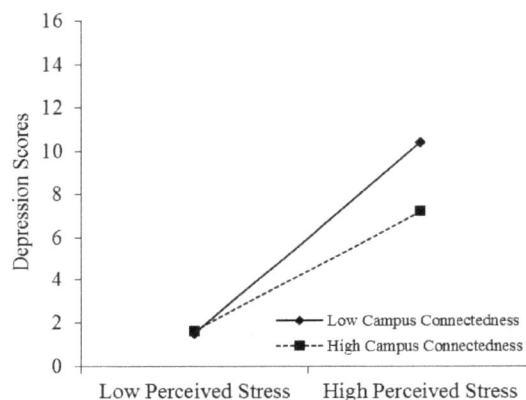

Figure 1. Campus connectedness moderated the relationship between perceived stress and depression.

Table 1. Model 1 investigating campus connectedness and perceived social support as moderating the relationships between perceived stress and depression.

	β	B	SE B	95% CI for B
Constant		4.14	1.10	[1.97, 6.30]
University	0.19	1.55***	0.56	[0.44, 2.65]
Constant		5.67	0.83	[4.02, 7.30]
Perceived stress	0.55	0.54***	0.06	[0.43, 0.66]
Perceived social support	−0.10	−0.06	0.04	[−0.13, 0.02]
Campus connectedness	−0.07	−0.07*	0.03	[−0.13, −0.02]
Constant		5.19	0.84	[3.53, 6.88]
Perceived stress ^{X} Campus connectedness	−0.13	−0.01**	0.00	[−0.12, −0.00]
Constant		10.71	7.45	[−3.99, 25.41]
Perceived stress ^{X} Perceived social support	−0.30	−0.00	0.01	[−0.02, 0.02]

Note: N = number of participants. CI = confidence intervals. *$p < 0.05$, **$p < 0.01$, ***$p < 0.001$.

Model 2. At Step 1 of the analysis, university was added to the regression equation and the overall model was non-significant, $F(1, 194) = 1.81$, $p = 0.180$. University explained a non-significant 1% of the variance in anxiety scores. Thus, university was non-significantly predictive of anxiety scores. At Step 2, after controlling for the effects of university, perceived stress, perceived social support, and campus connectedness were added to the regression equation and the overall model was significant, $F(4, 191) = 25.37$, $p < 0.001$. Perceived stress, perceived social support, and campus connectedness accounted for 34% of the variance in anxiety scores, $\Delta F (3, 191) = 32.93$, $p < 0.001$. At this step, perceived stress was a significant predictor of anxiety, $\beta = 0.44$ $p < 0.001$, indicating that a 1 SD increase in perceived stress resulted in a 0.44 SD increase in anxiety. Perceived social support at this step was a non-significant predictor of anxiety, $\beta = 0.13$, $p = 0.063$. Campus connectedness at this step was a significant negative predictor of anxiety, $\beta = -0.30$, $p < 0.001$, indicating that a 1 SD increase in campus connectedness resulted in a 0.13 decrease in anxiety. At Step 3 of the analysis, the perceived stress ^{X} campus connectedness interaction term was added to the regression equation and the overall model was significant, $F(5, 190) = 20.39$, $p < 0.001$. Inconsistent with hypothesis, the perceived stress ^{X} campus connectedness interaction term Therefore, the predictive relationship between perceived stress and anxiety did not vary according to campus connectedness. At Step 4, the perceived stress ^{X} perceived social support interaction term was added to the regression equation and the overall model was significant, $F(6, 189) = 17.39$, $p < 0.001$. Inconsistent with hypotheses, the perceived stress ^{X} perceived social support interaction term was non-significantly predictive of anxiety, explaining no further variance in scores on anxiety, $\Delta F(1, 189) = 1.92$, $p = 0.168$. Therefore the predictive relationship between perceived stress and anxiety did not vary according to perceived social support (**Table 2**).

4. Discussion

The aim of the current study was to examine psychosocial moderators of the relationships between perceived stress, anxiety, and depression in an international level in a sample of university students. It was firstly predicted that perceived social support would moderate the relationship between perceived stress and depression. Specifically, perceived social support would buffer the effects of perceived stress on depression, thereby reducing the strength of the relationship. The results of the moderation analysis did not support hypothesis two, as perceived social support did not moderate the relationship between perceived stress and depression. These findings do not support Cohen and Wills' [22] stress-buffering hypothesis. These results demonstrate perceived social support does not interact with perceived stress to protect university students from depression thus rejecting a buffering model of perceived social support.

Hypothesis two, evaluated the role of campus connectedness as a moderator in the relationship between perceived stress and depression. It was hypothesised that campus connectedness would buffer the relationship between perceived stress and depression, such that higher levels of campus connectedness would decrease the

Table 2. Model 2 investigating campus connectedness and perceived social support as moderating the relationships between perceived stress and anxiety.

	β	B	SE B	95% CI for B
Constant		5.42	1.07	[3.31, 7.54]
University	0.10	0.74	0.55	[−0.34, 1.82]
Constant		6.50	0.89	[4.75, 8.25]
Perceived stress	0.44	0.42***	0.06	[0.23, 0.54]
Perceived social support	0.13	0.07	0.04	[−0.00, 0.15]
Campus connectedness	−0.30	−0.14***	0.03	[−0.20, −0.70]
Constant		6.33	0.91	[4.53, 8.13]
Perceived stress ^{X} Campus connectedness	−0.05	−0.00	0.00	[−0.01, 0.01]
Constant		−4.77	8.06	[−20.68, 11.14]
Perceived stress ^{X} Perceived social support	0.62	0.01	0.01	[−0.02, 0.01]

Note: N = number of participants. CI = confidence intervals. *$p < 0.05$, **$p < 0.01$, ***$p < 0.001$.

strength of the positive association between perceived stress and depression. The results of the moderation analyses supported this hypothesis. A significant interaction of campus connectedness and perceived stress in predicting depression was found, with the interaction term accounting for 2% of the variance in depression scores. Again, this result is consistent with Chaplin's [35] review of the literature, in which interaction terms generally account for between 1% to 3% of the variance. The nature of this interaction appeared to be that campus connectedness at high levels buffered the relationship between perceived stress and depression, that is, campus connectedness reduced the strength of the association between the two variables. However, at low levels of campus connectedness the positive relationship between perceived stress and depression increased. These results demonstrate campus connectedness interacts with perceived stress to protect university students from depression.

Hypothesis three, in accordance with Cohen and Wills' [22] stress-buffering hypothesis examined whether perceived social support moderated the relationship between perceived stress and anxiety. It was predicted perceived social support would buffer the relationship between perceived stress and anxiety. This hypothesis was not supported, as the interaction term of perceived social support and perceived stress in predicting anxiety was non-significant. These findings do not support the stress-buffering hypothesis.

Hypothesis four, which investigated whether campus connectedness moderated the relationship between perceived stress and anxiety, was not supported. It was predicted that campus connectedness would buffer the relationship between perceived stress and anxiety. The interaction of campus connectedness and perceived stress in predicting anxiety was non-significant. To date no additional research has been conducted investigating the role of campus connectedness in moderating the relationship between perceived stress and anxiety. These findings demonstrate campus connectedness does not interact with perceived stress to provide a protective effect on anxiety. Although previous research supports associations among these variables, the results of the current study did not support a buffering model and only demonstrate support for a main effect model of campus connectedness on anxiety [29]. The findings from the current study suggest campus connectedness appears to make a beneficial contribution in reducing anxiety regardless of perceived stress levels. Although only one of the current study's four moderation analyses was significant, the results of the analysis demonstrating campus connectedness buffers the relationship between perceived stress and depression are noteworthy. The results make a valuable contribution to the body of knowledge and increase our understanding of the potential protective role of campus connectedness in preventing university students with high levels of perceived stress from the development of depression.

A number of limitations are noted with the current study. Firstly, the study did not control for social desirability biases and it is possible this may have influenced participants' responses. Future studies should consider the inclusion of a social desirability scale to avoid potential confounding of results. Another limitation of the current study was that a general measure of perceived stress was used and therefore it may not have fully encapsulated the unique stressors university students encounter. Future studies could use a measure of perceived stress that specifically assesses the stressors university students' experience. As the current study is the first to date to investigate the moderating role of campus connectedness, it is suggested future research is conducted to gain a further understanding of its protective utility in buffering the relationship between perceived stress, and depression. In addition, the moderating effects of variables such as resilience or optimism could be investigated to determine whether they can be fostered as protective factors in the university context.

The results from this study offer a valuable contribution to the literature in furthering our understanding of the utility of psychosocial factors in protecting university students on an international level from the adverse consequences of high levels of perceived stress, including the development of anxiety and depression. Cohen and Wills' [22] stress-buffering hypothesis was not supported within the current sample, suggesting that less emphasis should be placed on the protective role of perceived social support on perceived stress, anxiety, and depression among university students. However, the results from the current study provide support for both a main effect and buffering model of campus connectedness. Therefore, increasing campus connectedness in university students will result in deceases in levels of both depression and anxiety. Furthermore, recognising that psychosocial factors such as campus connectedness may protect university students from the development of stress-induced depression adds to the emerging body of literature surrounding connectedness within the university context. To reduce the high prevalence rates of mental health problems in university students, it seems likely that facilitating campus connectedness would provide positive outcomes for the mental health of university students. Future research should be directed towards examining the effectiveness of preventative programs and interventions that promote campus connectedness. Universities should remain committed to promoting campus connectedness in university students through the development of programs and activities that promote student diversity, cultural unity, and belonging, such as interest groups [30].

The present study has important implications for higher education, as findings indicate that university students who are more connected have lower levels of perceived stress, anxiety, and depression. These findings demonstrate it is important for students to become involved in and feel a part of their university communities in order to be protected against the effects of stress and, consequently, the occurrence of psychological distress. With the knowledge that campus connectedness buffers the relationship between perceived stress and depression, university students with higher levels of campus connectedness may be protected from the adverse effects of stress and the development of depression. The current study has provided insight into the benefits of increasing campus connectedness in university students internationally to promote psychological wellbeing and adjustment. This awareness should be used to initiate programs for universities in Australia, Hong Kong, and the United States to reduce the prevalence rates of mental health problems in university students.

References

[1] Lee, C., Dickson, D.A., Conley, C.S. and Holmbeck, G.N. (2014) A Closer Look at Self-Esteem, Perceived Social Support, and Coping Strategy: A Prospective Study of Depressive Symptomatology across the Transition to College. *Journal of Social and Clinical Psychology*, 33, 560-585. http://dx.doi.org/10.1521/jscp.2014.33.6.560

[2] Bewick, B., Koutsopoulou, G., Miles, J., Slaa, E. and Barkham, M. (2010) Changes in Undergraduate Students' Psychological Wellbeing as They Progress through University. *Studies in Higher Education*, 35, 633-645. http://dx.doi.org/10.1080/03075070903216643

[3] Andrews, B. and Wilding, J.M. (2004) The Relation of Depression and Anxiety to Life-Stress and Achievement in Students. *British Journal of Psychology*, 95, 509-521. http://dx.doi.org/10.1348/0007126042369802

[4] Chen, L., Wang, L., Qiu, X.H., Yang, X.X., Qiao, Z.X., Yang, Y.J. and Liang, Y. (2013) Depression among Chinese University Students: Prevalence and Socio-Demographic Correlates. *PLoS One*, 8, 667-672. http://dx.doi.org/10.1007/s00127-008-0345-x

[5] Wintre, M.G. and Yaffe, M. (2000) First-Year Students' Adjustment to University Life as a Function of Relationships with Parents. *Journal of Adolescent Research*, 15, 9-37. http://search.proquest.com/docview/211625077?accountid=26503 http://dx.doi.org/10.1177/0743558400151002

[6] Vaez, M., Kristenson, M. and Laflamme, L. (2004) Perceived Quality of Life and Self-Rated Health among First-Year University Students. *Social Indicators Research*, 68, 221-234. http://dx.doi.org/10.1023/B:SOCI.0000025594.76886.56

[7] Gruttadaro, D. and Crudo, D. (2012) College Students Speak: A Survey on Mental Health. National Alliance on Mental Health. www.nami.org/namioncampus

[8] Cohen, S. (2004) Social Relationships and Health. *The American Psychologist*, 59, 676-684. http://dx.doi.org/10.1037/0003-066X.59.8.676

[9] Dahlem, W.N., Zimet, D.G. and Walker, R.R. (1991) The Multidimensional Scale of Perceived Social Support: A Confirmation Study. *Journal of Clinical Psychology*, 47, 756-761.

[10] El Ansari, W., Stock, C., Snelgrove, S., Hu, X., Parke, S., Davies, S. and Mabhala, A. (2011) Feeling Healthy: A Survey of Physical and Psychological Wellbeing of Students from Seven Universities in the UK. *International Journal of Environmental Research and Public Health*, 8, 1308-23. http://dx.doi.org/10.3390/ijerph8051308

[11] Lee, R.M., Dean, B.L. and Jung, K.R. (2008) Social Connectedness, Extraversion, and Subjective Wellbeing: Testing a Mediation Model. *Personality and Individual Differences*, 45, 414-419. http://dx.doi.org/10.1016/j.paid.2008.05.017

[12] Eisenbarth, C.A., Champeau, D.A. and Donatelle, R.J. (2013) Relationship of Appraised Stress, Coping Strategies, and Negative Affect among College Students. *International Journal of Psychology and Behavioral Sciences*, 3, 131-138.

[13] Hammen, C., Brennan, P.A. and Shih, J.H. (2004) Family Discord and Stress Predictors of Depression and Other Disorders in Adolescent Children of Depressed and Nondepressed Women. *Journal of the American Academy of Child & Adolescent Psychiatry*, 43, 994-1002. http://dx.doi.org/10.1097/01.chi.0000127588.57468.f6

[14] Stewart-Brown, S., Evans, J., Patterson, J., Petersen, S., Doll, H., Balding, J. and Regis, D. (2000) The Health of Students in Institutes of Higher Education: An Important and Neglected Public Health Problem. *Journal of Public Health Medicine*, 22, 492. http://dx.doi.org/10.1093/pubmed/22.4.492

[15] Stallman, H.M. (2010) Psychological Distress in University Students: A Comparison with General Population Data. *Australian Psychologist*, 45, 249-257.

[16] Eisenberg, D., Speer, N. and Hunt, J.B. (2012) Attitudes and Beliefs about Treatment among College Students with

Untreated Mental Health Problems. *Psychiatric Services*, **63**, 711-713. http://dx.doi.org/10.1037/0002-9432.77.4.534

[17] Wong, J.G.W.S., Cheung, E.P.T., Chan, K.K.C., Ma, K.K.M. and Tang, S.W. (2006) Web-Based Survey of Depression, Anxiety and Stress in First-Year Tertiary Education Students in Hong Kong. *The Australian and New Zealand Journal of Psychiatry*, **40**, 777-782. http://dx.doi.org/10.1111/j.1440-1614.2006.01883.x

[18] Uchino, B.N. (2009) Understanding the Links between Social Support and Physical Health: A Life-Span Perspective with Emphasis on the Separability of Perceived and Received Support. *Perspectives on Psychological Science*, **4**, 236-255. http://dx.doi.org/10.1111/j.1745-6924.2009.01122.x

[19] Hyde, L.W., Gorka, A., Manuck, S.B. and Hariri, A.R. (2011) Perceived Social Support Moderates the Link between Threat-Related Amygdala Reactivity and Trait Anxiety. *Neuropsychologia*, **49**, 651-656. http://dx.doi.org/10.1016/j.neuropsychologia.2010.08.025

[20] Thoits, P.A. (2011) Mechanisms Linking Social Ties and Support to Physical and Mental Health. *Journal of Health and Social Behaviour*, **52**, 145-161. http://dx.doi.org/10.1177/0022146510395592

[21] Warner, R.M. (2013) Applied Statistics: From Bivariate through Multivariate Techniques. SAGE Publications, Thousand Oaks.

[22] Cohen, S. and Wills, T.A. (1985) Stress, Social Support, and the Buffering Hypothesis. *Psychological Bulletin*, **98**, 310-357. http://dx.doi.org/10.1037/0033-2909.98.2.310

[23] Lazarus, S.R. and Folkman, S. (1984) Stress, Appraisal, and Coping. Springer Publishing Company, New York.

[24] Skok, A., Harvey, D. and Reddihough, D. (2006) Perceived Stress, Perceived Social Support, and Wellbeing among Mothers of School-Aged Children with Cerebral Palsy. *Journal of Intellectual and Developmental Disability*, **31**, 53-57. http://dx.doi.org/10.1080/13668250600561929

[25] Chao, R.C.L. (2012) Managing Perceived Stress among College Students: The Roles of Social Support and Dysfunctional Coping. *Journal of College Counseling*, **15**, 5-21. http://dx.doi.org/10.1002/j.2161-1882.2012.00002.x

[26] Yarcheski, A. and Mahon, N.E. (1999) The Moderator-Mediator Role of Social Support in Early Adolescents. *Western Journal of Nursing Research*, 21, 685-698. http://dx.doi.org/10.1177/01939459922044126

[27] Williams, K.L. and Galliber, R.V. (2006) Predicting Depression and Self-Esteem from Social Connectedness, Support, and Competence. *Journal of Social and Clinical Psychology*, **25**, 855-874. http://dx.doi.org/10.1521/jscp.2006.25.8.855

[28] Lee, R.M. and Robbins, S.B. (1995) Measuring Belongingness: The Social Connectedness and the Social Assurance Scales. *Journal of Counselling Psychology*, **42**, 232. http://dx.doi.org/10.1037/0022-0167.45.3.338

[29] Leary, K.A. and DeRosier, M.E. (2012) Factors Promoting Positive Adaptation and Resilience during the Transition to College. *Psychology*, **3**, 1215-1222. http://dx.doi.org/10.4236/psych.2012.312A180

[30] Lee, R.M., Keough, K.A. and Sexton, J.D. (2002) Social Connectedness, Social Appraisal, and Perceived Life Stress in College Women and Men. *Journal of Counselling and Development*, **80**, 355-361. http://dx.doi.org/10.1002/j.1556-6678.2002.tb00200.x

[31] Townsend, K.C. and McWhirter, B.T. (2005) Connectedness: A Review of the Literature with Implications for Counseling, Assessment, and Research. *Journal of Counseling and Development*, **83**, 191-201. http://dx.doi.org/10.1002/j.1556-6678.2005.tb00596.x

[32] Rude, S.S. and Burnham, B.L. (1995) Connectedness and Neediness: Factors of the DEQ and SAS Dependency Scales. *Cognitive Therapy and Research*, **19**, 323-340. http://dx.doi.org/10.1007/BF02230403

[33] Cohen, S., Kamarck, T. and Mermelstein, R. (1983) A Global Measure of Perceived Stress. *Journal of Health and Social Behaviour*, **24**, 385-396. http://dx.doi.org/10.2307/2136404

[34] Lovibond, S.H. and Lovibond, P.F. (1995) Manual for the Depression Anxiety Stress Scales. 2nd Edition, Psychology Foundation, Sydney.

[35] Chaplin, W.F. (1991) The Next Generation of Moderator Research in Personality Psychology. *Journal of Personality*, **59**, 143-178. http://dx.doi.org/10.1111/j.1467-6494.1991.tb00772.x

[36] Evans, M.G. (1985) A Monte Carlo Study of the Effects of Correlated Method Variance in Moderated Multiple Regression Analysis. *Organisational Behaviour and Human Decision Processes*, **36**, 305-323. http://dx.doi.org/10.1016/0749-5978(85)90002-0

[37] Aiken, L.S. and West, S.G. (1991) Multiple Regression: Testing and Interpreting Interactions. Sage Publications, Inc., Thousand Oaks.

[38] Dawson, J.F. and Ritchter, A.Q. (2006) Probing Three-Way Interaction in Moderated Multiple Regression: Development and Application of a Slope Difference Test. *Journal of Applied Psychology*, **91**, 917-926. http://dx.doi.org/10.1037/0021-9010.91.4.917

4

Study on the Classification of Speech Anxiety Using Q-Methodology Analysis

SeoYoung Lee

GSI, Yonsei University, Seoul, Korea
Email: leeseoyoungann1004@gmail.com

Abstract

Public speaking is one of the cornerstones of mass communication, the influence of which has only been enhanced with the advent of the modern era. Yet despite its importance, up to 40% of the world's population feels anxious when faced with the prospect of presenting in front of an audience (Wilbur, 1981). However, public speaking anxiety is human condition that can be understood and with effort, overcome by sufferers. Based on theoretical research, this study presents an empirical investigation of speech anxiety. The research uses Q-methodology to generate categories of speakers and then draws on the PQ-method program to suggest ways for speakers to improve their speaking confidence based on these categories. This research is of a value to those who are interested in speech anxiety for therapeutic or pedagogical practice.

Keywords

Communication Apprehension, Trait Anxiety, State Anxiety, Anxious Arousal, Public Speaking, Q-Method, Stage Fright

1. Introduction

As society becomes more pluralistic, our social lives become more complicated which heightens the need for effective oratory skills.

This study provides a method of categorizing people according to their propensity to speech anxiety. It also aims to analyze the differences between each category in the factors of speech anxiety with the aim of deriving a typology of the components of the condition.

This study uses speech communication theory to derive practical solutions for dealing with speech anxiety. Effective communication is paramount in today's world where modern technologies offer numerous means for the exchanging of ideas and information. But verbal communication still remains the most important mode of human interaction. For example a professor's performance is evaluated not only by the content of his/her lecture but also by his/her speech delivery. The professor needs to be able to articulate clearly and in an inspiring manner as well.

In a pluralistic world where our social lives become ever more complex, the need for verbal communication of ideas and information remains vitally important. Yet 40% of the world's population feels some sort of anxiety about public speaking (Wilbur, 1981). Borkovec and O'Brien (1976) report that 25% of the adult population feels anxious about public speaking.

Most people have reported some feelings of public speaking anxiety. A wide body of academic literature attributes the causes of this condition to state or trait anxiety or a combination of the two. Based on my own theoretical research and teachings as a professor of speech communication as well as my experience in broadcasting, the researcher suggests using Q-methodology as instructional techniques to assist speakers in overcoming their anxiety.

2. Theoretical Background

2.1. Speech Anxiety

It was Spielberger (1966) who first suggested that anxiety is caused by a combination of the genetic disposition of a person (trait) and his emotional and mental state at a particular time. Spielberger's concept is applicable to a variety of situations and not just public speaking (Ayres & Hopf, 1993; Beatty, 1988; Beatty & Clair, 1990; McCroskey, 1997; McCroskey & Beatty, 1986) all sort to confirm that trait and state could explain why some people had such an aversion to public speaking.

When people are faced with a stressful situation, it has an impact on them physiologically, cognitively and behaviorally (Lang 1986). Fear or anxiety causes a number of physiological reactions such as increased heart rate, sweaty palms, numbness etc. Such autonomous reactions have been observed in speaking situations (Beatty & Dobos, 1997).

2.2. Trait Anxiety

Trait anxiety is a person's genetic predisposition to feeling anxious when faced with an uncomfortable or life threatening situations—such as the fear of being ridiculed in front of an audience. Beatty and McCroskey (2000) found that a person's communication apprehension is 80% genetically determined.

According to the Trait-State theory, highly anxious trait people are likely to experience heightened levels of state-anxiety, more seriously and more frequently, when faced with threats to self esteem (Spielberger, 1966).

Trait anxiety may also affect how a speaker interprets the non verbal responses of an audience (Hsu, 2009). Anxious individuals tend to have more negative opinions of their speech and will blame it on the audience. Less anxious individuals tend to view their own performances positively.

2.3. State Anxiety

State-anxiety contributes up to 20% of a person's adverse reaction. Trait anxiety is a good indicator of a person's state anxiety. State-anxiety can be decomposed into a person's reactivity—or the magnitude of his/or response to a stimuli plus his or her situation (Harris, Sawyer, & Behnke, 2006). The situation of a speech performance can be just as powerful as trait anxiety, if not more, in predicting state anxiety (Ayres, 1990; Beatty & Friedland, 1990; Harris, Sawyer, & Behnke, 2006; Keaten, Kelly, & Finch, 2004).

Klonowicz, Zawadzka, Zawadzki (1987) found that highly-reactive persons have elevated arousal levels even in the absence of stimuli. Thus they are likely to have a greater reaction to events around them. When aroused, they are likely to have a negative reaction to the stimuli. It is a cognitive process (Beatty, 1988) where the reaction to an arousal is viewed adversely. This psychological reaction only compounds the anxiety beyond the levels predicted by trait-anxiety. Conversely low reactive people may be aroused but are less likely to descend into anxiety.

Behnke & Sawyer (2001b) suggests that psychologically reactive people could benefit from public speaking practice sessions full of stress but with likelihood of a successful performance. Others like Beatty & McCroskey (2000) contend that it is difficult to utilize therapy to reduce psychological anxiety because so much of speech anxiety is genetically determined. Beatty and Valence (2000) showed that attempts to make classroom speeches less stressful did not prove effective. Still others like Kelly and Keaten (2000) suggest pedagogical means may provide effective cures.

Based on an experiment using bursting balloons to emulate stress, Behnke & Sawyer (2001b) found that psychological state anxiety reactivity contributed up to an additional 23% more state anxiety than the levels predicted by trait anxiety.

A speaker's anxiety is also affected by the situation in which he is asked to perform (Beatty, 1998). If the speaker is unfamiliar with the audience of the environment, he or she is more likely to be anxious, though the impact of familiarity is weak. This suggests that becoming accustomed to a speaking environment may not reduce speech anxiety. A speaker is also anxious if faced with speaking to superiors.

2.4. Behaviour Inhibition System

Anxiety is generated by our brain's Behaviour Inhibition System (BIS) (Gray & McNaughton, 2000; Gray, 1982). These neurological circuits are activated by situations such as public speaking where events are deviating from expectations and there is the possibility of punishment, non-reward or fear. This results in increased sensitivity to surroundings, speech disfluency, rigidity, heightened arousal, agitation and inhibited behavior. Those individuals with high trait anxiety disposition are particularly prone to a BIS reaction (Gray, 1982) and thus are more vulnerable to anxiety. This physiological reaction is the root cause of speech anxiety (Beatty, McCroskey, & Heisel, 1998).

2.5. The Four Stages of Speaker Apprehension

There are four stages of public speaker anxiety (Behnke & Sawyer, 2001a; Osorio, Crippa, & Loureiro, 2008). Stage 1 is the anticipatory stage when the speaker knows that the impending moment is imminent. This is followed by confrontational anxiety in the first few minutes of the speech. Anxiety adaptation occurs during the last minute of the speech and anxiety release after the speech is completed. Psychological anxiety peaks at the anticipatory stage while physiological anxiety peaks at the confrontational stage (Behnke & Sawyer, 2001a). After anxiety peaks, the speaker is more likely to adapt to the situation enabling speech anxiety to ease. The observation that state anxiety will ease with continuous exposure to fearful situation is known as Habituation (Finn, Sawyer, & Behnke, 2003; Gray, 1982, 1990; Gray & McNaughton, 2000). As habituation creeps in, the brain's BIS circuits will cease to exert influence over behaviour.

2.6. Q-Methodology

Q-Methodology is a research method used in psychology and in social sciences to study people's "subjectivity"—that is, their viewpoint. Q was developed by psychologist William Stephenson. It has been used both in clinical settings for assessing a patient's progress over time (intra-rater comparison) as well as in research settings that examines how people think about a topic (inter-rater comparisons).

Statistically, the variables of "R-research" are items or stimuli, whereas the variables of Q-methodology are people (Brown, 1980). The name "Q" comes from the form of factor analysis that is used to analyze the data. Normal factor analysis, called "R method", involves finding correlations between variables (e.g., height and age) across a sample of subjects. Q, on the other hand, looks for correlations between subjects across a sample of variables.

Q-factor analysis reduces the many individual viewpoints of the subjects down to a few "factors", which are claimed to represent shared ways of thinking. It is sometimes said that Q-factor analysis is R factor analysis with the data table turned sideways. While helpful as a heuristic for understanding Q, this explanation may be misleading, as most Q-methodologists argue that for mathematical reasons no one data matrix would be suitable for analysis with both Q and R.

2.6.1. Sorting the Statements in a Q-Sort

The data for Q-factor analysis come from a series of "Q-sorts" performed by one or more subjects. A Q-sort is a ranking of variables—typically presented as statements printed on small cards—according to some "condition of instruction". For example, in a Q study of people's views of a celebrity, a subject might be given statements like "He is a deeply religious man" and "He is a liar", and asked to sort them from "most like how I think about this celebrity" to "least like how I think about this celebrity". The use of ranking, rather than asking subjects to rate their agreement with statements individually, is meant to capture the idea that people think about ideas in relation to other ideas, rather than in isolation.

The sample of statements for a Q-sort is drawn from and claimed to be representative of a "concourse"—the sum of all things people say or think about the issue being investigated. Since concourses do not have clear membership lists (as would be the case in the population of subjects), statements cannot be drawn randomly so they do not meet R methodology expectations for statistically valid inferences. Commonly Q-methodologists use a structured sampling approach in order to try and represent the full breadth of the concourse.

One salient difference between Q and other social science research methodologies, such as surveys, is that it typically uses fewer subjects. This can be a strength, as Q is sometimes used with a single subject, and it makes research far less expensive. In such cases, a person will rank the same set of statements under different conditions of instruction. For example, someone might be given a set of statements about personality traits and then asked to rank them according to how well they describe herself, her ideal self, her father, her mother, etc. Working with a single individual is particularly relevant in the study of how an individual's rankings change over time and this was the first use of Q-methodology.

In studies of intelligence, Q-factor analysis can generate Consensus Based Assessment (CBA) scores as direct measures. Alternatively, the unit of measurement of a person in this context is his factor loading for a Q-sort he or she performs. Factors represent norms with respect to schemata. The individual who gains the highest factor loading on an operant factor is the person most able to conceive the norm for the factor. What the norm means is a matter, always, for conjecture and refutation (Popper, 1959). It may be indicative of the wisest solution, or the most responsible, the most important, or an optimized-balanced solution. These are all matters for future determination.

An alternative method that determines the similarity among subjects somewhat like Q-methodology, as well as the cultural 'truth" of the statements used in the test, is Cultural Consensus Theory.

The "Q-sort" data collection procedure is traditionally done using a paper template and the sample of statements or other stimuli printed on individual cards. However, there are also computer software applications for conducting online Q-sorts. For example, consulting firm Davis Brand Capital has created a proprietary online product, nQue, which is used to conduct online Q-sorts that mimic the analog, paper-based sorting procedure. However, the web-based software application that uses a drag-and-drop, graphical user interface to assist researchers is not available for commercial sale (Brown, 1980).

2.6.2. P-Samples

Stephenson (1953) said Q-methodology is based on small sample doctrine because large P-samples may cause statistical problems. Q-methodology trait is not jumping the logic or guessing. It has an experience based abduction trait (Plummar, 1974; Wells, 1975).

Participant selection in Q-methodology is not based on probability sampling (Aman, 2000) because the sampling is of the Q-set, not the participants (Stainton, Rogers, 1993). A large number of participants sometimes referred to as the P-set (van Excel, De Grand, 2005) are not required in Q-methodology as the aim of the process is to extricate key opinions of a selected participant group (Watts; Skenner, 2005). Accordingly, single cases came be the focus of Q-methodology research (Brown, 1993).

The reliability of each factor or cluster of beliefs is enhanced when 4 - 5 participants make up each factor. There are usually no more than 7 factors identified in a Q-sort (Brown, 1993). Accordingly, breadth and diversity of viewpoints is best achieved when a participant group contains between 40 - 80 participants (Stainton & Rogers, 2005). However reliable results can be obtained with far fewer participants (Watts and Stenner, 2006).

3. Methodology

3.1. Research Questions

A speaker's subjective experience of speech anxiety is amenable to Q-methodology and classification. Based on a speaker's subjective point of view, the traits of speakers who are susceptible to speech anxiety are classified according to their values, attitudes, assessment and orientation.

Research question 1: How to categorize people according to their speech anxiety and what are the characteristics of each classification?

Research question 2: What are the differences between the categories of speech anxiety?

Participants—P-Sample

The study sample consists of 20 graduates from the school of politics majoring in social science. Q studies can be very effective for studying small samples. Q studies are cost effective and take less time than an interview.

The most common participant to Q-sample ratio items found in other Q studies was roughly 1 to 1 (Watts &

Stenner, 2005). Therefore the number of participants should roughly match the number of Q-sample items.

3.2. Research, Design and Analysis

Q-samples are extracted from a concourse. Q-samples are respondents of a Q-sort and P-samples. The most important aim is how to structure the Q-samples. Respondents are usually interviewed to gain a deep understanding of their mindset. In this study P-samples are students of speech communication of which a subset of 20 interviewees were chosen. Each P-sample is normally distributed. We examine each sample to see the kind of classifications showing. The respondents are 20 graduate students majoring in social science (**Table 1**).

Interviews are referred to Q-sort. This data is analyzed by the Q-method program (**Table 2**).

The sort requires the use of software to analyze the data such as PQ-method. Interview participants score each statement in the survey. Correlations are then calculated between sorts to generate a correlation matrix.

Factors are then extracted from this correlation matrix. Factor analysis can then be either centroid factor analysis or principal components analysis. There is no conclusive evidence that one method is better than the other. Both methods produce similar results (Watts & Stener, 2005) (**Figure 1**).

Table 1. Distribution and numbers of statements.

Distribution	−4	−3	−2	−1	0	1	2	3	4
Numbers of Statements	1	2	3	4	5	4	3	2	1

Table 2. Q statements of interviewees and descending array of z scores.

Classification	Q Statements	Standard score of classification			
		I	II	III	IV
1	I feel nervous and anxious about making a speech.	1.966	2.005	2.263	2.011
2	I normally like to speak in front of an audience.	1.869	1.466	1.145	1.452
3	I am initially nervous. But as the speech progresses, I become relaxed and begin to enjoy speaking.	1.121	1.074	0.978	1.007
4	When I am making a speech, I think that the audience will laugh at me or think negatively of my speech.	0.877	0.89	0.927	0.894
5	I am very anxious because I lack experience in making speeches.	0.726	0.826	0.851	0.671
6	I am psychologically anxious in formal situations.	0.602	0.786	0.792	0.668
7	I think the audience is empathetic with me.	0.544	0.786	0.715	0.558
8	I display many nervous symptoms when doing presentations due to my speech phobia.	0.48	0.681	0.62	0.558
9	I am afraid of receiving negative feedback from the audience.	0.434	0.681	0.525	0.558
10	I am skilled in using gestures and voice tone to express myself.	0.401	0.394	0.435	0.449
11	I am good at speaking person to person but not in public.	0.262	0.287	0.376	0.445
12	I lack confidence in using gestures.	0.258	0.184	0.307	0.219
13	I lack confidence because I don't have presentation skills.	0.125	0.144	0.122	0.113
14	I am a natural at speaking in front of an audience.	0.066	0	−0.05	0.11
15	I am anxious because I cannot control my voice.	0	−0.144	−0.104	0
16	I feel very little anxiety about making speeches because I am attractive.	−0.175	−0.288	−0.217	0
17	I feel anxious about making speeches without the aid of power point.	−0.469	−0.537	−0.244	−0.336
18	I have very high self esteem so if I make a mistake, I get anxious about it.	−0.618	−0.681	−0.358	−0.445
19	I can overcome my anxiety about public speaking because my fears are derived from irrational thinking.	−0.754	−0.786	−0.57	−0.558
20	Speech anxiety is a common phenomenon.	−0.832	−0.787	−1.195	−0.558
21	I am very natural with eye contact.	−0.959	−0.825	−1.335	−1.339
22	If I was able to have more experience in making speeches, I will improve my speech making skills.	−1.08	−1.178	−1.38	−1.339
23	I am a very calm and introverted person, so I feel anxious about public speaking.	−1.102	−1.219	−1.407	−1.452
24	Public speaking is inherent so I cannot improve my skill.	−1.374	−1.756	−1.502	−1.452
25	I am not an eloquent person so I have a lot of anxiety about making speeches.	−2.37	−2.004	−1.693	−2.233

Issue to Investigate

Gathering of Opinions, Statements, Performance of Correspondence Among Them

Developments of Type Statements: Q Sampling

Ordering of Statement Rank Q Sort

Factor Analysis

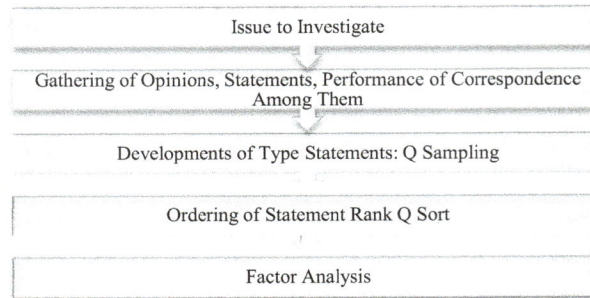

Figure 1. Stages of Q-factor analysis.

4. Research Results

4.1. Q-Factor Analysis

Type 1: Naturally Eloquent Speakers

Type 1 people are naturally eloquent speakers. They like to speak in front of an audience and they believe that it is an innate talent. They tend to think that their ability will always be available so they rarely feel anxious when speaking publicly nor do they care about a lack of experience. These are the traits of an innate naturally eloquent speaker. In addition they enjoy speaking in front of an audience but they tend not to make an effort. However their speech ability could be enhanced by practice and environmental factors so a lack of effort is a detriment. Yet compared to a type 2, type 1 persons are more anxious when making a speech (**Table 3**).

Type 2: Developed Professional Speakers

Type 2 people are professional speakers. They are developed speech professionals such as announcers, MCs and broadcasters. They like to speak in front of audiences, their speech is natural and their eye contact is natural. They are negative on speech anxiety, introverted characteristics, and the innate talent variables, so they are typically well trained in speech. Hence the name, developed speech professionals. Compared, to type 3 speakers, type 2 people conspicuously enjoy speaking in front of an audience. In addition, nonverbal messages, voice tone and body language are well executed so there is a big difference between type 2 and 3. Also compared with type 4, type 2 speakers deliver their speech naturally as well as nonverbal messages, voice tone and body language. Therefore there is also a marked difference between type 2 and 4 (**Table 4**).

Type 3: Introverted Speech Anxious Speakers

Type 3 persons are introverted with a high speech anxiety. They tend to believe that if they have more experience that they will improve. They are untrained speakers which is the greatest source of their anxiety. They are negative on the enjoyment for speaking in front audiences, voice tone, nonverbal expression, gestures, and the eye contact variables. They have an introverted personality so they are more concerned about their relative lack of experience. But when they are given more opportunities to speak in front of audiences they feel confident about improvement. When compared to type 4, a type 3 person experiences speech and presentation anxiety as an innate trait. This trait anxiety is typical of type 3 speakers. To overcome this, type 3 speakers need to improve their breath control. Such trait anxiety comes from timidity, shyness and sensitivity which emphasizes the importance of mind control and letting go of perfectionism. Other important ways to mitigate such anxiety include, using relaxation techniques and practicing positive thinking (**Table 5**).

Type 4: Speakers with Situational Stage Fright

The most prominent feature of type 4 speakers is they experience speech anxiety when they have speak in public as opposed to a one to one interaction in which they have no issues. They are positive on public speech anxiety, but are awkward when using gestures. In addition, they are negative on, a lack of confidence, experiencing psychological anxiety in formal situations, anxiety due to presentation skills, use of nonverbal communication, and the anxiety about making speeches variables. This type suffers from situational anxiety when they make a speech in public rather than anxiety over giving a speech itself. Situational anxiety sufferers can overcome their fears with experience and practice which leads to situational familiarity and increased confidence. Practice and experience clearly makes a significant difference to the skill levels of the practitioner. For example, Steve Jobs prepared 55 hours for a single presentation, so this type of person needs plenty of preparation to overcome this kind of anxiety (**Table 6**).

Table 3. Descending array of z scores and item description for type 1 (above and below +/−1).

	Q Statement	z score
Positive statements	2 I like to speak in front of audience.	1.966
	14 I am very natural with making speeches.	1.869
	24 Speech ability is natural or inherent so I cannot change my ability.	1.121
Negative statements	8 I have a lot of speech anxiety when doing presentations.	−1.08
	5 I am anxious because I lack experience.	−1.102
	4 The audience feels negative or will laugh at me.	−1.374
	1 I feel nervous and anxious about making a speech.	−2.37

Table 4. Descending array of z scores and item description for type 2 (above and below +/−1).

	Q Statement	z score
Positive statements	14 I am very natural with making speeches.	2.005
	2 I like to speak in front of audience.	1.466
	21 I am very natural with eye contact.	1.074
Negative statements	1 I feel nervous and anxious about making a speech.	−1.178
	23 I am a very calm and introverted person, so I feel anxious about public speaking.	−1.219
	24 Public speaking is inherent so I cannot improve my speech making skill.	−1.756
	25 I am not eloquent so I have high speech anxiety	−2.004

Table 5. Descending array of z scores and item description for type 3 (above and below +/−1).

	Q Statement	z score
Positive statements	23 I am a very calm and introverted person, so I feel anxious about public speaking.	2.263
	22 If I have more chances of making speeches, I will improve.	1.145
Negative Statements	3 Before I start my speech, I am very nervous. But as the speech progresses, I become relaxed and begin to enjoy speaking.	−1.195
	2 I like to speak in front of audience.	−1.335
	10 I am skilled in using gestures and voice tone to express myself.	−1.38
	21 I am very natural with eye contact.	−1.407
	16 I am very attractive so I am not afraid of making speeches.	−1.502
	1 I feel nervous and anxious about making a speech.	−1.693

Table 6. Descending array of z scores and item description for type 4 (above and below +/−1).

	Q Statement	z score
Positive statements	8 I have a lot of speech anxiety when doing presentations.	2.011
	11 I am very confident in speaking person to person but not in public.	1.452
	12 I am not confident with my gestures.	1.007
Negative statements	6 I feel psychologically anxious in formal situations.	−1.339
	5 I am very anxious because I lack experience in making speeches	−1.339
	13 I lack confidence because I don't have presentation skills	−1.452
	10 I am skilled in using gestures and voice tone to express myself	−1.452
	1 I feel nervous and anxious about making a speech.	−2.233

4.2. Comparison Analysis between the Main Types

Comparison between type 1 and type 2 speakers

Table 7 shows differences and similarities between the type 1 and type 2 speakers. Marked differences in attitudes are demonstrated in question 24 and 25. Statement 1 and 6 also showed some notable differences in attitudes. The results showed that professional speakers are more confident and like to speak in public while the results for type 1 speakers reflect some hesitancy and anxiety though not in all aspects of communication apprehension.

Comparison between type 1 and type 3 speakers

Table 8 shows differences in attitudes between naturally eloquent speakers (type 1) and introverted speech anxious types (type 3). When compared to type 1 speakers, type 3 speakers displayed larger differences in their

Table 7. Descending array of differences between factors type 1 and type 2.

No.	Statement	Type 1	Type 2	Difference
24	Public speaking is inherent so I think I cannot improve my speech making skill.	1.121	−1.756	2.877
25	I am not eloquent so I have high speech anxiety.	0.602	−2.004	2.606
23	I am a very calm and introverted person, so I feel anxious about public speaking.	0	−1.219	1.219
12	I am not confident with my gesture.	0.125	−0.681	0.806
2	I like to speak in front of audience.	1.966	1.466	0.499
15	I am very anxious because I cannot control my voice.	−0.469	−0.825	0.356
16	I am very attractive so I am not afraid of making speeches.	0.401	0.287	0.114
19	I can overcome speech anxiety because it comes from irrational thoughts.	0.726	0.786	−0.06
14	I am very natural with making speeches.	1.869	2.005	−0.136
17	I feel anxious about making speeches without the aid of powerpoint.	−0.175	0	−0.175
21	I am very natural with eye contact.	0.877	1.074	−0.197
7	I think the audience is empathetic with me.	0.48	0.681	−0.201
5	I am very anxious because I lack experience.	−1.102	−0.786	−0.316
3	Before I start my speech, I am very nervous. But as the speech progresses, I become relaxed and begin to enjoy speaking.	0.066	0.394	−0.328
22	If I have more chances of making speeches, I will improve.	0.544	0.89	−0.346
10	I am skilled in using gestures and voice tone to express myself.	0.434	0.826	−0.392
18	I have high self esteem so if I make a mistake, I am very anxious about it.	0.258	0.681	−0.423
20	speech anxiety is very common.	0.262	0.786	−0.524
8	I display many nervous symptoms when doing presentations due to my speech phobia.	−1.08	−0.537	−0.543
4	The audience feel negative or will laugh at me.	−1.374	−0.787	−0.587
11	I am very confident in speaking person to person but not in public.	−0.754	−0.144	−0.61
13	I lack confidence because I don't have presentation skills.	−0.959	−0.288	−0.671
9	I am afraid of negative feedback from the audience.	−0.618	0.144	−0.762
6	I feel psychologically anxious in the formal situations.	−0.832	0.184	−1.015
1	I feel nervous and anxious about making a speech.	−2.37	−1.178	−1.191

Table 8. Descending array of differences between factors type 1 and type 3.

No.	Statement	Type 1	Type 3	Difference
2	I like to speak in front of audience.	1.966	−1.335	3.301
21	I am very natural with eye contact.	0.877	−1.407	2.284
16	I am very attractive so I am not afraid of making speeches.	0.401	−1.502	1.903
10	I am skilled in using gestures and voice tone to express myself.	0.434	−1.38	1.814
24	Public speaking is inherent so I think I cannot improve my skill.	1.121	−0.244	1.365
3	First time anxious and then enjoy the speech.	0.066	−1.195	1.261
14	I am very natural with making speeches.	1.869	0.851	1.018

Continued

7	I think the audience is empathetic with me.	0.48	−0.358	0.838
25	I am not eloquent so I have high speech anxiety.	0.602	−0.104	0.706
19	I can overcome speech anxiety because it came from irrational thoughts.	0.726	0.307	0.419
17	If I cannot use speech aids like PPT, I am anxious with making speech.	−0.175	−0.57	0.394
18	I have high self esteem and if I make a mistake, I am very anxious about it.	0.258	−0.05	0.309
12	I am not confident with my gesture.	0.125	0.62	−0.495
22	If I have more chances of making speeches, I will improve.	0.544	1.145	−0.6
6	I feel psychologically anxious when I am in the formal situation.	−0.832	−0.217	−0.614
20	speech anxiety is very common.	0.262	0.927	−0.665
1	I feel nervous and anxious about making a speech.	−2.37	−1.693	−0.677
11	I am very confident in speaking person to person but not in public.	−0.754	0.122	−0.876
15	I am very anxious because I cannot control my voice.	−0.469	0.525	−0.993
9	I am very afraid of negative feedback from the audience.	−0.618	0.715	−1.333
5	I am very anxious because I am lack of experience.	−1.102	0.435	−1.537
4	The audience feel negative or laugh at me.	−1.374	0.376	−1.75
8	I have a lot of speech anxiety when doing presentations.	−1.08	0.792	−1.872
13	I am very anxious with my presentation skills.	−0.959	0.978	−1.936
23	I am a very introverted and calm person. I have high speech.	0	2.263	−2.263

public speaking attitudes than that was shown for type 2 speakers in **Table 2**. As expected, type 3 speakers showed less confidence in their public speaking ability compared to type 1 speakers—as reflected in statements 2, 21, 16, 8, 13 & 23.

Comparison between type 1 and type 4 speakers

Type 4 speakers are confident speaking person to person but not in public and this attitude is reflected in the positive score (1.452) shown for statement 11. Interesting to note however that type 1 speakers are negative on this aspect. As expected, type 4 speakers are not confident in doing presentations (statement 8). Statements 10, 14 and 2 all reflect notable difference in ability attitudes between type 1 and 4 speakers (**Table 9**).

Comparison between type 2 and 3 speakers

There are more notable differences in attitudes between these two types of speakers than in the three previous tables. Statement 23, 2, 21 and 10 all reflect the differences that we would expect between the two speaker types. It is interesting to note that type 3 speakers still felt a moderate level of ability in their public speaking ability (statement 14) (**Table 10**).

Comparison between the type 2 and type 4 speakers

Similar to the previous table, there are numerous differences in the attitudes, confidence and abilities between type 2 and type 4 speakers. Again, it is interesting to note is that type 4 speakers don't feel anxious (statement 6). The biggest differences (statement 10, 14, 6, 8, 12, 24 and 25) are all in line with what we would expect between these groups of people (**Table 11**).

Comparison between type 3 and type 4 speakers

Type 3 and type 4 speakers are the two groups with the least confidence in their public speaking ability. But the following table shows that type 3 speakers are considerably less confident than type 4 speakers about their speech making abilities–as reflected in statement 23, 24, 6, 16, 21, 3, and 2. Once more, it is interesting to note that both groups don't feel nervous about making a speech (statement 1) but they admit to feeling speech anxiety (statement 8). In addition, the groups don't feel confident about their non-verbal communication skills (statement 10) (**Table 12**).

Table 9. Descending array of differences between factors type 1 and type 4.

No.	Statement	Type 1	Type 4	Difference
10	I can speak non-verbally with my tone of voice and body language.	0.434	−1.452	1.886
14	I am very natural with making speeches.	1.869	0.11	1.76
2	I like to speak in front of audience.	1.966	0.668	1.298
24	Speech ability is natural or inherent so I cannot improve my skill.	1.121	0.113	1.008
18	I have high self esteem so if I make a mistake, I get anxious about it.	0.258	−0.336	0.594
23	I am a very calm and introverted person, so I feel anxious about public speaking.	0	−0.558	0.558
6	I feel psychologically anxious in the formal situations.	−0.832	−1.339	0.508
13	I lack confidence because I don't have presentation skills.	−0.959	−1.452	0.494
7	I think the audience is empathetic with me.	0.48	0	0.48
21	I am very natural with eye contact.	0.877	0.445	0.432
16	I am very attractive so I am not afraid of making speeches.	0.401	0	0.401
5	I am very anxious because I lack experience.	−1.102	−1.339	0.237
15	I am very anxious because I cannot control my voice.	−0.469	−0.558	0.09
25	I am not eloquent so I have high speech anxiety.	0.602	0.558	0.044
22	If I have more chances of making speeches, I will improve.	0.544	0.558	−0.014
1	I feel nervous and anxious about making a speech.	−2.37	−2.233	−0.136
19	I can overcome speech anxiety because it came from irrational thoughts.	0.726	0.894	−0.168
9	I am afraid of negative feedback from the audience.	−0.618	−0.445	−0.173
20	Speech anxiety is very common.	0.262	0.558	−0.296
3	I am initially nervous. But as the speech progresses, I become relaxed and begin to enjoy speaking.	0.066	0.671	−0.606
17	I feel anxious about making speeches without the aid of power point.	−0.175	0.449	−0.624
12	I am not confident with my gesture.	0.125	1.007	−0.882
4	The audience feel negative or will laugh at me.	−1.374	0.219	−1.593
11	I am very confident in speaking person to person but not in public.	−0.754	1.452	−2.206
8	I display many nervous symptoms when doing presentations due to my speech phobia.	−1.08	2.011	−3.09

Table 10. Descending array of differences between factors type 2 and type 3.

No.	Statement	Type 2	Type 3	Difference
2	I like to speak in front of audience.	1.466	−1.335	2.802
21	I am very natural with eye contact.	1.074	−1.407	2.481
10	I am skilled in using gestures and voice tone to express myself.	0.826	−1.38	2.206
16	I am very attractive so I am not afraid of making speeches.	0.287	−1.502	1.789
3	I am initially nervous. But as the speech progresses, I become relaxed and begin to enjoy speaking.	0.394	−1.195	1.589
14	I am very natural with making speeches.	2.005	0.851	1.154
7	I think the audience is empathetic with me.	0.681	−0.358	1.039
18	I have high self esteem and if I make a mistake, I am very anxious about it.	0.681	−0.05	0.732
17	I feel anxious about making speeches without the aid of power point.	0	−0.57	0.57
1	I feel nervous and anxious about making a speech.	−1.178	−1.693	0.515
19	I can overcome speech anxiety because it came from irrational thoughts.	0.786	0.307	0.479

Continued

6	I feel psychologically anxious in formal situations.	0.184	−0.217	0.401
20	speech anxiety is very common.	0.786	0.927	−0.142
22	If I have more chances of making speeches, I will improve.	0.89	1.145	−0.255
11	I am very confident in speaking person to person but not in public.	−0.144	0.122	−0.266
9	I am very afraid of negative feedback from the audience.	0.144	0.715	−0.571
4	The audience feel negative or will laugh at me.	−0.787	0.376	−1.163
5	I am very anxious because I lack experience.	−0.786	0.435	−1.221
13	I lack confidence because I don't have presentation skills.	−0.288	0.978	−1.265
12	I am not confident in using gestures.	−0.681	0.62	−1.301
8	I display many nervous symptoms when doing presentations due to my speech phobia.	−0.537	0.792	−1.33
15	I am very anxious because I cannot control my voice.	−0.825	0.525	−1.35
24	Public speaking is inherent so I cannot improve my skill.	−1.756	−0.244	−1.512
25	I am not eloquent so I have high speech anxiety.	−2.004	−0.104	−1.9
23	I am a very calm and introverted person, so I feel anxious about public speaking.	−1.219	2.263	−3.481

Table 11. Descending array of differences between factors type 2 and type 4.

No.	Statement	Type 2	Type 4	Difference
10	I am skilled in using gestures and voice tone to express myself.	0.826	−1.452	2.278
14	I am very natural with making speeches.	2.005	0.11	1.895
6	I feel psychologically anxious in formal situations.	0.184	−1.339	1.523
13	I lack confidence because I don't have presentation skills.	−0.288	−1.452	1.165
1	I feel nervous and anxious about making a speech.	−1.178	−2.233	1.055
18	I have high self esteem so if I make a mistake, I get very anxious about it.	0.681	−0.336	1.017
2	I like to speak in front of audience.	1.466	0.668	0.798
7	I think the audience is empathetic with me.	0.681	0	0.681
21	I am very natural with eye contact.	1.074	0.445	0.629
9	I am very afraid of negative feedback from the audience.	0.144	−0.445	0.59
5	I am very anxious because I lack experience.	−0.786	−1.339	0.553
22	If I have more chances of making speeches, I will improve.	0.89	0.558	0.332
16	I am very attractive so I am not afraid of making speeches.	0.287	0	0.287
20	speech anxiety is very common.	0.786	0.558	0.227
19	I can overcome speech anxiety because it came from irrational thoughts.	0.786	0.894	−0.108
15	I am very anxious because I cannot control my voice.	−0.825	−0.558	−0.267
3	I am initially nervous. But as the speech progresses, I become relaxed and begin to enjoy speaking.	0.394	0.671	−0.278
17	I feel anxious about making speeches without the aid of power point.	0	0.449	−0.449
23	I am a very calm and introverted person, so I feel anxious about public speaking.	−1.219	−0.558	−0.66
4	The audience feel negative or will laugh at me.	−0.787	0.219	−1.006
11	I am very confident speaking person to person but not in public.	−0.144	1.452	−1.596
12	I am not confident with my gestures.	−0.681	1.007	−1.688
24	Public speaking is inherent so I cannot improve my skill.	−1.756	0.113	−1.869
8	I have a lot of speech anxiety when doing presentations.	−0.537	2.011	−2.548
25	I am not eloquent so I have high speech anxiety.	−2.004	0.558	−2.563

Table 12. Descending array of differences between factors type 3 and type 4.

No.	Statement	Type 3	Type 4	Difference
23	I am a very calm and introverted person, so I feel anxious about public speaking.	2.263	−0.558	2.821
13	I lack confidence because I don't have presentation skills.	0.978	−1.452	2.43
5	I am very anxious because I lack experience.	0.435	−1.339	1.774
9	I am very afraid of negative feedback from the audience.	0.715	−0.445	1.161
6	I feel psychologically anxious when I am in formal situations.	−0.217	−1.339	1.122
15	I am very anxious because I cannot control my voice.	0.525	−0.558	1.083
14	I am very natural with making speeches.	0.851	0.11	0.742
22	If I have more chances of making speeches, I will improve.	1.145	0.558	0.586
1	I feel nervous and anxious about making a speech.	−1.693	−2.233	0.54
20	speech anxiety is very common.	0.927	0.558	0.369
18	I have high self esteem and if I make a mistake, I get very anxious about it.	−0.05	−0.336	0.285
4	The audience feel negative or will laugh at me.	0.376	0.219	0.157
10	I am skilled in using gestures and voice tone to express myself.	−1.38	−1.452	0.072
24	Public speaking is inherent so I cannot improve my skill.	−0.244	0.113	−0.357
7	I think the audience is empathetic with me.	−0.358	0	−0.358
12	I lack confidence in using gesture.	0.62	1.007	−0.387
19	I can overcome speech anxiety because it came from irrational thoughts.	0.307	0.894	−0.587
25	I am not eloquent so I have high speech anxiety.	−0.104	0.558	−0.662
17	I feel anxious about making speeches without the aid of powerpoint.	−0.57	0.449	−1.018
8	I have a lot of speech anxiety when doing presentations.	0.792	2.011	−1.218
11	I am very confident in speaking person to person but not in public.	0.122	1.452	−1.33
16	I am very attractive so I am not afraid of making speeches.	−1.502	0	−1.502
21	I am very natural with eye contact.	−1.407	0.445	−1.852
3	I am initially nervous. But as the speech progresses, I become relaxed and begin to enjoy speaking.	−1.195	0.671	−1.866
2	I like to speak in front of audience.	−1.335	0.668	−2.003

5. Discussion

This paper derived methods to overcome speech anxiety by analyzing the personal traits of speakers, the characteristics of communication apprehension, a speaker's self perception and their public speaking experience. A person's speech ability depends on how fast they can overcome their speech anxiety. The speaker has to come to terms with their speech apprehension and alter their speech style. From an academic perspective, there is a plethora of research on this discipline but this paper is the first to use Q-methodology to examine the problem. The classification of speech anxiety has pragmatic value.

Recent research indicates that "speaking in from of others is rated as the largest cause of anxiety in people" (Anwan, Azher, Anwar, & Naz, 2010).

Current research suggests three techniques to reduce public speaking anxiety. First, systematic desensitization involves relaxation, deep breathing, and visualization (Friedrich, Goss, Cunconan, & Lane, 1997). This technique can be practiced in group settings or alone.

Second, cognitive restructuring requires participants to create a negative self-talk list, identify irrational beliefs embedded in each thought, develop a coping statement for each irrational belief, and practice the coping statements until they become second nature (Ayres, Hopf, & Peterson, 2000).

The third technique, skills training, refers to learning and practicing techniques targeted toward improving individual speaking behaviours (Kelly, 1997). Skill training usually involves participating in a course where the student learns and practices public speaking skills.

Berkun (2009) suggests being prepared by practicing will assist in overcoming speech anxiety. Memorize key points but don't recite the speech word for word like a robot. Visualisation techniques such as imagining standing in front of an audience will prepare a speaker to deal with the adverse situation. Perfecting your presentation through practice will also provide you with confidence and a mental picture of how to proceed throughout different points of the speech. It also makes it easier to improvise should the audience behave badly like falling asleep or if someone heckles you.

Other strategies recommended by Berkun for calming nerves include: arriving early to avoid being flustered, checking the sound and audio visual equipment to avoid hiccups, pacing up and down the stage whilst speaking helps to calm nerves, sitting with the audience beforehand to obtain a feel of what they are seeing and eat early but not before your talk. Speaking with members of the audience beforehand puts your mind in the mood for talking–similar to overcoming the initial nerves of talking to strangers when arriving at a party.

Some people find that exercise will burn off their nervous energy before a talk. They then become too tired to worry about nerves. Exercise also puts you in a natural high so you will be more relaxed on stage.

Anxious people will also need to deal with irrational thoughts such as being laughed at, saying something silly or putting people to sleep. Berkun (2009) believes that if you are comfortable talking to people in a social situation, then you should be comfortable talking to an audience. A speaker should apply this logic when dealing with this irrational thought. Most audiences are polite and will not judge you badly if you make an embarrassing mistake. President George Bush was infamous for making silly statements on camera and the media would ridicule him. But despite these verbal transgressions, he managed to be re-elected for a second term. Compare your irrationality to the verbal mistakes Bush committed during his presidency and you realize how irrelevant your worries are.

6. Conclusion

Using Q-methodology, I have categorized four types of people according to their speech anxiety. Type 1 persons are eloquent natural speakers. They enjoy speaking in front of an audience and they don't believe that practicing will improve their natural ability. However, I find that naturally gifted speakers could improve their skills by practicing.

Type 2 persons are professional speakers such as broadcasters who have gotten accustomed to speaking publicly by constantly practicing in front of a camera or in front of an audience.

Type 3 persons are introverted person. They are genetically predisposed to trait-anxiety. They would benefit from systematic desensitization, positive thinking and relaxation therapy to mitigate their fear of public speaking. The treatment would involve continual exposure to a series of situations which cause anxiety (like giving a speech). In addition, the patient would be attempting to relax via deep muscle relaxation exercises. The initial stimuli do not provoke a lot of anxiety but gradually increased throughout the therapy session. Thus the introvert is trained to relax whilst being exposed to anxious stimuli. In this manner the bond between these stimuli and the anxiety responses will be weakened (Wolpe, 1958: p. 71).

There are other desensitization techniques such as reactive inhibition therapy which involves teaching introverts to deliberately evoke all the unpleasant feelings associated with speech anxiety (Malleson, 1959: p. 226). The basis of this therapy is that a person is always trying to escape from these unpleasant feelings but if he was made to face his fears, the cycle of anxiety would be broken.

Type 4 is situational fright person. They suffer from speech anxiety because of the lack of experience. It is a psychological condition triggered by the situation. Such speakers would benefit from exercising mind control—such as imagining that they are communicating in a one to one situation instead being in front of an audience. These people will improve their skills if they practice very hard.

Therefore I recommend cognitive behaviour therapy involving systematic desensitization and cognitive restructuring procedures as effective means for reducing worry and emotional responses in anxious situations.

Constant practice and skills training will enable speech anxiety sufferers to overcome their fears. I also suggest using instructional techniques to improve the speaking confidence of speech anxiety sufferers for pedagogical and therapeutic practice.

References

Anwan, R., Azher, M., Anwar, M. N., & Naz, A. (2010). An Investigation of Foreign Language Classroom Anxiety and Its Relationship with Students' Achievement. *Journal of College Teaching and Learning, 7*, 33-40.

Ayres, J., & Hopf, T. (1993). *Coping with Speech Anxiety*. Norwood, NJ: Ablex.

Ayres, J., Hopf, T. S., & Peterson, E. (2000). A Test of Communication-Orientation Motivation (COM) Therapy. *Communication Reports, 13*, 35-44. http://dx.doi.org/10.1080/08934210009367721

Beatty, M. J. (1988). Public Speaking Apprehension, Decision-Making Errors in the Selection of Speech Introduction Strategies and Adherence to Strategy. *Communication Education, 37*, 297-311. http://dx.doi.org/10.1080/03634528809378731

Beatty, M. J., & Dobos, J. A. (1997). Physiological Assessment. In J. A. Day, J. C. McCroskey, H. Ayres, T. Hopf, & D. M. Ayres (Eds.), *Avoiding Communication Shyness, Reticience and Communication* (2nd ed., pp. 216-230). Creskill, NJ. Hampton Press.

Beatty, M., & Friedland, M. (1990). Public Speaking State Anxiety as a Function of Selected Situational and Predispositional Variables. *Communication Education, 39*, 142-147. http://dx.doi.org/10.1080/03634529009378796

Beatty, M. J., & Clair, R. P. (1990). Decision Rule Orientation and Public Speaking Apprehension. *Journal of Social Behavior and Personality, 5*, 105-116.

Beatty, M. J., & Dobos, J. A. (1997). Psychological Assessment. In J. A. Daly, J. C. McCroskey, H. Ayres, T. Hopf, & D. M. Ayres (Eds.), *Avoiding Communication Shyness, Reticence and Communication Apprehension* (pp. 217-229). Cresskill, NJ: Hampton Press.

Beatty, M. J., McCroskey, J. C., & Heisel, A. D. (1998). Communication Apprehension as Temperamental Expression: A Communibiological Paradigm. *Communication Monographs, 65*, 197-219. http://dx.doi.org/10.1080/03637759809376448

Beatty, M. J., & McCroskey, J. C. (2000). The Communibiological Perspective: Implications for Communication in Instruction. *Communication Education, 49*, 1-6. http://dx.doi.org/10.1080/03634520009379187

Behnke R., & Sawyer, C. R. (2001a). Patterns Of Psychological State Anxiety in Public Speaking as a Function of Anxiety Sensitivity. *Communication Quarterly, 49*, 84-94. http://dx.doi.org/10.1080/01463370109385616

Behnke R., & Sawyer, C. R. (2001b). Public Speaking Arousal as a Function of Anticipatory Activation and Autonomic Reactivity. *Communication Reports, 14*, 73-85. http://dx.doi.org/10.1080/08934210109367740

Berkun, S. (2009). *Confessions of a Public Speaker*. California: O'Reilly Media Inc.

Borkovec, T. D., & O'Brien, G. T. (1976). Methodological and Target Issues in Analogue Therapy Outcome Research. In Hersen, E. Eisler, & P. Miller (Eds.), *Progrees in Behaviour Modification* (p. 3). New York: Academic Press.

Finn, A. N., Sawyer, C. R., & Behnke, R. (2003). Audience-Perceived Anxiety Patterns of Public Speakers. *Communication Quarterly, 51*, 470-481. http://dx.doi.org/10.1080/01463370309370168

Friedrich, G., Goss, B., Cunconan, T., & Lane, D. R. (1997). Systematic Desensitization. In *Avoiding Communication: Shyness, Reticence, and Communication Apprehension* (pp. 305-330). Cresskill, NJ: Hampton Press.

Gray, J. A. (1982). *The Neuropsychology of Anxiety: An Enquiry into the Functions of the Septo-Hippocampal System*. Oxford: Oxford University Press.

Gray, J. A. (1990). Brain Systems that Mediate both Emotion and Cognition. *Cognition & Emotion, 4*, 269-288. http://dx.doi.org/10.1080/02699939008410799

Gray, J. A., & McNaughton, N. (1982). *The Neuropsychology of Anxiety: An Enquiry into the Functions of the Septo-Hippocampal System* (2nd ed.). Oxford: Oxford University Press.

Gray, J. A., & McNaughton, N. (2000). Anxiolytic Action on the Behavioural Inhibition System Implies Multiple Types of Arousal Contribute to Anxiety. *Journal of Affective Disorders, 61*, 161-176. http://dx.doi.org/10.1016/S0165-0327(00)00344-X

Harris, K. B., Sawyer, C., & Behnke, R. R. (2006). Predicting Speech State Anxiety from Trait Anxiety, Reactivity, and Situational Influences. *Communication Quarterly, 54*, 213-226. http://dx.doi.org/10.1080/01463370600650936

Hsu, C. F. (2009). The Relationship of Trait Anxiety, Audience Nonverbal Feedback and Attributions to Public Speaking State Anxiety. *Communication Research Reports, 26*, 237-246. http://dx.doi.org/10.1080/08824090903074407

Kelly, L. (1997). Skills Training as a Treatment for Communication Problems. In J. A. Daly, J. C. McCroskey, H. A. Ayres, T. Hopf, & D. M. Ayres (Eds.), *Avoiding Communication: Shyness, Reticence, and Communication Apprehension* (2nd ed., pp. 331-336). Cresskill, NJ: Hampton.

Kelly, L., & Keaten, J. A. (2000). Treating Communication Anxiety: Implications of the Commuibiological Paradigm. *Communication Education, 49,* 45-47. http://dx.doi.org/10.1080/03634520009379192

Kelly, L., Keaten, J. A., & Finch, C. (2004). Reticent and Non-Reticent College Students' Preferred Communication Channels for Communicating with Faculty. *Communication Research Reports, 21,* 197-209. http://dx.doi.org/10.1080/08824090409359981

Klonowicz, T., Zawadzka, G., & Zawadzki, B. (1987). Reactivity, Arousal, and Coping with Stress. *Personality and Individual Differences, 8,* 793-798. http://dx.doi.org/10.1016/0191-8869(87)90132-2

Lang, P. J. (1986). The Cognitive Psychophysiology of Emotion: Fear and Anxiety. In A. H. Tuma, & J. D. Maser (Eds.), *Anxiety and the Anxiety Disorders* (pp. 130-179). Hillside, NJ: Erlbaum.

McCroskey, J. C., & Beatty, M. J. (1986). Oral Communication Apprehension. In W. H. Jones, J. M. Cheek, & S. R. Briggs (Eds.), *Shyness: Perspectives on Research and Treatment* (pp. 279-293). New York: Plenum Press.

McCroskey, J. C. (1997). Willingness to Communicate, Communication Apprehension, and Self Perceived Communication Competence: Conceptualizations and Perspectives. In J. A. Daly, J. C. McCroskey, J. Ayres, T. Hopf, & D. M. Sonadre (Eds.), *Avoiding Communication: Shyness, Reticence, and Communication Apprehension* (2nd ed.). Cresskill, NJ: Hampton.

Malleson, N. (1959). Panic and Phobia: A Possible Method of Treatment. *The Lancet, 273,* 225-227. http://dx.doi.org/10.1016/S0140-6736(59)90052-2

Osorio, F., Crippa, J. A., & Loureiro, S. R. (2008). Experimental Models for the Evaluation of Speech and Public Speaking Anxiety: A Critical Review of the Designs Adopted. *The Journal of Speech-Language Pathology and Applied Behavior Analysis, 2,* 97.

Popper, K. (1959). *The Logic of Scientific Discovery.* English Edition, London: Hutchison & Co.

Spielberger, C. D. (1966). *Anxiety and Behavior.* New York: Academic Press.

Stephenson, T. D. (1985). Q-Methodology in Communication Science: An Introduction. *Communication Quarterly, 33,* 193-208. http://dx.doi.org/10.1080/01463378509369598

Watts, S., & Stenner, P. (2005*).* Doing Q-Methodological Research: Theory, Method & Interpretation. *Qualitative Research in Psychology, 2,* 67-91. http://dx.doi.org/10.1191/1478088705qp022oa

Wilbur, P. K. (1981). *Stand up, Speak up, or Shut up: A Practical Guide to Public Speaking.* New York: Dembner Books.

Wolpe, J. (1958). *Psychotherapy by Reciprocal Inhibition.* Palo Alto, CA: Stanford University Press.

5

Depression, Anxiety and Stress among Undergraduate Students: A Cross Sectional Study

Choon Khim Teh[*], **Choon Wei Ngo, Rashidatul Aniyah binti Zulkifli, Rammiya Vellasamy, Kelvin Suresh**

Melaka Manipal Medical College, Melaka, Malaysia
Email: [*]choonkhim91@hotmail.com

Abstract

Background: The prevalence of moderate to extremely severe level of depression, anxiety and stress among undergraduate students in Malaysia was ranging from 13.9% to 29.3%, 51.5% to 55.0% and 12.9% to 21.6% respectively. Medical students have been shown to be more inclined to emotional disorders, especially stress and depression, as compared to their non-medical peers. Therefore, the objective of this cross-sectional study was to determine the prevalence of depression, anxiety and stress among undergraduate students in Melaka Manipal Medical College. Methods: Self-administered questionnaires consisted of 3 sections: demographic data, socioeconomic data and DASS 21 questions. Data processing was performed using Microsoft Excel 2010. The psychological status was categorized according to the presence or absence of depression, anxiety and stress. The data were analyzed using Epi Info™ 7.1.4 and SPSS. Student's t-test, Fisher Exact and Chi-square test were used to analyze the associations. P-value of <0.05 was considered as statistically significant. Multiple logistic regression was used to calculate the adjusted Odd Ratio. Results: A total of 397 undergraduates participated in this study. The prevalence of the depression, anxiety and stress, ranging from moderate to extremely severe, was 30.7%, 55.5%, and 16.6% respectively. Multiple logistic regression shows significant associations between relationship status, social life and total family income per month with depression. Only ethnicity has been shown to be significantly associated with anxiety. There are significant associations between ethnicity and total family income per month with stress. No other factors have been found to be significantly associated. Conclusion: Depression, anxiety and stress have a high detrimental effect to individual and society, which can lead to negative outcomes including medical dropouts, increased suicidal tendency, relationship and marital problems, impaired ability to work effectively, burnout and also existing problems of health care provision. With that, there is a need for greater attention to the psychological wellbeing of undergraduate students to improve their quality of life.

[*]Corresponding author.

Keywords

Prevalence, Depression, Anxiety, Stress, Undergraduates, Melaka Manipal Medical College

1. Introduction

According to WHO definition, "Health is a state of complete physical, mental and social well-being and not merely the absence of disease or infirmity" [1]. Many people perceive health as being physically well and free of any diseases, and thus they have neglected the importance of mental health. Therefore, mental health is an irreplaceable aspect of health. Poor mental health will lead to many life threatening diseases such as cardiovascular disease deaths, deaths from external causes or even cancer deaths, which was only associated with psychological distress at higher levels [2].

Depression, anxiety and stress levels in the community are considered as important indicators for mental health. Failure to detect and address to these emotional disorders will unfortunately lead to increased psychological morbidity with undesirable impacts all through their professions and lives [3].

In public medical universities, the prevalence of depression and anxiety ranged from 10.4% to 43.8% and 43.7% to 69% respectively. However, the prevalence of depression and anxiety among private medical students has been estimated to be 19% to 60% and 29.4% to 60% respectively [4]. In Hong Kong, a web-based survey of stress among the first-year tertiary education students found that 27% of the respondents were having stress with moderate severity or above [5]. While in India, a study was conducted to focus on the prevalence of current depression, anxiety, and stress-related symptoms among young adults, ranging from mild to extremely severe, which was 18.5%, 24.4%, and 20% respectively. Clinical depression was present in 12.1% and generalized anxiety disorder in 19.0%. Co-morbid anxiety and depression were high, with about 87% of those having depression also suffering from anxiety disorder [6].

A research conducted in Malaysia showed that the prevalence of moderate to extremely severe level of depression, anxiety and stress among undergraduate students was ranging from 13.9% to 29.3%, 51.5% to 55.0% and 12.9% to 21.6% respectively [7] [8].

With respect to the source of stressors, the top ten stressors chosen by the students were mainly academic and personal factors [9]. As indicated by Porter, there were up to 60% of university dropouts recorded; the majority of these students leave within the first two years. Steinberg and Darling specified that 50% of university students who consulted mental health service complained of challenges in study, anxiety, tension, and depression which contributed to poor grades in courses [10].

In Malaysia, tertiary learning institutions offering medical degrees have expanded in numbers in the previous couple of years to meet the nation's demand for more graduate doctors and medical personnel. All things considered, the environment of medical education and practice has long been viewed as a distressing factor [11]. Medical students have been shown to be more inclined to emotional disorders, especially stress and depression, as compared to their non-medical peers.

Therefore, we conducted the cross-sectional study to determine the prevalence of depression, anxiety and stress among undergraduate students in Melaka Manipal Medical College.

2. Methodology

This cross-sectional study was done among undergraduate students, from September to October 2014 in Melaka Manipal Medical College (Melaka Campus), Malaysia.

We calculated the sample size using prevalence of 55.0% [7]. With the 95% CI and precision of 5%, we require a total sample size of 384 students. After accommodate the non-response rate of 10%, we distributed 430 sets of the questionnaires. A total of 397 undergraduate students participated in this study. Written informed consent was taken from every participant. The students who were absent for class on the day of data collection were excluded from this study.

This study helps to arbitrate the differences in psychological distress with respect to the demographic variables among MMMC students. There are several stress reducing factors (stress busters) and are divided into 6 groups: friends, gym workouts, physical factors, co-curricular activities, teacher's patronage and personal hobbies.

Self-administered questionnaires consisted of 3 sections: Demographic data, socioeconomic data and DASS 21 questions. Demographic data consists of 8 questions based on personal details: age, gender, ethnicity, study course, residence, relationship status, academic performance and social life status. The socioeconomic data include parental marital status and total family income per month.

The Depression Anxiety Stress Scale (DASS 21, Psychology Foundation of Australia) was used to screen mental health problems among the population [12]. The DASS 21 is a 21 item self report questionnaire devised to measure and assesses the severity of a range of symptoms common to depression, anxiety and stress. However, it is not a categorical measure of clinical diagnoses of the said conditions [13].

In completing the DASS 21 questionnaire, the individual is required to indicate the presence of a symptom over the previous week. DASS 21 consists of 21 questions in total which was designated for participants to specify their emotional level for each statement. In total, there are 7 items for each depression, anxiety and stress assessment [14]. Each item is scored from 0 (did not apply to me at all over the last week) to 3 (applied to me very much or most of the time over the past one week) [15]. Because the DASS 21 is a short form version of the DASS (the Long Form has 42 items), the final score of each item groups (depression, anxiety and stress) must be multiplied by two ($\times 2$) [12]. The minimum score is zero and the maximum score is 42. The final score of DASS can be categorized as in **Table 1**.

Studies have shown that the DASS 21 score have validity in the measurement of the degree of depression, anxiety and stress in the person. It also has high reliability in terms of usage in a clinical and non-clinical setting [16] [17].

Data processing was performed using Microsoft Excel 2010. The psychological status was categorized according to the presence or absence of depression, anxiety and stress. Data was analyzed using Epi Info™ 7.1.4 and SPSS. Descriptive statistics such as frequency (%), mean and standard deviation (SD) were also described. The Student's t-test, Fisher's exact test and Chi-square test were used for bivariate analysis. The variables which had P-value < 0.1 were included in multiple logistic regression analysis. P-value of <0.05 was considered as statistically significant.

The study was carried out by giving a brief introduction on the purpose of the research and the procedures involved prior to distribution of questionnaire. Participants were then informed about their rights to not participate in the study and written consent was taken before they answered the questionnaire. Confidentiality of participants' information given was preserved. This study was conducted under the permission of the research committee of Melaka Manipal Medical College (MMMC).

3. Results

Table 2 shows the descriptive statistics of demographic and socioeconomic factors among respondents. The average age of the respondents is 21.9 years old with a range of 18 to 24 years old. 63.2% of the respondents are female and the remaining 36.8% are male respondents. Chinese contribute to the largest portion of the ethnic group (34.5%), followed by Malay (33.3%), Indian (28.5%) and lastly others (3.8%). Many of the respondents are single (73.8%), followed by those who are in the relationship (26.2%). For the academic performance, 2.8% and 28.0% of the respondents are very satisfied and satisfied with their results respectively. However, most of the respondents (69.3%) have least satisfaction with their performance. Besides, 7.1% respondents are very satisfied with their social life, 49.1% are just satisfied, while 43.8% has least satisfaction.94.5% of the respondents'

Table 1. Severity of depression, anxiety and stress.

Rating	Depression	Anxiety	Stress
Normal	0 - 9	0 - 7	0 - 14
Mild	10 - 13	8 - 9	15 - 18
Moderate	14 - 20	10 - 14	19 - 25
Severe	21 - 27	15 - 19	26 - 33
Extremely Severely	28+	20+	37+

parents are happily married, 3.5% respondents are either orphan or from single parent family.

Table 3 shows the prevalence of depression, anxiety and stress among undergraduates. Depression, anxiety and stress are divided into 5 categories, which are normal, mild, moderate, severe and extremely severe. In depression, 54.2% of the respondents are normal while 15.1%, 20.9%, 6.3% and 3.5% of the respondents have mild, moderate, severe and extremely severe depression respectively. Mean ± Standard Deviation for depression score is 9.8 ± 7.9. For the anxiety status, 36.0% of the respondents are free from it while the rest, ranging from

Table 2. Descriptive statistics of socio-demographic factors among medical undergraduates (n = 397).

Variables	Numbers (%)
Age (Mean ± Std Deviation)	21.9 ± 2.2
Gender	
Female	251 (63.2)
Male	146 (36.8)
Ethnicity	
Chinese	137 (34.5)
Malay	132 (33.3)
Indian	113 (28.5)
Others	15 (3.8)
Relationship Status	
In a relationship	104 (26.2)
Single	293 (73.8)
Academic Performance	
Satisfied	111 (28.0)
Least satisfied	275 (69.3)
Very satisfied	11 (2.8)
Social Life	
Satisfied	195 (49.1)
Least satisfied	174 (43.8)
Very satisfied	28 (7.1)
Parental Status	
Married	375 (94.5)
Orphan/Single parent	22 (3.5)

Table 3. Prevalence of depression, anxiety and stress among undergraduates (n = 397).

Variables	Number (%)
Depression	
Normal	215 (54.2)
Mild	60 (15.1)
Moderate	83 (20.9)
Severe	25 (6.3)
Extremely severe	14 (3.5)
Mean ± Std Deviation	9.8 ± 7.9
Anxiety	
Normal	143 (36.0)
Mild	34 (8.6)
Moderate	121 (30.5)
Severe	4.0 (10.1)
Extremely severe	59 (14.9)
Mean ± Std Deviation	11.0 ± 7.7
Stress	
Normal	270 (68.0)
Mild	61 (15.4)
Moderate	43 (10.8)
Severe	20 (5.0)
Extremely severe	3 (0.8)
Mean ± Std Deviation	12.7 ± 12.8

8.6% to 30.5% have mild to extremely severe anxiety. Mean ± Standard Deviation for anxiety score is 11.0 ± 7.7. Moreover, 68.0% of the respondents do not have any stress. Those who are with mild level of stress consist of 15.4%, followed by moderate level of stress (10.8%), severe level of stress (5.0%) and lastly extremely severe level of stress (0.8%). Mean ± Standard Deviation for stress score is 12.7 ± 12.8.

Table 4 shows the association between socio-demographic factors and depression, anxiety and stress among the respondents. There are no significant association between socio-demographic factors and depression. However, the students who are least satisfied to social life (Unadjusted OR 2.0; 95% CI 1.3 - 3.1) and the students who have total family income of <RM1000 per month (Unadjusted OR 3.4; 95% CI 1.0 - 11.3) are significantly more likely to have depression. Regarding anxiety, there are no significant association between socio-demographic factors and anxiety, but Malay students are significantly more likely to have anxiety (Unadjusted OR 2.1; 95% CI 1.2 - 3.4). Regarding stress, there are no significant association between socio-demographic factors and stress. However, the students who are least satisfied to social life (Unadjusted OR 1.6; 95% CI 1.0 - 2.4) and the students who have total family income of <RM1000 per month (Unadjusted OR 6.2; 95% CI 1.9 - 20.7) are significantly more likely to have stress.

The variables which had P-value < 0.1 in bivariate analysis were included in multiple logistic regression analysis. **Table 5** shows the multiple logistic regression analysis of socio-demographic factors and depression,

Table 4. Bivariate analysis of socio-demographic factors and depression, anxiety and stress.

Variables	Depression (n = 182) Unadjusted OR (95% CI)	Anxiety (n = 256) Unadjusted OR (95% CI)	Stress (n = 127) Unadjusted OR (95% CI)
Age^t (Mean ± SD)	22.1 ± 2.0	22.0 ± 2.3	22.1 ± 2.0
Sex^C			
Female	1 (Reference)	1 (Reference)	1 (Reference)
Male	1.0 (0.7 - 1.6)	0.9 (0.6 - 1.4)	0.8 (0.5 - 1.2)
Ethnicity^C			
Chinese	1 (Reference)	1 (Reference)	1 (Reference)
Malay	1.5 (0.9 - 2.4)	2.1 (1.2 - 3.4)**	1.8 (1.1 - 3.1)
Indian	1.4 (0.8 - 2.3)	1.6 (0.9 - 2.7)	1.4 (0.8 - 2.4)
Others	1.3 (0.4 - 3.8)	0.9 (0.3 - 2.7)	1.5 (0.5 - 4.6)^F
Study Course^C			
FIS	1 (Reference)	1 (Reference)	1 (Reference)
MBBS	1.6 (1.0 - 2.6)	0.9 (0.6 - 1.5)	1.3 (0.8 - 2.3)
Residence^C			
Non-hostelile	1 (Reference)	1 (Reference)	1 (Reference)
Hostelite	1.0 (0.6 - 1.4)	1.0 (0.7 - 1.5)	0.8 (0.5 - 1.2)
Relationship Status^C			
In a relationship	1 (Reference)	1 (Reference)	1 (Reference)
Single	1.4 (0.9 - 2.1)	1.5 (1.0 - 2.4)	0.9 (0.6 - 1.5)
Academic Performance^C			
Satisfied	1 (Reference)	1 (Reference)	1 (Reference)
Least satisfied	1.5 (1.0 - 2.4)	1.4 (0.9 - 2.2)	1.2 (0.8 - 2.0)
Very satisfied^F	1.3 (0.4 - 4.6)	0.8 (0.2 - 3.0)	1.4 (0.4 - 5.1)
Social Life^C			
Satisfied	1 (Reference)	1 (Reference)	1 (Reference)
Least satisfied	2.0 (1.3 - 3.1)***	1.5 (0.9 - 2.2)	1.6 (1.0 - 2.4)*
Very satisfied	0.6 (0.3 - 1.5)	0.6 (0.3 - 1.4)	0.7 (0.3 - 1.8)
Parental Status^C			
Married	1 (Reference)	1 (Reference)	1 (Reference)
Orphan/Single parent	0.8 (0.3 - 1.9)	0.5 (0.2 - 1.3)	0.6 (0.2 - 1.7)
Total Family Income per Month^C			
>RM6000	1 (Reference)	1 (Reference)	1 (Reference)
<RM1000	3.4 (1.0 - 11.3)*	2.0 (0.5 - 7.5)^F	6.2 (1.9 - 20.7)^{F***}
RM1000 - RM3000	1.1 (0.6 - 1.9)	1.1 (0.6 - 1.9)	1.1 (0.6 - 2.0)
RM3001 - RM6000	1.3 (0.8 - 2.1)	0.8 (0.5 - 1.3)	1.2 (0.8 - 2.0)

^{t}Student's t-test; ^{C}Chi-square; ^{F}Fisher exact; *P value < 0.05; **P value < 0.01; ***P value < 0.001.

Table 5. Multiple logistic regression analysis of socio-demographic factors and depression, anxiety and stress.

Variables	Depression Adjusted OR (95% CI)	Anxiety Adjusted OR (95% CI)	Stress Adjusted OR (95% CI)
Ethnicity			
Chinese	1 (Reference)	1 (Reference)	1 (Reference)
Malay	1.5 (0.9 - 2.4)	2.1 (1.2 - 3.6)**	2.0 (1.2 - 3.5)*
Indian	1.6 (1.0 - 2.8)	1.5 (0.9 - 2.6)	1.5 (0.8 - 2.6)
Others	2.0 (0.6 - 6.0)	1.0 (0.3 - 2.9)	1.8 (0.5 - 5.8)
Study Course			
FIS	1 (Reference)	1 (Reference)	1 (Reference)
MBBS	1.7 (1.0 - 3.2)	0.7 (0.4 - 1.3)	1.1 (0.6 - 2.1)
Relationship Status			
In a relationship	1 (Reference)	1 (Reference)	1 (Reference)
Single	1.6 (1.0 - 2.7)*	1.5 (0.9 - 2.4)	1.0 (0.6 - 1.6)
Academic Performance			
Satisfied	1 (Reference)	1 (Reference)	1 (Reference)
Least satisfied	0.9 (0.5 - 1.6)	1.3 (0.7 - 2.23)	0.9 (0.5 - 1.6)
Very satisfied	1.8 (0.4 - 7.0)	1.3 (0.4 - 4.9)	2.0 (0.5 - 7.9)
Social life			
Satisfied	1 (Reference)	1 (Reference)	1 (Reference)
Least satisfied	2.1 (1.3 - 3.5)**	1.5 (0.9 - 2.4)	1.6 (1.0 - 2.7)
Very satisfied	0.5 (0.2 - 1.3)	0.6 (0.2 - 1.3)	0.5 (0.2 - 1.4)
Total Family Income per Month			
>RM6000	1 (Reference)	1 (Reference)	1 (Reference)
<RM1000	3.8 (1.0 - 13.8)*	2.8 (0.7 - 11.2)	7.7 (2.1 - 28.2)**
RM1000 - RM3000	1.0 (0.5 - 1.8)	1.0 (0.5 - 1.8)	1.0 (0.6 - 2.0)
RM3001 - RM6000	1.3 (0.8 - 2.0)	0.8 (0.5 - 1.2)	1.2 (0.7 - 2.0)

*P value < 0.05; **P value < 0.01; ***P value < 0.001.

anxiety and stress. Regarding depression, the students who are single (Adjusted OR 1.6; 95% CI 1.0 - 2.7), least satisfied to social life (Adjusted OR 2.1; 95% CI 1.3 - 3.5) and having total family income <RM1000 per month (Adjusted OR 3.8; 95% CI 1.0 - 13.8) are significantly more likely to have depression. However, there are no significant association between other socio-demographic factors and depression. Similarly, there are no significant association between socio-demographic factors and anxiety, but Malay students are significantly more likely to have anxiety (Adjusted OR 2.1; 95% CI 1.2 - 3.6). Regarding stress, Malay students are significantly more likely to have stress (Adjusted OR 2.0; 95% CI 1.2 - 3.5) and having total family income <RM1000 per month (Adjusted OR 7.7; 95% CI 2.1 - 28.2). There are no significant association between other socio-demographic factors and stress.

4. Discussion

The objective of the study is to determine the prevalence of depression, anxiety and stress among undergraduate students in Malaysia. In the present study, prevalence for moderate to extremely severe depression, anxiety and stress are 30.7%, 55.5%, and 16.6% respectively. This is lower than one study done among Malaysian university students whereby the percentages are 37.2%, 63.0%, and 23.7% for depression, anxiety and stress [18]. A higher prevalence of depression, anxiety and stress could be attributed to the fact that enormous syllabus has to be covered in a limited time period, sudden change in their style of studying, thought of appearing or failing in exams, inadequate time allocated to clinical posting have become the main factors. Furthermore, social stress such as relationship with peer groups, hostel friends, displacement from home and financial problem have also potentially psychologically influence undergraduate students greatly. This study is conducted done to determine the differences in elevated psychological distress with respect to the demographic variables among MMMC students.

To the best of our knowledge, no study has found association between relationship status and depression. We hypothesised that single individuals are more likely to have depression due to the fact that they may lack a partner to express their daily stressors, thereby lacking social support and social buffer. Social life has invariably been associated with depression. It has been shown that individuals, who are satisfied with their social life and thus, a good social support, has a good social support, has shown more resilience to stressors in life, hence acting as a life buffer. This minimizes the risk of developing depression [19] [20]. In the present study, students with total family income per month of less than RM1000 are more likely to have depression. This is consistent with studies which also shows that lower socioeconomic status are strongly associated with major depressive disorder and depressive symptomatology [21]. Lefkowitz *et al.* also found that lower family income are associated with higher prevalence of childhood depression [22]. Students with lower total family income per month may encounter problem with everyday's expenses and thus contributing to the precipitating factors for depression.

Malay ethnicity has been shown to be significantly more likely in developing anxiety and stress. According to Khadijah Shamsuddin *et al.*, they found that Malay ethnicity has a higher stress score on DASS as compared to their other ethnic counterparts [18]. This could be due to cultural differences. We postulate that Malays are more susceptible to stress due to cultural factors. However, this is in contradiction to an earlier study on medical students in a Malaysian university, which reported no difference in emotional distress among Malays, Chinese, Indians and students from other ethnicity [23]. Total family income per month less than RM1000 is significantly associated with risk of having stress. We postulate that this to be due to addition of stressors to the lives of students, particularly to sustain everyday's living expenditures as well as the already-costly medical education. One study has also shown that socioeconomic status, especially parents' education and income, indirectly relates to children's academic achievement through parents' belief and behaviours [24].

Our study did not find any significant association between age, sex, study course, residence, academic performance and parental status with depression, anxiety and stress.

To pinpoint some limitations of our study, we had chosen an analytical cross-sectional study which has the disadvantage of being unable to establish the incidence rate of the mental health status of MMMC students. We can only determine the prevalence of the psychological distress among the students. Besides, lack of baseline information concerning mental status of medical students has become a limitation of our study. Since our study was done only among the medical students from a single private medical college, who are more likely to have high levels of stress, selection bias might be present. Associations among all these might not be representative of the general population because this study is only focus on undergraduates.

Other than this, the students may not remember the events happened last week which might disturb their emotion. Also, the life events happen might not cause an immediate change in an individual's mental status. Hence, to understand the temporal relationship and the mechanism of how these risk factors may affect one's mental state, it will require not only longitudinal data throughout the lifetime but also regular assessment of individual's mental health with the consistent measurement of level of exposure to each risk factor intermittently.

Emotional disturbances in the form of depression, anxiety and stress exist are existing in high rate among undergraduate science students that require early intervention [25]. We recommend that to achieve a healthy life as per define by WHO [1], students are encouraged to spend adequate time on their social and personal lives and emphasize the importance of health promoting coping strategies which might be helpful in overcoming stress throughout their medical condition. Academy management-wise, a student counseling centre with adequate facilities and qualified staff should be established in the campus to provide a medium for students to seek appropriate help for mental health problems. Also, preventive programming efforts should be introduced and begin early in medical education and address a wide variety of concerns from academic to interpersonal relationship and financial worries. Early signs of depressive symptoms among students should be addressed. Intervention will help students to cope with stress to make a smooth transition through medical college and also to adjust to different learning environments during different phases of medical education.

5. Conclusion

In conclusion, depression, anxiety and stress have a high detrimental effect to individual and society, which can lead to negative outcomes including medical dropouts, increased suicidal tendency, relationship and marital problems, impaired ability to work effectively, burnout and also existing problems of health care provision. With that, there is a need for greater attention to the psychological wellbeing of undergraduate students to improve their quality of life.

Acknowledgements

We would like to thank undergraduate students for their kind volunteering for the research and also to our college, Melaka Manipal Medical College, for the approval for research. Our gratitude to Associate Professor Dr. Htoo Htoo Kyaw Soe, Department of Community Medicine, Melaka Manipal Medical College for her valuable advice on the statistical analysis and interpretation of the data. Also, we would like to express gratitude to Professor Dr. Adinegara bin Lutfi Abas, Head of Department, Department of Community Medicine, Melaka Manipal Medical College, for his guidance and approval for the conduct of the study, without which would have been proved difficult for us. Lastly, we would like to thank Tay Geng Yi, Mohd Adi Zafri bin Jasmani and Muhammad Syahid bin Jafri for helping in data collection.

References

[1] World Health Organization (2013) WHO Definition of Health. WHO, Geneva. http://www.who.int/about/definition/en/print.html

[2] Russ, T.C., Stamatakis, E., Hamer, M., Starr, J.M., Kivimaki, M. and Batty, G.D. (2013) Association between Psychological Distress and Mortality: Individual Participant Pooled Analysis of 10 Prospective Cohort Studies. *British Medical Journal*, **345**, e4933. http://dx.doi.org/10.1136/bmj.e4933

[3] Al-Naggar, R.A. and Al-Naggar, D.H. (1987) Prevalence and Associated Factors of Emotional Disorders among Malaysian University Students. *International Journal of Collaborative Research on Internal Medicine & Public Health*, **4**. http://internalmedicine.imedpub.com/prevalence-and-associated-factors-of-emotional-disorderamong-malaysian-university-students.pdf

[4] Saravanan, C. and Wilks, R. (2014) Medical Students' Experience of and Reaction to Stress: The Role of Depression and Anxiety. *The Scientific World Journal*, **2014**, Article ID 737382. http://dx.doi.org/10.1155/2014/737382

[5] Wong, J.G.W.S., Cheung, E.P.T., Chan, K.K.C., Kamela, K.M. and Tang, S.W. (2006) Web-Based Survey of Depression, Anxiety and Stress in First-Year Tertiary Education Students in Hong Kong. *Australian and New Zealand Journal of Psychiatry*, **40**, 777-782. http://dx.doi.org/10.1080/j.1440-1614.2006.01883.x

[6] Saddichha, S. and Christoday, K.R.J. (2010) Prevalence of Depression, Anxiety, and Stress among Young Male Adults in India: A Dimensional and Categorical Diagnoses-Based Study. *Journal of Nervous & Mental Disease*, **198**, 901-904. http://dx.doi.org/10.1097/NMD.0b013e3181fe75dc

[7] Gan, W.Y., Mohd Nasir, M.T., Shariff, Z.M. and Hazizi, A.S. (2011) Disordered Eating Behaviours, Depression, Anxiety and Stress among Malaysian University Students. *College Student Journal*, **45**, 296. http://connection.ebscohost.com/c/articles/61863660/disordered-eating-behaviors-depression-anxiety-stress-among-malaysian-university-students

[8] Al-Ani, Radeef, A.S. and Ghazi, F.G. (2015) Depression, Anxiety and Stress among Undergraduate Science Students in Malaysia. 17th *Johor Mental Health Conference*, Malaysia, 17-18 April 2015, Unpublished. http://irep.iium.edu.my/42809/

[9] Radeef, A.S., Faisal, G.G., Ali, S.M. and Ismail, M.K.H.M. (2014) Source of Stressors and Emotional Disturbances among Undergraduate Science Students in Malaysia. *International Journal of Medical Research & Health Sciences*, **3**, 401-410. http://dx.doi.org/10.5958/j.2319-5886.3.2.082

[10] Safree, M.A., Yasin, M. and Dzulkifli, M.A. (2011) Differences in Depression, Anxiety and Stress between Low- and High-Achieving Students. *Journal of Sustainability Science and Management*, **6**, 169-178. http://jssm.umt.edu.my/files/2012/01/19.June11.pdf

[11] Zaid, Z.A., Chan, S.C. and Ho, J.J. (2007) Emotional Disorders among Medical Students in a Malaysian Private Medical School. *Singapore Medical Journal*, **48**, 895-899. http://www.researchgate.net/publication/5934756_Emotional_disorders_among_medical_students_in_a_Malaysian_private_medical_school

[12] Ronk, F.R., Korman, J.R., Hooke, G.R. and Page, A.C. (2013) Assessing Clinical Significance of Treatment Outcomes Using the DASS-21. *Psychological Assessment*, **25**, 1103-1110. http://www.researchgate.net/publication/237015113_Assessing_Clinical_Significance_of_Treatment_Outcomes_Using_the_DASS-21 http://dx.doi.org/10.1037/a0033100

[13] Gomez, F. A Guide to the Depression, Anxiety and Stress Scale. http://www.iwsml.org.au/images/mental_health/Frequently_Used/Outcome_Tools/Dass21.pdf

[14] Anonymous (2014) Overview of the DASS and Its Uses. http://www2.psy.unsw.edu.au/Groups/Dass/over.htm

[15] Anonymous (2013) Depression Anxiety Stress Scale-21 (DASS-21).
http://www.scireproject.com/outcome-measures-new/depression-anxiety-stress-scale-21-dass-21

[16] Henry, J.D. and Crawford, J.R. (2010) The Short-Form Version of the Depression Anxiety Stress Scales (DASS-21): Construct Validity and Normative Data in a Large Non-Clinical Sample. *British Journal of Clinical Psychology*, **44**, 227-239.
http://onlinelibrary.wiley.com/doi/10.1348/014466505X29657/abstract;jsessionid=FD33C9C042CDCB1E17BCE4861 51CFAC6.f03t02?userIsAuthenticated=false&deniedAccessCustomisedMessage=
http://dx.doi.org/10.1348/014466505X29657

[17] Nieuwenhuijsen, K., de Boer, A.G.E.M., Verbeek, J.H.A.M., Blonk, R.W.B. and vanDijk, F.J.H. (2002) The Depression Anxiety Stress Scales (DASS): Detecting Anxiety Disorder and Depression in Employees Absent from Work Because of Mental Health Problems. *Occupational & Environmental Medicine*, **60**, i77-i82.
http://oem.bmj.com/content/60/suppl_1/i77.short
http://dx.doi.org/10.1136/oem.60.suppl_1.i77

[18] Shamsuddin, K., Fadzil, F., Wan Ismail, W.S., Azhar Shah, S., Omar, K., Muhammad, N.A., *et al.* (2013) Correlates of Depression, Anxiety and Stress among Malaysian University Students. *Asian Journal of Psychiatry*, **6**, 318-323.
http://www.researchgate.net/publication/243966318_Correlates_of_depression_anxiety_and_stress_among_Malaysian _university_students
http://dx.doi.org/10.1016/j.ajp.2013.01.014

[19] Cohen, S. and Wills, T.A. (1985) Stress, Social Support, and the Buffering Hypothesis. *Psychological Bulletin*, **98**, 310-357. http://psycnet.apa.org/journals/bul/98/2/310/
http://dx.doi.org/10.1037/0033-2909.98.2.310

[20] Cohen, S. and Hoberman, H.M. (1983) Positive Events and Social Supports as Buffers of Life Change Stress. *Journal of Applied Social Psychology*, **13**, 99-125.
http://repository.cmu.edu/cgi/viewcontent.cgi?article=1264&context=psychology
http://dx.doi.org/10.1111/j.1559-1816.1983.tb02325.x

[21] Everson, S.A., Maty, S.C., Lynch, J.W. and Kaplan, G.A. (2002) Epidermiological Evidence for the Relation between Socioeconomic Status and Depression, Obesity, and Diabetes. *Journal of Psychosomatic Research*, **53**, 891-895.
http://deepblue.lib.umich.edu/handle/2027.42/51444
http://dx.doi.org/10.1016/S0022-3999(02)00303-3

[22] Monroe, M.L., Edward, P.T. and Neal, H.G. (1980) Childhood Depression, Family Income, and Locus of Control. *Journal of Nervous & Mental Disease*, **168**, 732-735.
http://journals.lww.com/jonmd/Abstract/1980/12000/Childhood_Depression,_Family_Income,_and_Locus_of.4.aspx

[23] MohdSidik, S., Rampal, L. and Kaneson, N. (2003) Prevalence of Emotional Disorders among Medical Students in a Malaysian University. *Asia Pacific Family Medicine*, **2**, 213-217.
http://onlinelibrary.wiley.com/doi/10.1111/j.1444-1683.2003.00089.x/abstract
http://dx.doi.org/10.1111/j.1444-1683.2003.00089.x

[24] Kean, D. and Pamela, E. (2005) The Influence of Parent Education and Family Income on Child Achievement: The Indirect Role of Parental Expectations and the Home Environment. *Journal of Family Psychology*, **19**, 294-304.
http://psycnet.apa.org/journals/fam/19/2/294/
http://dx.doi.org/10.1037/0893-3200.19.2.294

[25] Radeef, A.S., Faisal, G.G., Ali, S.M. and Ismail, M.K.H.M. (2014) Source of Stressors and Emotional Disturbances among Undergraduate Science Students in Malaysia. *International Journal of Medical Research & Health Sciences*, **3**, 401-410.
http://ijmrhs.com/source-of-stressors-and-emotional-disturbances-among-undergraduate-science-students-in-malaysia/
http://dx.doi.org/10.5958/j.2319-5886.3.2.082

6

Does Early Improvement in Anxiety Symptoms in Patients with Major Depressive Disorder Affect Remission Rates? A Post-Hoc Analysis of Pooled Duloxetine Clinic Trials

Murat Altin[1]*, Eiji Harada[2], Alexander Schacht[3], Lovisa Berggren[3], Daniel Walker[4], Hector Dueñas[5]

[1]Eli Lilly-Turkey, Istanbul, Turkey
[2]Lilly Research Laboratories Japan, Eli Lilly Japan K.K., Kobe, Japan
[3]Eli Lilly and Company, Health Technology Appraisal Group, Bad Homburg, Germany
[4]Lilly USA, LLC, Indianapolis, USA
[5]Eli Lilly de México, Mexico City, Mexico
Email: *altin_murat@lilly.com

Abstract

Objectives: Patients with major depressive disorder (MDD) and a comorbid anxiety disorder or significant anxiety symptoms have decreased functioning, increased risk of suicidality, and worse post-treatment outcomes. This pooled analysis of 8 duloxetine MDD trials was designed to determine whether early improvement in anxiety symptoms predicts MDD remission. Methods: Eight trials were pooled. Patients with a baseline 17-item Hamilton Rating Scale for Depression (HA-MD$_{17}$) anxiety/somatization factor score ≥ 7 were considered to have anxious depression. Early response on the HAMD$_{17}$ total score was defined as a 20% reduction at weeks 2 or 4, a 30% reduction at weeks 2 or 4, or a 50% reduction at weeks 2 or 4 in the HAMD$_{17}$ anxiety subscale. Each category was analyzed separately for all patients. MDD remission is a score of ≤ 7 on the HAMD$_{17}$ total score at study endpoint. Results: The early responder group in each analysis showed greater numerical improvement at endpoint on the HAMD$_{17}$ total score than the nonresponder group. Duloxetine showed statistically significantly greater improvement than placebo in most nonresponder and responder subgroups. There were no statistically significant interaction effects for the difference between duloxetine and placebo for any of the anxious categories. Conclusion: Although patients who responded in the various response categories had greater numerical improvement and greater remission rates than nonresponding patients, the response and nonresponse groups did not differ statistically regarding the treatment effect of duloxetine. Therefore, early improve-

---

*Corresponding author.

ment in anxiety symptoms was not a predictor of greater endpoint remission of depressive symptoms for duloxetine treatment.

Keywords

Anxiety, Clinical Trials, Duloxetine, Early Response, Major Depressive Disorder, Remission

---

1. Introduction

Depression affects more than 350 million people worldwide and has a lifetime prevalence range of 10% to 15% (Lépine & Briley, 2011; World Health Organization, 2012). Depression is the leading cause of disability worldwide and by 2020 is predicted to be second only to cardiovascular disease in overall disease burden worldwide (Lopez & Murray, 1998; World Health Organization, 2008). Unfortunately, treatment of depression is often either nonexistent or inadequate in the majority of people with major depressive disorder (MDD) (Kessler et al., 2003; Lépine, Gastpar, Mendlewicz, & Tylee, 1997). The percentage of people with MDD in the National Comorbidity Survey Replication study who were treated was only 51.6%; furthermore, only 41.9% of those patients received adequate levels of treatment (Kessler et al., 2003). The majority of patients who are not adequately treated for their symptoms will relapse (Bakish, 2001). Studies have shown that relapse rates are much higher in patients with partial remission than in those who experience complete remission (Bakish, 2001; Pintor, Gastó, Navarro, Torres, & Fañanas, 2003). In the treatment of depression, early symptom improvement may be a clinically useful indicator for successful treatment or treatment failure (Nierenberg, Qyitkin, Kremer, Keller, & Thase, 2004; Wade & Friis Anderson, 2006). Some analyses have suggested that early drug-specific symptom improvement is predictive of greater overall response and symptom resolution at endpoint (Nierenberg et al., 2004; Wade & Friis Anderson, 2006).

Anxious depression has been defined as people with MDD having a comorbid anxiety disorder or having high levels of anxiety symptoms (Fava et al., 2004). The frequency of a comorbid anxiety disorder or significant levels of anxious symptoms in people with MDD is approximately 50% (Fava et al., 2004; Kessler et al., 1996, 2003). A significant percentage of patients with MDD have comorbid anxiety disorders, such as generalized anxiety disorder (GAD), social phobia, and posttraumatic stress disorder (Rush et al., 2005; Zimmerman, Chelminski, & McDermut, 2002). Anxious depression has been shown to be associated with increased symptom severity, worse functioning, greater risk of suicidality, and higher rates of unemployment (Farabaugh et al., 2012; Nelson, 2008). People with anxious depression tend to have worse outcomes than patients with nonanxious depression, including a reduced likelihood of response and remission, increased rate of side effects, and slower rate of recovery from an MDD episode (Fava et al., 2008; Nelson, 2008). Among other variables, residual anxiety symptoms, high baseline levels of anxiety, or having a comorbid anxiety disorder have been shown to predict relapse or recurrence of MDD (Dombrovski et al., 2007; Parker, Wilhelm, Mitchell, & Gladstone, 2000; Wilhelm, Parker, Dewhurst-Savellis, & Asghari, 1999; Yang et al., 2010).

A recent study found that the severity of anxiety at baseline adversely affected depression severity at 12 months and that a reduction of anxiety within the first 3 months leads to additional improvement in depression (Bair et al., 2013). Few studies in MDD patients have evaluated whether early onset of improvement in anxiety symptoms results in higher rates of remitted depression. A 12-week study of active treatment in patients with MDD found that early change (1 week) in items of the 17-item Hamilton Rating Scale for Depression ($HAMD_{17}$) (Hamilton, 1960) anxiety/somatization factor was predictive of achieving remission at endpoint for only item 13 (general somatic symptoms) but not for the other items (Farabaugh et al., 2005). In a post-hoc analysis of a different study, only early improvement in item 12 (gastrointestinal somatic symptoms) was significantly predictive of MDD remission, although item 13 just missed reaching statistical significance (Farabaugh et al., 2010). A study by Davidson, Meoni, Haudiquet, Cantillon and Hackett (2002) found that the serotonin-norepinephrine reuptake inhibitor (SNRI) venlafaxine was significantly better than placebo in achieving remission in severely anxious-depressed patients, whereas the selective serotonin reuptake inhibitor (SSRI) fluoxetine did not separate from placebo. Similarly, another study showed that venlafaxine improved psychic anxiety better than SSRIs (Silverstone, Entsuah, & Hackett, 2002).

Katz and colleagues (2004) found that antidepressant drugs with pharmacologically different mechanisms of action produced different early therapeutic effects. Duloxetine is an SNRI that has been approved for the treatment of MDD and GAD in many countries worldwide. Duloxetine has shown early separation from placebo (within the first 2 weeks of treatment) on core depressive systems, including depressed mood, guilt, suicidal ideation, psychomotor retardation, and psychic anxiety (Hirschfeld, Mallinckrodt, Lee, & Detke, 2005; Shelton et al., 2007). In a post-hoc analysis of a double-blind, placebo- and active-controlled study of duloxetine in patients with MDD, several items and factors of the $HAMD_{17}$ that showed early improvement were predictors of sustained MDD remission (Katz, Meyers, Prakash, Gaynor, & Houston, 2009). However, the analysis was done in all patients and not separately in anxious and nonanxious patients. In the current post-hoc analysis, 8 randomized, placebo-controlled, duloxetine trials in MDD having a duration of 4 to 12 weeks were pooled to assess whether early improvement in anxiety symptoms resulted in greater rates of MDD remission. In this analysis, patients were considered to have anxious depression if they had a $HAMD_{17}$ anxiety/somatization factor subscale score of ≥ 7 at baseline (Fava et al., 2008). This definition of anxious depression has been used in previous studies, including analyses of the Sequenced Treatment Alternatives to Relieve Depression (STAR*D) trial (Farabaugh et al., 2012; Fava et al., 2008). Using this definition of anxious depression, patients from the 8 pooled duloxetine MDD trials were assigned to either having or not having anxious depression. The primary objective of this study was to determine whether early improvement in anxiety symptoms predicted remission of MDD.

2. Materials and Methods

2.1. Study Design

Data were pooled from 8 randomized, double-blind, placebo-controlled trials of duloxetine for the treatment of MDD conducted by Eli Lilly and Company (**Table 1**). The 8 studies took place from November 2000 to March 2011. Data were taken from short-term studies and from the acute-treatment phase of those studies that had extensions. Relapse studies are not included in the analysis set. Although patients were randomized to the 60 to 120 mg/day arm of duloxetine in some studies, patients randomized to duloxetine arms >60 mg/day were excluded from these analyses. The $HAMD_{17}$ scale had to have been included in the study. These 8 studies comprised the full set of appropriate and available placebo-controlled studies at the time this work was initiated.

All study protocols were developed in accordance with the ethical standards of Good Clinical Practice and the Declaration of Helsinki. Before studies began, all patients provided written informed consent, and each clinical study site's institutional review board approved the protocol

2.2. Patient Population

Patients were ≥ 18 years, male or female outpatients with MDD as defined by criteria from the *Diagnostic and Statistical Manual of Mental Disorders*, Fourth Edition (DSM-IV) or DSM, Fourth Edition Text Revision (DSM-IV-TR). Patients were excluded from each study if they had any current primary psychiatric or neurologic diagnosis other than MDD, including any anxiety disorder (1 study allowed mild dementia); had a serious

Table 1. Summary of the 8 randomized, double-blind, placebo-controlled studies in major depressive disorderused in the analyses.

Study Identifier	Study Phase	Placebo (n)	Duloxetine [n (dosage; mg/day)]	Treatment Duration (wk)	Primary Disclosure
HMBHa	III	115	121 (60)	9	Detke, Lu, Goldstein, McNamara, & Demitrack, 2002[a]
HMBHb	III	136	123 (60)	9	Detke, Lu, Goldstein, Hayes, & Demitrack, 2002[b]
HMBV	IV	102	201 (60)	8	Raskin et al., 2007
HMCB	IIIb	136	132 (60)	7	Brannan et al., 2005
HMCR	IIIb	135	262 (60 - 120)	8	Nierenberg et al., 2007
HMFA	IV	121	246 (60)	12	Robinson et al., 2014
HMFS	IV	248	501 (60 - 120)	36	Oakes et al., 2012
HQAC	II	34	17 (60, 120)	4	Mundt, DeBrota, & Greist, 2007

HMFS: only first 12 weeks of study included in the analyses. b. Patients randomized to duloxetine arms greater than 60 mg/day were excluded from these analyses.

medical illness; had a history of substance abuse or dependence within 1 year of study entry; or had a positive urine drug screen. Details for each study can be found in the primary publication (**Table 1**). A total of 2630 patients from the 8 studies were included in the present study. Patients were analyzed (grouped) based on whether they were considered to have anxious depression. Anxious depression in the current analyses was defined as a $HAMD_{17}$ anxiety/somatization factor score ≥ 7 at baseline (Fava et al., 2008).

2.3. Outcome Measures

The primary outcome measure for these analyses is the $HAMD_{17}$ total score. Response was defined as $\geq 50\%$ improvement from baseline to endpoint on the $HAMD_{17}$ total score. Remission was defined as a score of ≤ 7 on the $HAMD_{17}$ total score at endpoint. The 6-item $HAMD_{17}$ anxiety/somatization subscale consists of the sum of items 10 (psychic anxiety), 11 (somatic anxiety), 12 (gastrointestinal somatic symptoms), 13 (general somatic symptoms), 15 (hypochondriasis), and 17 (insight). Several other scales were measured at baseline to determine whether there were significant differences between the anxious and nonanxious subgroups. These included the following $HAMD_{17}$ subscales: Maier, Retardation, Sleep, Bech, and Mood. Other scales included the Montgomery-Åsberg depression rating scale (MADRS) (Montgomery & Asberg, 1979), the Sheehan Disability Scale (SDS) (Sheehan, Harnett-Sheehan, & Raj, 1996) to assess functional impairment, the Brief Pain Inventory (BPI) (Cleeland & Ryan, 1994) to assess pain and functioning, the Clinical Global Impression of Severity (CGI-S) (Guy, 1976) to measure overall improvement, and the Hamilton Anxiety Rating Scale (HAMA) (Hamilton, 1959).

2.4. Statistical Analyses

The continuous endpoints were analyzed using analysis of covariance (ANCOVA) via the following approach: one ANCOVA model was calculated for each study with the fixed effects including treatment, anxious (y/n), treatment by anxious (y/n) interaction, and baseline score of the endpoint evaluated as covariates. For logistic regression analyses, an additional model included all 2- and 3-way interactions between treatment, study, and anxious (y/n) to check for heterogeneity. Effect sizes in each model were calculated for least squares (LS) mean differences, divided by the standard deviation (SD) of the residuals provided by the model of this study. Overall LS mean estimates and effect sizes were calculated as a weighted mean of the corresponding estimates in all studies, with weights based on within-study variance, assuming a fixed study effect. The binary outcomes were analyzed using logistical regression adjusting for study within the anxious and nonanxious patients. The impact of anxiety being present or not at baseline on the treatment response of the endpoints will be described. The mean changes in $HAMD_{17}$ total score, items, and subscales were assessed via last observation carried forward to endpoint. Early response on the $HAMD_{17}$ total score was defined as one of the following: a 20% reduction at weeks 2 or 4, a 30% reduction at weeks 2 or 4, or a 50% reduction at weeks 2 or 4 in the $HAMD_{17}$ anxiety/somatization subscale score. Each of these 6 categories was analyzed separately for all patients. Remission of MDD is a score of ≤ 7 on the $HAMD_{17}$ total score at endpoint.

Fixed effects using ANCOVA for mean changes in $HAMD_{17}$ total score, subscales, and items and logistic regression for binary endpoints, including study, treatment, anxious (y/n), and baseline score of the endpoint, were evaluated. An additional logistic regression model included all 2- and 3-way interactions between treatment, study, and anxious (y/n). Because this was a post-hoc analysis, no adjustment for multiplicity was made and results should be interpreted as being exploratory in nature. All confidence intervals (CIs) presented were 95% CIs, and statistical significance was defined as a *p*-value <5%. All analyses were performed using SAS software version 9.2 software (SAS Institute, Cary, NC).

3. Results

The mean age of patients (N = 2630) was 50.1 years (SD = 17.5 years), with the majority of patients being female (64%) and Caucasian (75%). Baseline patient characteristics for anxious and nonanxious-depressed patients are shown in **Table 2**. There were statistically significant differences between the groups for gender, race, geography, and all efficacy measures. The percentage of patients completing the studies in which they were enrolled was not significantly different between the anxious and nonanxious groups (**Table 3**). The most common overall reasons for discontinuing the study were adverse event (8%) and subject decision (6%).

Table 2. Baseline patient characteristics.

Characteristic	Nonanxious Depression N = 1331	Anxious Depression N = 1299	p-value
Age, y, mean (SD)	50.3 (17.5)	49.9 (17.5)	
Range	18 - 90	18 - 90	0.555
Gender, n (%)			
Female	813 (61.1)	856 (65.9)	0.010
Male	518 (38.9)	443 (34.1)	
Race, n (%)			
Caucasian	1033 (77.6)	940 (72.4)	
Black/African American	129 (9.7)	143 (11.0)	
Hispanic	144 (10.8)	190 (14.6)	0.050
Asian	14 (1.1)	15 (1.2)	
Native American	1 (0.1)	1 (0.1)	
Other	10 (0.8)	10 (0.8)	
Geography, n (%)			
USA	1265 (95.0)	1204 (92.7)	
Europe	5 (0.4)	16 (1.2)	0.010
Other	61 (4.6)	79 (6.1)	
Prior Tx with antidepressant, n (%)			
Any antidepressant	728 (54.7)	745 (57.4)	0.170
Duration of current MDD episode, mo, mean (SD)	18.9 (38.6)	17.3 (38.0)	0.441
Number of previous episodes of MDD, n, mean (SD)	5.1 (22.0)	5.5 (26.1)	0.628
CGI-S, mean (SD)	4.2 (0.7)	4.5 (0.7)	<0.0001
MADRS total score, mean (SD)	29.4 (4.6)	32.1 (4.9)	<0.0001
HAMD$_{17}$, mean (SD)			
Total score	17.6 (4.3)	23.6 (3.9)	<0.0001
Maier	9.5 (2.8)	11.7 (2.2)	<0.0001
Retardation	6.8 (2.1)	7.8 (1.7)	<0.0001
Sleep	3.3 (1.8)	3.8 (1.7)	<0.0001
Bech	10.1 (2.8)	12.5 (2.0)	<0.0001
Mood	7.7 (2.5)	9.0 (2.0)	<0.0001
Anxiety/Somatization	4.7 (1.3)	8.3 (1.4)	<0.0001
HAMA total score, mean (SD)	12.7 (4.6)	18.3 (4.6)	<0.0001
BPI Average Pain, mean (SD)	3.4 (2.3)	4.5 (2.2)	<0.0001
BPI Interference Summary, mean (SD)	2.6 (2.5)	3.9 (2.8)	<0.0001
SDS total score, mean (SD)	17.8 (6.5)	20.0 (6.4)	<0.0001

Abbreviations: BPI = Brief Pain Inventory; CGI-S = Clinical Global Improvement of Severity; HAMA = Hamilton Anxiety Scale Scores; HAMD$_{17}$ = 17-item Hamilton Rating Scale for Depression; MADRS = Montgomery-Åsberg depression rating scale; MDD = major depressive disorder; SD = standard deviation; SDS = Sheehan Disability Scale; Tx = treatment; USA = United States of America.

Table 3. Patient disposition.

Reason, n (%)	Nonanxious Depression N = 1331	Anxious Depression N = 1299	p-value
Completed	980 (73.6)	927 (71.4)	0.193
Discontinued any reason	351 (26.4)	372 (28.6)	
Adverse event	104 (7.8)	98 (7.5)	
Subject decision	80 (6.0)	87 (6.7)	
Lost to follow up	80 (6.0)	69 (5.3)	
Lack of efficacy	59 (4.4)	69 (5.3)	
Protocol violation	21 (1.6)	29 (2.2)	
Physician decision	4 (0.3)	13 (1.0)	
Sponsor decision	2 (0.2)	4 (0.3)	
Other	1 (0.1)	1 (0.1)	
Death	0	2 (0.2)	

Overall, the percentage of patients attaining a 50% response rate at endpoint was 38.2% (duloxetine, 42.9%; placebo, 30.3%) in the nonanxious group and 38% (duloxetine, 41.7%; placebo, 32.6%) in the anxious group. The percentage of patients attaining remission status at endpoint was 32.5% (duloxetine, 36.2%; placebo, 26.3%) in the nonanxious group and 20.3% (duloxetine, 22.9%; placebo, 16.6%) in the anxious group. The LS mean difference between duloxetine and placebo on the $HAMD_{17}$ total score was -1.94 (standard error [SE] = 0.39) for the nonanxious group (duloxetine, -7.70; placebo, -5.77) and -2.26 (SE = 0.40) for the anxious subgroup (duloxetine, -8.30; placebo, -6.31). The LS mean change treatment difference within each group was statistically significant (both $p < 0.0001$), but the interaction effect between treatment and anxious group was nonsignificant ($p = 0.575$). The odds ratio (95% CI) of duloxetine versus placebo for achieving a 50% response rate at week 8 was 1.740 (95% CI: 1.371, 2.209) for the nonanxious group and 1.508 (95% CI: 1.192, 1.909) for the anxious group. The odds ratio (95% CI) for reaching remission at week 8 was 1.596 (95% CI: 1.240, 2.054) for the nonanxious group and 1.589 (95% CI: 1.187, 2.127) for the anxious group. The interaction effect between the treatment and anxious group was nonsignificant for both the response and remission rates.

The mean change in the $HAMD_{17}$ total score based on response status and week is shown in **Figure 1**. The responder subgroup in each analysis showed greater improvement at endpoint than the nonresponder subgroup. Moreover, duloxetine showed statistically significantly greater improvement than placebo in most (9 of 12) of the nonresponder and responder subgroups (**Figure 1**). However, there were no statistically significant interaction effects for the difference between duloxetine and placebo for any of the response categories. That is, the difference between duloxetine and placebo for nonresponder and responder subgroups was not significantly different within each of the 6 early-response categories.

Table 4 presents the odds of whether placebo- or duloxetine-treated patients (early responders and nonresponders) have a greater chance of obtaining a 50% response rate at endpoint. In all cases, duloxetine-treated patients had greater odds of achieving response at endpoint compared with placebo, although only a few reached statistical significance. **Figure 2** shows the percentage of patients (early responders and nonresponders) who reached a 50% response rate at endpoint for each of the response categories. The odds ratios for early responders and nonresponders in reaching remission showed that duloxetine had numerically greater odds of doing so than placebo in all categories, although only 5 were statistically significant (**Table 5**). **Figure 3** shows the percentage

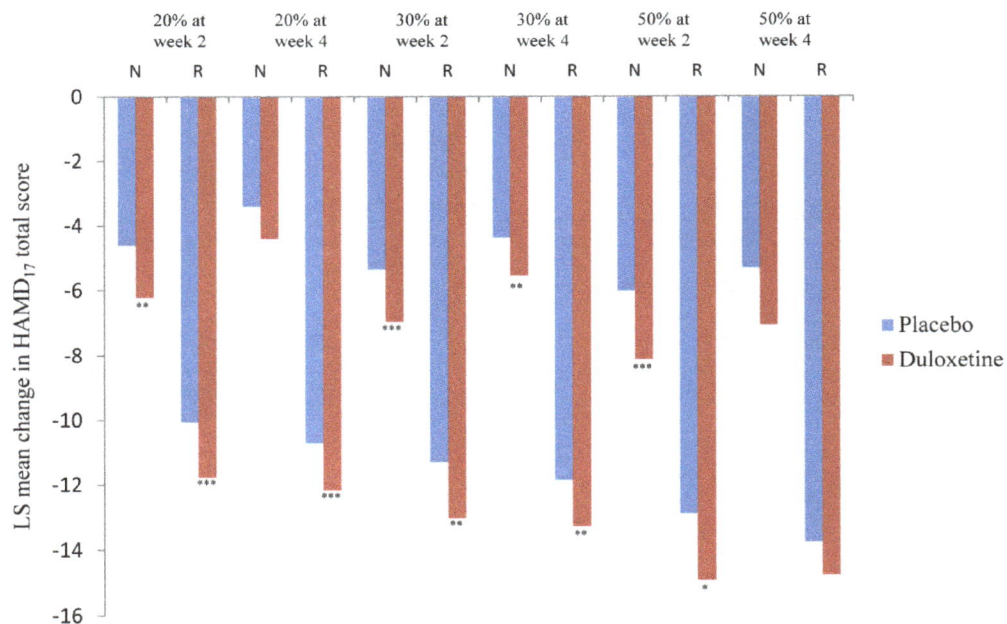

Figure 1. Mean changes in 17-item Hamilton Rating Scale for Depression ($HAMD_{17}$) total score by response status for anxious-depression group at endpoint (week 8). ***$p < 0.001$, **$p < 0.01$, *$p < 0.05$ versus placebo. Total number of patients: placebo = 525, duloxetine = 774. Number of patients per response status varies for each analysis. Abbreviations: LS = least squares; N = nonresponder; R = responder.

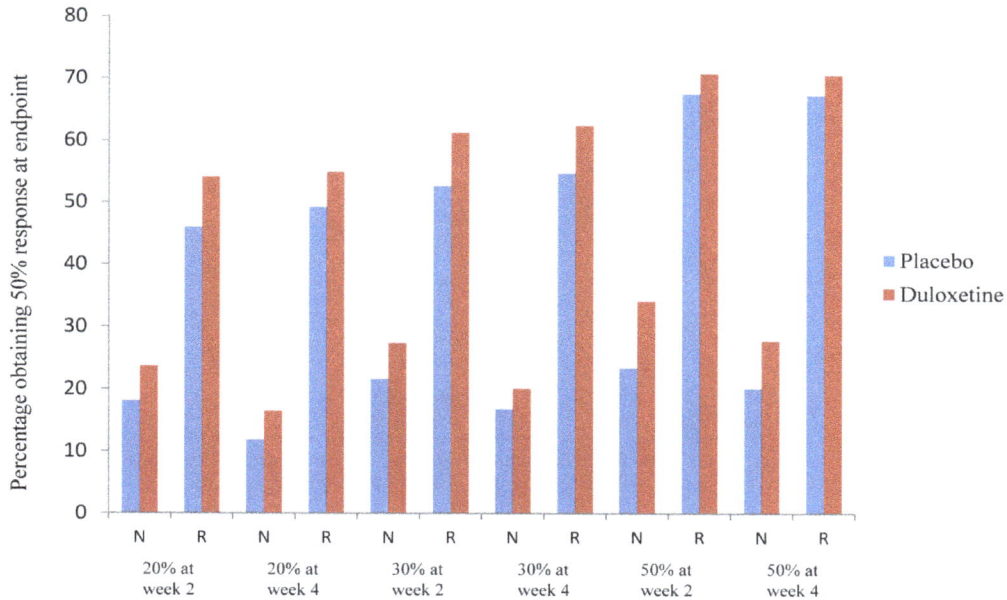

Figure 2. Frequency of 50% response at week 8 by response status as measured by the 17-item Hamilton Rating Scale for Depression. Total number of patients: placebo = 525, duloxetine = 774. Number of patients per response status varies for each analysis. Abbreviations: N = nonresponder; R = responder.

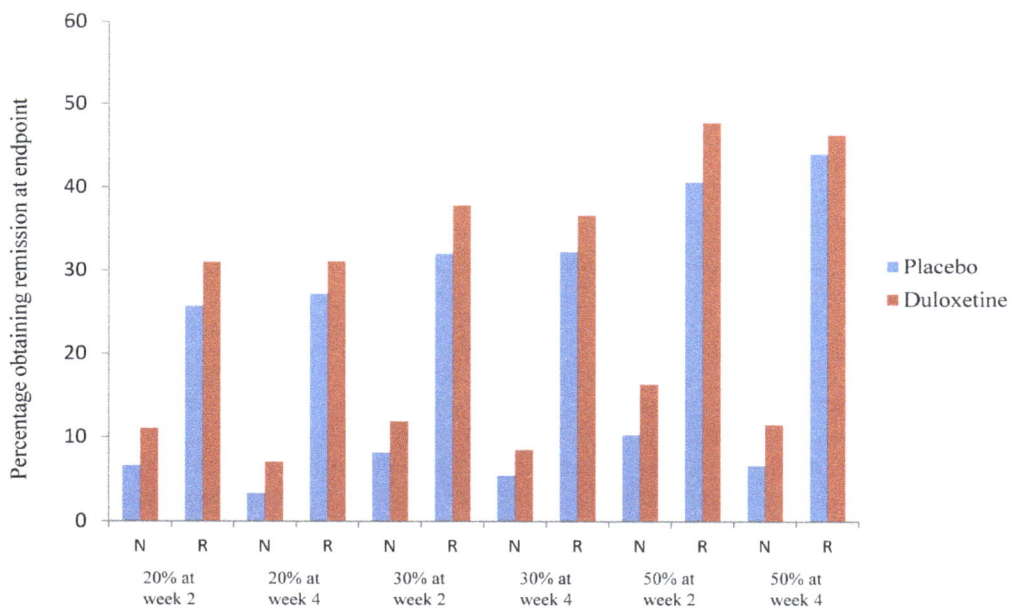

Figure 3. Frequency of remission at week 8 by response status as measured by the 17-item Hamilton Rating Scale for Depression. Total number of patients: placebo = 525, duloxetine = 774. Number of patients per response status varies for each analysis. Abbreviations: N = nonresponder; R = responder.

of patients that achieved remission at endpoint for each of the response categories.

4. Discussion

Overall, there was not a significant interaction effect between the treatment and anxious group for both response and remission. That is, the difference between placebo and duloxetine in the 2 groups was similar; thus, having

Table 4. Odds ratios of duloxetine versus placebo in patients achieving or not achieving a 50% response rate at endpoint.

HAMD$_{17}$ Anxiety Subscale Improvement/Week	Patients	Odds Ratio (95% CI)
20% at week 2	Nonresponder	1.421 (0.937, 2.154)
	Responder	1.420 (1.045, 1.928)[a]
20% at week 4	Nonresponder	1.484 (0.888, 2.481)
	Responder	1.269 (0.945, 1.705)
30% at week 2	Nonresponder	1.394 (0.995, 1.952)
	Responder	1.436 (0.992, 2.078)
30% at week 4	Nonresponder	1.253 (0.845, 1.858)
	Responder	1.393 (0.990, 1.960)
50% at week 2	Nonresponder	1.721 (1.293, 2.292)[a]
	Responder	1.164 (0.683, 1.984)
50% at week 4	Nonresponder	1.524 (1.109, 2.093)[a]
	Responder	1.189 (0.754, 1.874)

Abbreviations: CI = confidence interval; HAMD$_{17}$ = 17-item Hamilton Rating Scale for Depression. Total number of patients: duloxetine = 774; placebo = 525. Odds ratio is based on duloxetine versus placebo. [a]Duloxetine is statistically significantly more likely than placebo to achieve a 50% response rate at endpoint.

Table 5. Odds ratios of duloxetine versus placebo in patients achieving or not achieving remission at endpoint.

HAMD$_{17}$ Anxiety Subscale Improvement/Week	Patients	Odds Ratio (95% CI)
20% at week 2	Nonremitter	1.858 (1.006, 3.428)[a]
	Remitter	1.423 (1.006, 2.013)[a]
20% at week 4	Nonremitter	2.296 (0.980, 5.376)
	Remitter	1.330 (0.956, 1.851)
30% at week 2	Nonremitter	1.652 (1.011, 2.699)[a]
	Remitter	1.402 (0.946, 2.078)
30% at week 4	Nonremitter	1.647 (0.891, 3.046)
	Remitter	1.375 (0.956, 1.977)
50% at week 2	Nonremitter	1.835 (1.242, 2.712)[a]
	Remitter	1.477 (0.889, 2.454)
50% at week 4	Nonremitter	1.865 (1.147, 3.033)[a]
	Remitter	1.285 (0.833, 1.983)

Abbreviations: CI = confidence interval; HAMD$_{17}$ = 17-item Hamilton Rating Scale for Depression. Total number of patients: duloxetine = 774; placebo = 525. Odds ratio is based on duloxetine versus placebo. [a]Duloxetine is statistically significantly more likely than placebo to achieve remission at endpoint.

anxious depression did not result in significantly lower response and remission rates than patients without anxious depression under duloxetine treatment. Similar to previous studies (Fava et al., 2008), patients with anxious depression were significantly more depressed as measured on both the MADRS and HAMD$_{17}$ depression scales than patients with nonanxious-depression. Anxious patients also experienced worsened functioning, global impairment, and significantly higher levels of pain. It has been shown that longer duration of an MDD episode (Judd et al., 2000; Keller, Lavori, Rice, Coryell, & Hirschfeld, 1986) and/or a greater number of previous MDD episodes (Bulloch, Williams, Lavorato, & Patten, 2014; Kessing, Hansen, Andersen, & Angst, 2004; Lin et al., 1998) may result in patients being harder to treat. However, this does not necessarily imply that the difference between active and placebo treatment is changed, as observed in a recent analysis of pooled duloxetine studies (Dodd, Berk, Kelin, Mancini, & Schacht, 2013). In our pooled analysis, the anxious-depressed group showed nonsignificant differences from the nonanxious group for both of these baseline illness parameters. Pain levels were significantly higher in the anxious-depression group compared with the nonanxious group. Pain has been shown to be a predictor of relapse (Montgomery & Asberg, 1979) and predictor of longer time to remission (Karp et al., 2005). However, response and remission rates were similar between the anxious and nonanxious groups, although it is unknown whether relapse rates would have differed between the 2 groups based on the acute studies included in the current analysis.

Although anxious-depressed patients who met response criteria at each of the cutoffs showed much higher response and remission rates than those anxious-depressed patients who did not meet the response criteria, none of the early-response categories was found to predict significantly better endpoint remission rates under duloxetine treatment. That is, the difference between placebo and duloxetine for the responder groups was not significantly different from the comparable nonresponder group. Thus, patients with anxious depression meeting response criteria was a prognostic factor for greater mean change in depression scores, as well as better response and remission rates at endpoint, but it was not predictive of improved depressive outcomes (duloxetine vs. placebo).

The anxious-depressed patients in these analyses had a mean $HAMD_{17}$ anxiety/somatization score of 8.3. The amount of anxiety these patients experienced may not be high enough to observe increased remission rates in early responders. Many patients with MDD often have much higher levels of anxiety symptoms or have a comorbid anxiety disorder (Fava et al., 2004; Kessler et al., 1996, 2003), and these patients might be a better population to study to answer the question of whether an early response in anxiety symptoms leads to increased remission rates of MDD. A mean score of 8 (24 is maximum) on the $HAMD_{17}$ anxiety/somatization score is actually fairly low even though a score of ≥ 7 is considered to qualify a patient as having anxious depression (Fava et al., 2008).

One limitation of this study was that these were post-hoc analyses. The clinical trials had a number of exclusions, such as comorbid psychiatric disorders and various other medical illnesses. Thus, one should be cautious in extrapolating these results to the general population of patients with MDD. However, there are several strengths to these analyses, including that the pooled data all came from randomized, double-blind, placebo-controlled trials. The analyses contained a sizable number of patients, including 1331 patients without anxious depression and 1299 patients with anxious depression. Importantly, the study designs of the 8 clinical trials used in these pooled analyses were similar, including most of the inclusion and exclusion criteria.

5. Conclusion

In this pooled analysis of duloxetine MDD studies, anxious-depressed patients who responded early in their anxiety symptoms showed higher rates of response and remission compared with patients who did not show early improvement in anxiety symptoms. However, the differences between placebo and duloxetine were not significantly different in the response and nonresponse subgroups; thus early response in anxiety symptoms was a prognostic factor for greater endpoint remission of MDD symptoms, but it was not a predictor of greater endpoint remission for duloxetine. This was true for each of the 6 response categories.

Acknowledgements

The authors thank Renee Granger for editing and proofreading the manuscript.

Role of Funding Source

This project was funded by Eli Lilly and Company.

Contributors

Authors MA, EH, AS, and HD designed the project. Authors DW, MA, EH, HD, and AS managed the literature searches. Authors AS and LB managed the statistical analyses and authors DW and MA wrote the first draft of the manuscript. All authors contributed to and have approved the final manuscript.

Conflict of Interest

This project was funded by Eli Lilly and Company. MA, EH, AS, DW, and HD are employees of Eli Lilly and Company. LB is a contractor working for Lilly.

References

Bair, M. J., Poleshuck, E. L., Wu, J., Krebs, E. K., Damush, T. M., Tu, W., & Kroenke, K. (2013). Anxiety but Not Social Stressors Predict 12-Month Depression and Pain Severity. *Clinical Journal of Pain, 29,* 95-101. http://dx.doi.org/10.1097/AJP.0b013e3182652ee9

Bakish, D. (2001). New Standard of Depression Treatment: Remission and Full Recovery. *Journal of Clinical Psychiatry, 62,*

5-9.

Brannan, S. K., Mallinckrodt, C. H., Brown, E. B., Wohlreich, M. M., Watkin, J. G., & Schatzberg, A. F. (2005). Duloxetine 60 mg Once-Daily in the Treatment of Painful Physical Symptoms in Patients with Major Depressive Disorder. *Journal of Psychiatric Research, 39,* 43-53. http://dx.doi.org/10.1016/j.jpsychires.2004.04.011

Bulloch, A., Williams, J., Lavorato, D., & Patten, S. (2014). Recurrence of Major Depressive Episodes Is Strongly Dependent on the Number of Previous Episodes. *Depression and Anxiety, 31,* 72-76. http://dx.doi.org/10.1002/da.22173

Cleeland, C. S., & Ryan, K. M. (1994). Pain Assessment: Global Use of the Brief Pain Inventory. *Annals of Academic Medicine Singapore, 23,* 129-138.

Davidson, J. R. T., Meoni, P., Haudiquet, V., Cantillon, M., & Hackett, D. (2002). Achieving Remission with Venlafaxine and Fluoxetine in Major Depression: Its Relationship to Anxiety Symptoms. *Depression and Anxiety, 16,* 4-13. http://dx.doi.org/10.1002/da.10045

Detke, M. J., Lu, Y., Goldstein, D. J., Hayes, J. R., & Demitrack, M. A. (2002). Duloxetine, 60 mg Once Daily, for Major Depressive Disorder: A Randomized Double-Blind Placebo-Controlled Trial. *Journal of Clinical Psychiatry, 63,* 308-315. http://dx.doi.org/10.4088/JCP.v63n0407

Detke, M. J., Lu, Y., Goldstein, D. J., McNamara, R. K., & Demitrack, M. A. (2002). Duloxetine 60 mg Once Daily Dosing Versus Placebo in the Acute Treatment of Major Depression. *Journal of Psychiatric Research, 36,* 383-390. http://dx.doi.org/10.1016/S0022-3956(02)00060-2

Dodd, S., Berk, M., Kelin, K., Mancini, M., & Schacht, A. (2013). Treatment Response for Acute Depression Is Not Associated with Number of Previous Episodes: Lack of Evidence for a Clinical Staging Model For Major Depressive Disorder. *Journal of Affective Disorders, 150,* 344-349. http://dx.doi.org/10.1016/j.jad.2013.04.016

Dombrovski, A. Y., Mulsant, B. H., Houck, P. R., Mazumdar, S., Lenze, E. J., Andreescu, C. et al. (2007). Residual Symptoms and Recurrence during Maintenance Treatment of Late-Life Depression. *Journal of Affective Disorders, 103,* 77-82. http://dx.doi.org/10.1016/j.jad.2007.01.020

Farabaugh, A., Mischoulon, D., Fava, M., Wu, S. L., Mascarini, A., Tossani, E., Alpert, J. E. (2005). The Relationship between Early Changes in the HAMD-17 Anxiety/Somatization Factor Items and Treatment Outcome among Depressed Outpatients. *International Clinical Psychopharmacology, 20,* 87-91. http://dx.doi.org/10.1097/00004850-200503000-00004

Farabaugh, A. H., Bitran, S., Witte, J., Alpert, J., Chuzi, S., Clain, A. J. et al. (2010). Anxious Depression and Early Changes in the HAMD-17 Anxiety-Somatization Factor Items and Antidepressant Treatment Outcome. *International Clinical Psychopharmacology, 25,* 214-217. http://dx.doi.org/10.1097/YIC.0b013e328339fbbd

Farabaugh, A., Alpert, J., Wisniewski, S. R., Otto, M. W., Fava, M., Baer, L. et al. (2012). Cognitive Therapy for Anxious Depression in STAR*D: What Have We Learned? *Journal of Affective Disorders, 142,* 213-218. http://dx.doi.org/10.1016/j.jad.2012.04.029

Fava, M., Alpert, J. E., Carmin, C. N., Wisniewski, S. R., Trivedi, M. H., Biggs et al. (2004). Clinical Correlates and symptom patterns of anxious depression among patients with Major Depressive Disorder in STAR*D. *Psychological Medicine, 34,* 1299-1308. http://dx.doi.org/10.1017/S0033291704002612

Fava, M., Rush, A. J., Alpert, J. E., Balasubramani, G. K., Wisniewski, S. R., Carmin, C. N. et al. (2008). Difference in Treatment Outcome in Outpatients with Anxious Versus Nonanxious Depression: A STAR*D Report. *American Journal of Psychiatry, 165,* 342-351. http://dx.doi.org/10.1176/appi.ajp.2007.06111868

Guy, W. (1976). ECDEU Assessment Manual for Psychopharmacology, Revised. US Department of Health, Education, and Welfare Publication (ADM). Rockville, MD: National Institute of Mental Health, 76-338.

Hamilton, M. (1959). The Assessment of Anxiety States by Rating. *British Journal of Medical Psychology, 32,* 50-55. http://dx.doi.org/10.1111/j.2044-8341.1959.tb00467.x

Hamilton, M. (1960). A Rating Scale for Depression. *Journal of Neurology, Neurosurgery, and Psychiatry, 23,* 56-62. http://dx.doi.org/10.1136/jnnp.23.1.56

Hirschfeld, R. M., Mallinckrodt, C., Lee, T. C., & Detke, M. J. (2005). Time Course of Depression-Symptom Improvement during Treatment with Duloxetine. *Depression and Anxiety, 21,* 170-177. http://dx.doi.org/10.1002/da.20071

Judd, L. L., Paulus, M. J., Schettler, P. J., Akiskal, H. S., Endicott, J., Leon, A. C. et al. (2000). Does Incomplete Recovery from First Lifetime Major Depressive Episode Herald a Chronic Course of Illness? *The American Journal of Psychiatry, 157,* 1501-1504. http://dx.doi.org/10.1176/appi.ajp.157.9.1501

Karp, J. F., Scott, J., Houck, P., Reynolds 3rd, C. F., Kupfer, D. J., & Frank, E. (2005). Pain Predicts Longer Time to Remission during Treatment of Recurrent Depression. *Journal of Clinical Psychiatry, 66,* 591-597. http://dx.doi.org/10.4088/JCP.v66n0508

Katz, M. M., Tekell, J. L., Bowden, C. L., Brannan, S., Houston, J. P., Berman, N., & Frazer, A. (2004). Onset and Early Behavioral Effects of Pharmacologically Different Antidepressants and Placebo in Depression. *Neuropsychopharmacology, 29*, 566-579. http://dx.doi.org/10.1038/sj.npp.1300341

Katz, M. M., Meyers, A. L., Prakash, A., Gaynor, P. J., & Houston, J. P. (2009). Early Symptom Change Prediction of Remission in Depression Treatment. *Psychopharmacology Bulletin, 42*, 94-107.

Keller, M. B., Lavori, P. W., Rice, J., Coryell, W., & Hirschfeld, R. M. (1986). The Persistent Risk of Chronicity in Recurrent Episodes of Nonbipolar Major Depressive Disorder: A Prospective Follow-Up. *American Journal of Psychiatry, 143*, 24-28.

Kessing, L. V., Hansen, M. G., Andersen, P. K., & Angst, J. (2004). The Predictive Effect of Episodes on the Risk of Recurrence in Depressive and Bipolar Disorders—A Life-Long Perspective. *Acta Psychiatrica Scandinavica, 109*, 339-344. http://dx.doi.org/10.1046/j.1600-0447.2003.00266.x

Kessler, R. C., Nelson, C. B., McGonagle, K. A., Liu, J., Swartz, M., & Blazer, D. G. (1996). Comorbidity of DSM-III-R Major Depressive Disorder in the General Population: Results from the US National Comorbidity Survey. *British Journal of Psychiatry, 168*, 17-30.

Kessler, R. C., Berglund, P., Demler, O., Jin, R., Koretz, D., Merikangas, K. R. et al. (2003). The Epidemiology of Major Depressive Disorder: Results from the National Comorbidity Survey Replication (NCS-R). *Journal of the American Medical Association, 289*, 3095-3105. http://dx.doi.org/10.1001/jama.289.23.3095

Lépine, J. P., Gastpar, M., Mendlewicz, J., & Tylee, A. (1997). Depression in the Community: The First Pan-European Study DEPRES (Depression Research in European Society). *International Clinical Psychopharmacology, 12*, 19-29. http://dx.doi.org/10.1097/00004850-199701000-00003

Lépine, J. P., & Briley, M. (2011). The Increasing Burden of Depression. *Neuropsychiatric Disease Treatment, 7*, 3-7.

Lin, E. H. B., Katon, W. J., VonKorff, M., Russo, J. E., Simon, G. E., Bush, T. M. et al. (1998). Relapse of Depression in Primary Care: Rate and Clinical Predictors. *Archives of Family Medicine, 7*, 443-449. http://dx.doi.org/10.1001/archfami.7.5.443

Lopez, A. D., & Murray, C. C. (1998). The Global Burden of Disease, 1990-2020. *Nature Medicine, 4*, 1241-1243. http://dx.doi.org/10.1038/3218

Montgomery, S. A., & Asberg, M. (1979). A New Depression Scale Designed to Be Sensitive to Change. *British Journal of Psychiatry, 134*, 382-389. http://dx.doi.org/10.1192/bjp.134.4.382

Mundt, J. C., DeBrota, D. J., & Greist, J. H. (2007). Anchoring Perceptions of Clinical Change on Accurate Recollection of the Past: Memory Enhanced Retrospective Evaluation of Treatment (MERET®). *Psychiatry, 4*, 39-45.

Nelson, J. C. (2008). Anxious Depression and Response to Treatment. *American Journal of Psychiatry, 165*, 297-299. http://dx.doi.org/10.1176/appi.ajp.2007.07121927

Nierenberg, A. A., Qyitkin, F. M., Kremer, C., Keller, M. B., & Thase, M. E. (2004). Placebo-Controlled Continuation Treatment with Mirtazapine: Acute Pattern of Response Predicts Relapse. *Neuropsychopharmacology, 29*, 1012-1018. http://dx.doi.org/10.1038/sj.npp.1300405

Nierenberg, A. A., Greist, J. H., Mallinckrodt, C. H., Prakash, A., Sambunaris, A., Tollefson, G. D., & Wohlreich, M. M. (2007). Duloxetine Versus Escitalopram and Placebo in the Treatment of Patients with Major Depressive Disorder: Onset of Antidepressant Action, a Non-Inferiority Study. *Current Medical Research and Opinion, 23*, 401-416. http://dx.doi.org/10.1185/030079906X167453

Oakes, T. M., Myers, A. L., Marangell, L. B., Ahl, J., Prakash, A., Thase, M. E., & Kornstein, S. G. (2012). Assessment of Depressive Symptoms and Functional Outcomes in Patients with Major Depressive Disorder Treated with Duloxetine versus Placebo: Primary Outcomes from Two Trials Conducted under the Same Protocol. *Human Psychopharmacology: Clinical and Experimental, 27*, 47-56. http://dx.doi.org/10.1002/hup.1262

Parker, G., Wilhelm, K., Mitchell, P., & Gladstone, G. (2000). Predictors of 1-Year Outcome in Depression. *The Australian and New Zealand Journal of Psychiatry, 34*, 56-64. http://dx.doi.org/10.1046/j.1440-1614.2000.00698.x

Pintor, L., Gastó, C., Navarro, V., Torres, X., & Fañanas, L. (2003). Relapse of Major Depression after Complete and Partial Remission during a 2-Year Follow-Up. *Journal of Affective Disorders, 73*, 237-244. http://dx.doi.org/10.1016/S0165-0327(01)00480-3

Raskin, J., Wiltse, C. G., Siegal, A., Sheikh, J., Xu, J., Dinkel, J. J. et al. (2007). Efficacy of Duloxetine on Cognition, Depression, and Pain in Elderly Patients with Major Depressive Disorder: An 8-Week, Double-Blind, Placebo-Controlled Trial. *American Journal of Psychiatry, 164*, 900-909. http://dx.doi.org/10.1176/appi.ajp.164.6.900

Robinson, M., Oakes, T. M., Raskin, J., Liu, P., Shoemaker, S., & Nelson, J. C. (2014). Acute and Long-Term Treatment of Late-Life Major Depressive Disorder: Duloxetine versus Placebo. *American Journal of Geriatric Psychiatry, 22*, 34-45. http://dx.doi.org/10.1016/j.jagp.2013.01.019

Rush, A. J., Zimmerman, M., Wisniewski, S. R., Fava, M., Hollon, S. D., Warden, D. et al. (2005). Comorbid Psychiatric

Disorders in Depressed Outpatients: Demographic and Clinical Features. *Journal of Affective Disorders, 87,* 43-55. http://dx.doi.org/10.1016/j.jad.2005.03.005

Sheehan, D. V., Harnett-Sheehan, K., & Raj, B. A. (1996). The Measurement of Disability. *International Clinical Psychopharmacology, 11,* 89-95. http://dx.doi.org/10.1097/00004850-199606003-00015

Shelton, R. C., Prakash, A., Mallinckrodt, C. H., Wohlreich, M. M., Raskin, J., Robinson, M. J., & Detke, M. J. (2007). Patterns of Depressive Symptom Response in Duloxetine-Treated Outpatients with Mild, Moderate or More Severe Depression. *International Journal of Clinical Practice, 61,* 1337-1348. http://dx.doi.org/10.1111/j.1742-1241.2007.01444.x

Silverstone, P. H., Entsuah, R., & Hackett, D. (2002). Two Items on the Hamilton Depression Rating Scale Are Effective Predictors of Remission: Comparison of Selective Serotonin Reuptake Inhibitors with the Combined Serotonin/Norepinephrine Reuptake Inhibitor, Venlafaxine. *International Clinical Psychopharmacology, 17,* 273-280. http://dx.doi.org/10.1097/00004850-200211000-00002

Wade, A., & Anderson, H. F. (2006). The Onset of Effect for Escitalopram and Its Relevance for the Clinical Management of Depression. *Current Medical Research and Opinion, 22,* 2101-2110. http://dx.doi.org/10.1185/030079906X148319

Wilhelm, K., Parker, G., Dewhurst-Savellis, J., & Asghari, A. (1999). Psychological Predictors of Single and Recurrent Major Depressive Episodes. *Journal of Affective Disorders, 54,* 139-147. http://dx.doi.org/10.1016/S0165-0327(98)00170-0

World Health Organization (2008). The Global Burden of Disease: 2004 Update. http://www.who.int/healthinfo/global_burden_disease/2004_report_update/en/

World Health Organization (2012). Depression, Fact Sheet. http://www.who.int/mediacentre/factsheets/fs369/en/

Yang, H., Chuzi, S., Sinicropi-Yao, L., Johnson, D., Chen, Y., Clain, A. et al. (2010). Type of Residual Symptom and Risk of Relapse during the Continuation/Maintenance Phase Treatment of Major Depressive Disorder with the Selective Serotonin Reuptake Inhibitor Fluoxetine. *European Archives of Psychiatry and Clinical Neuroscience, 260,* 145-150. http://dx.doi.org/10.1007/s00406-009-0031-3

Zimmerman, M., Chelminski, I., & McDermut, W. (2002). Major Depressive Disorder and Axis I Diagnostic Comorbidity. *Journal of Clinical Psychiatry, 63,* 187-193. http://dx.doi.org/10.4088/JCP.v63n0303

7

Validation of a Tunisian Version of the French Scale State Anxiety in Competition (EEAC): Sport and Exercise Context

Driss Boudhiba[1], Najoua Moalla[2], Yassine Arfa[2], Noureddine Kridis[3]

[1]High Institute of Sport and Physical Education, University of Sfax, Sfax, Tunisia
[2]High Institute of Sport and Physical Education of Ksar Saïd, University of Manouba, Manouba, Tunisia
[3]Faculty of Humanities and Social Sciences, University of Tunis, Tunis, Tunisia
Email: dr.boudhiba@gmail.com

Abstract

This study aims to adapt the CSAI-2 in the French version (EEAC), among 156 Tunisian athlete boys and girls one hour before competition. Therefore, our purpose is to refine the factorial analysis and get a shorter but stronger structure of the EECA version. Our study proposes a new Tunisian version of 13 items with (α = 0.85) instead of the first twenty three French version.

Keywords

CSAI-2, EEAC, Cognitive Anxiety, Somatic Anxiety, Self Confidence, Sport Psychology

1. Introduction

Subject practicing semi professional or professional sport activity or those playing regular competitions are exposed frequently to the competitive stress causing different mood states and shooting behavioral troubles among athletes. Therefore, willing to explore the impact of the competitive stress on the state of humor and because of the lack of adapted scales in Tunisian library, we try to verify a very famous instrument, the French version of CSAI-2 (the EEAC; Cury, F., Sarrazin, P., Pérès, C., and Famose, J.P, 1999) by realizing this study [1], consisting of twenty-three items measuring the following three components: self-confidence, cognitive anxiety, somatic anxiety and evaluating the intensity of cognitive anxiety (characterized by negative expectations and self-doubts) dominated by somatic anxiety symptoms such as increased heart rate and muscle tension while that plus a third component of self-confidence. Anxiety is the most studied variable in psychology including sports psychology.

In fact, Marten's *et al.* (1990) [2] define somatic anxiety as "emotional and physiological components of anxious experience directly from a state of autonomic arousal". Moreover, the cognitive anxiety comes in signs of negative expectations related to performance. Thus, state anxiety is considered as predictors of state cognitive and somatic anxiety (Gould *et al.* 1984; Crocker *et al.*, 1988) [3] [4], expectancy of success and achievement of a goal predicted essentially cognitive anxiety (Lane *et al.*, 1995) [5]. The age and the expertise are also identified as indicative of state anxiety (Hammermeister and Burton, 1995; Jones and Swain, 1995) [6] [7].

There are an English version CSAI-2R (Cox *et al.*, 2003) [8], a Greek version (Tsorbadzoudis *et al.*, 2002) [9], a Swedish version (Lunqvist *et al.*, 2006) [10] and a French version with 23 items (Scale State Anxiety in Competition; Cury, Sarrazin, Peres, and Famose (1997) [1]. Moreover, the CSAI-2 is subject to a confirmatory factor analysis to develop a Portuguese version. On the other hand, Coelho *et al.* (2007) [11] have set themselves the goal of measuring the factor structure of CSAI-2. They are administered to two subgroups of footballers; the first consists of 266 players at the regional level. The results of the confirmatory analysis reveal a better two-factor version of 18 items adapted to the Brazilian footballing population (p < 0.057). The authors of this study confirm that their version is better compared to the version of Cox *et al.* (2003) [8] and three factors and 17 items. Terry *et al.* (2008) [12] have conducted research to reassess the psychometric properties of the CSAI-2R release to 17 items proposed by Cox *et al.* (2003) [8]. Repeated measures data collected from 92 tennis players performed at five pre-competitive are the subject of a principal factor analysis (promax rotation). The results confirm the three-factor model measures.

2. Method

The purpose of this study is an adaptation of a French version of the rating scale of competitive anxiety (EECA).

2.1. Participants

To achieve this, we selected 156 athletes from practicing all the various types of sports; team and individual all young athletes' schoolchildren. (Age: 18.66 ± 2.87 years) and licensed in their specialty (see **Table 1**).

Table 1. Descriptive statistics.

	Male	Female	Total
Sample size	109	47	156
Age	18.59 (2.26)	18.81 (3.90)	18.66 (2.87)
Level of instruction	12.53 (2.72)	12.98 (3.65)	12.76 (2.80)

Table 1 shows a normal distribution of the sample composed by 156 athletes all semi professional, 109 males and 47 females. Analyses revealed a normal distribution and no significant difference p > 0.20.

Figure 1 shows clearly a normal distribution of the level of instruction indicating a homogeneity perceived in the red gauss curve.

Figure 2 shows also a regular normal distribution of the nominal variable age and non significant difference between males and females of the sample.

2.2. Procedures

The linguistic validation method of the instrument includes the steps proposed by Vallerand (1989). The first concerns the development of a preliminary version which consists of a type evaluation committee, and an assessment of the clarity of items pretest on the target population. The second step involves assessing the accuracy and validity of the instrument consists of factor analysis known as "exploratory" and a search for internal consistency. We translated the scale into Arabic, simple-translation and reverse (forward/backward translation) then applied concurrent assessments and analyzed the content and reliability and construct validity by investigating the factor structure to assess, in the end, consistency internally.

2.3. Data Collection

To attend the meaning of interaction between the different variables and the significance of the eventual rela-

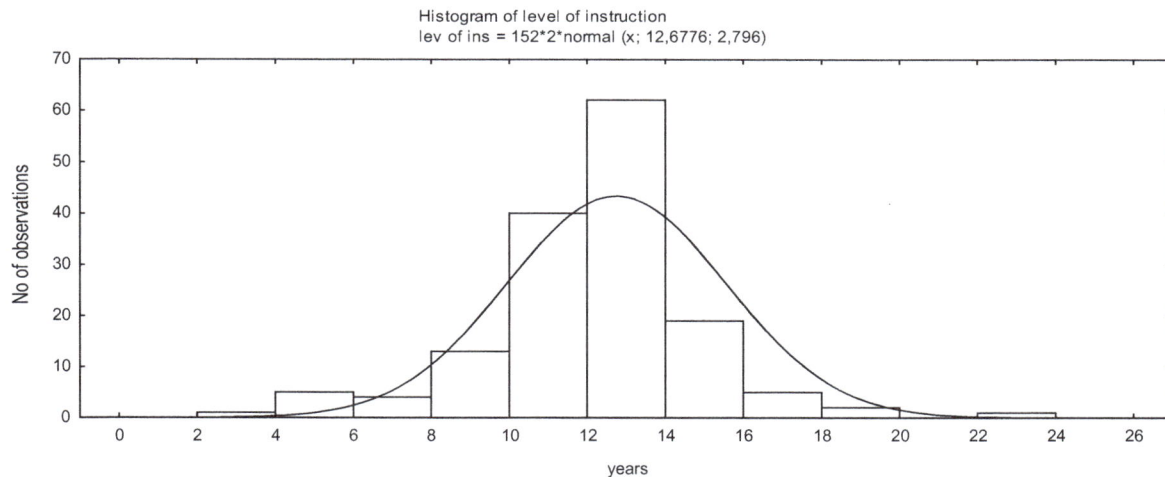

Histogram of level of instruction
lev of ins = 152*2*normal (x; 12,6776; 2,796)

Figure 1. Distribution by level of instruction.

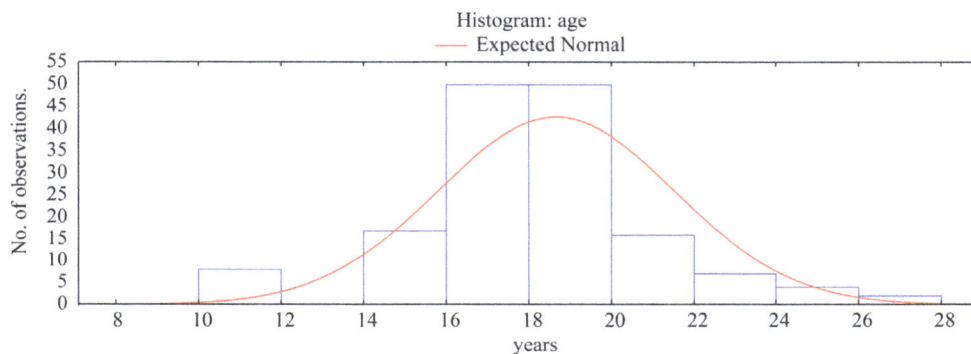

Histogram: age
— Expected Normal

Figure 2. Distribution by age.

tions we used the statistica 8 [13] program applying the basic statistics, the parametric and non parametric methods using tables and adequate figures to achieve the ultimate analysis of the collected data.

3. Results

The exploratory analysis aims to formulate a first version of the instrument from the responses of a sample of athletes. Only items whose loadings are above (0.45) and only factors with Eigen values greater than 1 were retained.

3.1. Main Analysis

Factor structures features are represented and then subjected to analysis of internal consistency by calculating Cronbach's alpha coefficient for judging the homogeneity of the subscales comprising the two questionnaires. The index ranges from 0 to 1. Consistency is considered acceptable when the alpha is between 0.60 and 0.90.

Table 2 shows a normal distribution of the results obtained among our sample and no significant difference was revealed. In the first dimension of cognitive anxiety males n = 109 obtain a mean of 17.19 with standard deviation 3.67 however females n = 47 got a mean of 16.38 and standard deviation 6.07. Total mean in this dimension is 16.95 and standard deviation 4.40. On the other hand males obtain in the second dimension measuring the somatic anxiety a mean of 22.93 and standard deviation 2.64. Females have a mean of 19.80 with standard deviation of 5.09 and total score in this dimension was 21.88 with standard deviation 5.09. In the last dimension self confidence, results are as follows: males obtain a mean of 16.45 and standard deviation 4.45. Females got a mean of 15.33 and standard deviation 6.96. Finally, total mean for males is 56.27 with standard

Table 2. Descriptive statistics per dimension.

	Male n = 109	Female n = 47	Total N = 156
Cognitive Anxiety	17.19 (3.67)	16.38 (6.07)	16.95 (4.40)
Somatic Anxiety	22.62 (3.96)	19.80 (7.13)	21.88 ((5.09)
Self confidence	16.45 (4.45)	15.33 (6.96)	16.16 (5.20)
Total	56.27 (9.44)	51.52 (18.21)	55.02 (6.50)

Table 3. Factorial respective dimensions of the Tunisian version.

Factor DIMENSION	1	2	3	4	5	6
COGNITIVEANXIETY						
3				0.65		
6	0.64					
9	0.68					
12	0.77					
15	0.72					
18	0.70					
20	0.80					
SOMATIC ANXIETY						
1						
4					0.78	
7					0.49	
10				0.72	0.46	
13			−0.75			
16				0.66		
22				0.55		
SELF CONFIDENCE						
2						
5		−0.75	−0.55			
8		−0.70				
11						
14		0.70				
17						
19						.60
21			−0.60			
23						

Table 4. Hierarchial multiple regression analysis predicting mood and self confidence interactions.

Predictor	R	R^2 Change	B	SE B	β
Gender	0258	0.029*			
Cognitive Anxiety			0.012	0.017	0.125
Somatic Anxiety			0.025	0.011	−0.291*
Self Confidence			−0.004*	0.013	0.056

Note N = 156, *$p < 0.05$, R = simple regression, R^2 = adjusted regression, SE B = Standard Estimation of B.

Table 5. Confirmatory analysis of Tunisian version of EEAC.

N	Mean	SD	α Crombach	α Standerdized	Other quest
156	57.17	5.99	0.44	0.40	0.05

N = sample size, *SD = standard deviation.*

Table 6. Comparison between the French and the Tunisian versions of CSAI-2.

	French Version of Csai-2	Tunisian Version of Csai-2
Cognitive Anxiety	3-6-9-12-5-18-20	6-9-12-15-18-20
Somatic Anxiety	1-4-7-10-13 inversed-16-22	1-4-7-10-16-22
Self-Esteem	2-5-8-11-14-17-19-21-23	2-5-8-11-14-19+13

deviation 9.44. Females obtain a mean 51.52 and standard deviation of 18.21. However total score is 55.02 with a standard deviation 6.50.

3.2. Factorial Analysis

Factorial analysis performed on data collected after the award with 156 athlete boys and girls practitioners of different sports: Team, individual and combat (contact), in pre-competitive situation is thirty minutes to an hour before the competition has led us to identify six factors (**Table 3**). As to the different dimensions the results showed that: 1) Dimension of Cognitive Anxiety as measured by test (F = 0.11; p < 0.05). 2) The dimension of somatic anxiety (F = 0.10; p < 0.10). 3) And the third dimension Self-confidence (F = 0.09; p < 0.20). Thus we can present the factors of Tunisian version with respective items as follows: Following distribution of items per factor, we find that the three dimensions that measure the CSAI-2 have emerged in the Tunisian version of a separate and very clear. The only remark is the fact that you can delete items 21 and 23. The item 21: I am confident because I see myself succeed. The item 23: I am sure not yield to pressure. These two items not mentioned in any of the six factors identified.

Table 3 shows a big similarity in factor distribution between the French CSAI-2 version twenty three item scale and the Tunisian version of the same scale. Analysis of Inter-items correlations were subjected to principal components factor analysis, followed by Varimax orthogonal rotation procedure for isolating items saturating the best studied factors reveals a coefficient Crombach ($\alpha = 0.44$). A second analysis was performed on selected items. In order to provide the best possible compromise between the extent of the scale and its internal consistency, we note that 13 items ($\alpha = 0.84$) to three factors instead of seven factors for the version with 23 items could fit better.

Moreover, regression summary, as shows (**Table 4**) for dependant variable gender shows; R = 0.258 and $R^2 = 0.066$, an adjusted $R^2 = 0.029$, F (3.76) = 1.80, p < 0.05. Standard deviation of estimate = 0.4361.

So, for simple regression analysis of the first dimension, cognitive anxiety examination of the coefficients indicate (B = 0.012, SE = 0.017, $\beta = 0.125$, p = 0.66).

Concerning the somatic anxiety, simple regression analysis examination of the coefficients indicate (B= −0.025, SE = 0.011, $\beta = -0.291$, p = 0.034).

In the last dimension self confidence (B = −0.004, SE = 0.013, $\beta = 0.056$, p = −0.05).

The objective of our study is to develop a Tunisian version of the factorial validity of the (23 items) French version of CSAI-2. The purpose is to be as objective as possible assessing emotional and mood competitive dimensions trying the best to determine their Tunisian cultural specificities. Results are as following, look **Table 5**).

Table 6 shows clearly the consistency and the robustness of both of the French and Tunisian version of the structure and the reliability of CSAI-2 despite the cultural differences proving the uniformity of human being and the biological determinations such as the emotions and especially anxiety and self confidence.

4. Discussion

Lane [5] by managing the scale an hour before the competition has come from the fact that for the two subgroups, measures of the robustness index benchmarking are as follows: group A = 0.82, Group B = 0.84 and simultaneously measuring the comparative index 0.83 suggesting that the model assumed a low index showing the factor structure proposed by Martens [2] is low. The results these authors have managed can lead to the conclusion that the low level of cognitive anxiety is related to the translation of items in the world precisely the "concerned" instead of "anxious". Lane et al. (1999) [5] emphasize the fact that the item "in English" concerned being affected by an impending performance does not necessarily mean that the athlete has dark thoughts and negative but recognizes that the athlete recognizes the importance and difficulty of the challenge and tries to mobilize his or her resources to cope. Thus, Lane [5] questions the use of the CSAI-2 as a valid measure of anxiety-state competitive. By applying structures suggested by previous study, with two samples, 287 students in physical education and sports, and 323 individual sport athletes. Results indicate according to certain authors [2]-[5] of work poor posture of the model. Other structures have been suggested by various other authors who are analyzed showing levels of acceptable values of good index and some others are not adequate. The authors propose a new model, scale-free awakening, showing an adequate fit calibration sample and its capacity has been validated by the second sample. The authors reveal a double negative correlation scales (negativity and self-confidence).

The study confirms the psychometric properties of the CSAI-2R [8] which he considers satisfactory squaring results of Lane *et al.* (1999) [5] who considers those of the original version (CSAI-2) [2] as defective and to which our results are not in line. Terry *et al.* [13] invite to use version CSAI-2R [8] instead the 27 items (CSAI-2) [2]. We can criticize the English version [2] while supporting the French version of the EEAC [1], even if results don't agree with the findings of Lane [5] concerning the factorial or structural robustness of the CSAI-2. We confirm the three factorial construct of the French version (23 items) [1]. However, our findings agree the fact that the confusion can be caused by the translation of the item "concerned" which should be "anxious" and not "interested".

In conclusion, it is an opportunity for future scientific studies to light on this aspect improving the conditions of such assessments in very special competitive circumstances, characterized by the rapid changes.

References

[1]   Cury, F., Sarrazin, P., Pérès, C. and Famose, J.P. (1999) Mesurer l'anxiété du sportif en compétition: Présentation de l'échelle d'état d'anxiété en compétition (EEAC), in Christine Le Scanff et Jean Pierre Famose. *La gestion du Stress*, Dossier EPS n°43, Paris, Eds Revue EPS.

[2]   Martens, R., Burton, D., Vealey, R.S., Bump, L.A. and Smith, D.E. (1990) Development and Validation of the Competitive State Anxiety Inventory-2 (CSAI-2). In: Martens, R., Vealey, R.S. and Burton, D., Eds., *Competitive Anxiety in sport*, Human Kinetics, Chapaign, 117-190.

[3]   Gould, D., Petlichkoff, L. and Weinberg, R.S. (1984) Antecedents of Temporal Changes in, and Relationships between CSAI-2 Subcomponents. *Journal of Sport Psychology*, **6**, 289-304.

[4]   Crocker, P.R.E., Alderman, R.B. and Smith, F.M.R. (1988) Cognitive-Affective Stress Management Training with His Performance Youth Volleyball Players: Effects on Affect, Cognition and Performance. *Journal of Sport and Exercise Psychology*, **10**, 448-460.

[5]   Lane, A.M., Sewell, D.F., Terry, P.C., Bartam, D. and Nesti, A.S. (1999) Confirmatory Factor Analysis of the Competitive State Anxiety Inventory-2. *Journal of Sport Sciences*, **17**, 505-512. http://dx.doi.org/10.1080/026404199365812

[6]   Hammermeister, J. and Burton, D. (1995) Anxiety and the Ironman: Investigating the Antecedents and Consequences of Endurance Athletes' State Anxiety. *The Sport Psychologist*, **9**, 29-40.

[7]   Jones, G. and Swain, A.B.J. (1995) Predispositions to Experience Debilitative and Facilitative Anxiety in Elite and Non-Elite Performers. *The Sport Psychologist*, **99**, 201-211.

[8]   Cox, R.H., Martens, M.P. and Russell, W.D. (2003) Measuring Anxiety in Athletes: The Revised Competitive Anxiety Inventory-2. *Journal of Sport Psychology*, **25**, 519-533.

[9]   Tsoubatroudis, H., Barkoukis, V., Kaissidis-Rodafinos, G. and Grouios, G. (2002) Confirmatory Factor Analysis of the Greek Version of the Competitive State Anxiety Inventory-2 (CSAI-2). *International Journal of Sport Psychology*, **33**, 182-194.

[10]   Lunqvist, C. (2006) Competing under Pressure. US-AB Stokholm.

[11]   Coelho, E.M., Vasconcelos-Raposo, J. and Fernandes, H.M. (2007) Confirmatory Factor Analysis of the Portuguese Version of the CSAI-2. *Motricidade.*

[12]   Terry, P.C. and Munro, A. (2008) Psychometric Re-Evaluation of the Revised Version of the Competitive State Anxiety Inventory-2. *43rd Australian Psychological Society Annual Conference*, Hobart, 23-27 September 2008.

[13]   StatSoft STATISTICA 8.0.360-English Edition.

8

Shoulda' Put a Ring on It: Investigating Adult Attachment, Relationship Status, Anxiety, Mindfulness, and Resilience in Romantic Relationships

Aileen M. Pidgeon, Alexandra C. Giufre

Bond University, Gold Coast, Australia
Email: alexandragiufre@live.com

Abstract

This study aimed to investigate the predictive ability of relationship status, anxiety, mindfulness, and resilience in relation to the two orthogonal dimensions of adult attachment: attachment anxiety and attachment avoidance. 156 participants completed measures assessing relationship status, adult attachment, anxiety, mindfulness and resilience. The results showed that resilience and the relationship status of single significantly predicted attachment anxiety, whereas anxiety and being either single or divorced significantly predicted attachment avoidance. A significant mediating role of resilience in the prediction of attachment anxiety from being single was also observed. The main implications of this study provided preliminary support for the significant predictive value of resilience in attachment anxiety.

Keywords

Attachment, Romantic Relationships, Relationship Status, Anxiety, Mindfulness, Resilience

1. Introduction

Romantic relationships are one of the most important relationships formed in many people's lives with interpersonal communication being central to romantic relationships. The way two people interact when they first meet can either ignite or extinguish hopes of future romance [1]-[3]. Although numerous benefits emerge from engaging in romantic relationships [4] [5], challenges such as relationship conflict can also arise [3]. For many individuals, the costs of a successful relationship can sometimes far outweigh the benefits, resulting in many men and women terminating their romantic relationship. Relationship termination can represent the end of a relationship resulting in singlehood, separation from a partner, or divorce. Extensive research has shown that separation, divorce, and singlehood can increase the risk of negative emotions, behaviours, and health concerns [6] [7]. Such negative consequences warrant extending upon previous research to further our understanding of the modifiable factors that predict a successful and high quality romantic relationship.

The theory of adult attachment styles has its roots in Bowlby [8], and offers a promising theoretical framework for understanding variations in the quality of romantic relationships [3] [9]. Research on adult attachment indicates the importance of secure attachments for well-being and interpersonal functioning [2]. Individuals with different attachments differ greatly in the nature and quality of their close relationships [3]. Adult attachment in romantic relationships can be reliably assessed by self-report measures that examine two orthogonal dimensions: attachment anxiety and attachment avoidance [10] [11]. The Experiences in Close Relationship Scale [11] which measures these dimensions has been criticized by its problematic length, and thus a psychometrically sound shorter version of the measure was developed named the Experiences in Close Relationships Scale-Short Form [12]. However to date, no study has utilised this shortened measure of adult attachment. This current study will investigate the predictive factors of romantic relationships in regards to both attachment anxiety and attachment avoidance assessed by the ECR-S.

2. Relationship Status

A paucity of research to date has directly examined the issue of the association between adult attachment and relationship status. For example, research by Adamczyk and Bookwala [13] investigated the association between adult attachment and relationship status (single vs. partnered) in a Polish university sample. Within their study, adult attachment was determined based on a three-dimensional measure conceptualised by Collins and Read [14]. These three dimensions captured an individual's confidence that a partner would be loving (anxiety dimension), belief of a partner's availability and responsiveness (depend dimension), and desire for close contact with a partner (close dimension). In terms of scoring, the "depend" and "close" dimensions were combined in order to create one factor that incorporated the two factors. Collins and Reads' three-dimensional model is similar to that of Brennan *et al.* [11] as both contain an anxiety dimension, with the combined factor of "depend" and "close" equating to the avoidance dimension. The results of Adamczyk and Bookwala's study showed that individuals classified as single reported higher levels of worry about being rejected or feeling unloved (anxiety dimension), lower levels of comfort with closeness (close dimension), and lower levels of comfort with depending on other people (depend dimension) compared to partnered individuals. This current study will add to the body of knowledge by examining whether individuals who are single will score significantly higher on both attachment anxiety and attachment avoidance dimensions, as determined by the ECR-S.

Additionally, a study that investigated relationship status in regards to both the orthogonal dimensions of adult attachment was conducted by Noftle and Shaver (2006) [15]. The results demonstrated that relationship status was a significant predictor of both attachment anxiety and attachment avoidance, where individuals who were not in a relationship scored significantly higher on both these dimensions. However, although Noftle and Shaver investigated people who were single (*i.e.*, those who were not currently dating, in a committed relationship, or married), a limitation of their study was that the predictive ability of individuals who were separated or divorced was not examined. Therefore, the current study will expand upon Noftle and Shavers' study by addressing this limitation and examining adult attachment amongst individuals who are single, defacto, married, separated, and divorced.

2.1. Anxiety

Close relationships play a vital role with the onset, duration, and treatment of anxiety [16]. As such, the presence of anxiety can have detrimental long-term effects on romantic relationships. For instance, a study by Schachner *et al.* [7] within a community sample of single and coupled adults identified an association between the orthogonal dimensions of adult attachment and anxiety. In particular, significant main effects for anxiety were found where individuals who scored high on attachment anxiety and attachment avoidance also scored significantly higher on anxiety. As Schachner and Colleagues established that attachment anxiety and avoidance significantly predicted higher levels of anxiety, the present study will aim to determine whether this relationship is bi-directional, by determining whether high scores of anxiety will significantly predict attachment anxiety and avoidance.

2.2. Mindfulness

A predictor of adult attachment that has not been extensively examined in the literature is mindfulness. Bowlby [8] initially raised awareness that some of the most intense emotions experienced are those concerned with close relationships. This concept has since been investigate by Barnes Brown, Krusemark, Campbell, and Roggee (2007) [17] who examined whether mindfulness was associated with greater satisfaction in romantic relationships, in addition to the capacity of mindfulness to manage relationship related stress. Their results showed that individuals who scored higher on mindfulness reported greater levels of satisfaction, and better capacities to respond to relationship stress. Additionally, Barnes and Colleagues noted that because their sample was comprised of only dating university students, it was not established whether their results were generalisable to married couples. Conversely, it can also be assumed that their results did not generalize to single, separated, or divorced individuals.

Additionally, a recent study by Leigh and Anderson [18] investigated the potential contribution of adult attachment to self-reported mindfulness. In particular, the researchers were interested in examining how university students who had not received mindfulness training developed the mindfulness tendencies that they reported. The researchers investigated whether attachment theory assisted in understanding the development of mindfulness and concluded that the orthogonal dimensions of attachment anxiety and avoidance did in fact negatively predict mindfulness. In terms of methodological considerations, Leigh and Anderson measured mindfulness and attachment from the Five Facet Mindfulness Questionnaire [19] and the Experiences in Close Relationships [11] respectively, and it is therefore of interest to the present study to determine if the findings from Leigh and Andersons [18] study can be replicated using the Freiburg Mindfulness Inventory [20] and the ECR-S [12].

2.3. Resilience

An additional variable of interest in relation to adult attachment that has limited empirical evidence available is resilience. To date, the relationship between resilience and adult attachment as determined by the ECR-S has not been directly investigated. However, a study by Caldwell and Shaver (2012) [21] investigated the relationship between attachment anxiety, attachment avoidance, rumination, negative affect, mood repair, and ego resiliency. The authors defined ego resiliency as a "positive adjustment by fostering an open, flexible, and optimistic approach to life's diverse and often unpredictable challenges" [21], which appears to be a similar definition of resilience used in the present study. Although Caldwell and Shavers' study found that both attachment anxiety and attachment avoidance predicted lower ego-resiliency, a structural equation model was utilized which may have influenced the results by taking into account other variables of rumination, negative affect, and mood repair. Therefore, this study will address this issue by investigating the predictive ability of resilience in relation to attachment anxiety and avoidance without the combination of additional variables.

2.4. The Current Study

The current study aimed to examine the association of relationship status, anxiety, mindfulness, and resilience to changes in attachment anxiety and attachment avoidance.

H_1: It was hypothesised that in regards to attachment anxiety:

a   Being single, separated, and divorced would be significant predictors of attachment anxiety, where individuals who are classified as single, separated, or divorced will score higher on attachment anxiety than individuals who are in a relationship.

b   Mindfulness and resilience would be significant predictors of attachment anxiety, where individuals with lower scores of mindfulness and resilience will have higher scores of attachment anxiety.

c   Anxiety would be a significant predictor of adult attachment, where individuals who score higher on anxiety will have higher scores of attachment anxiety.

H_2: It was hypothesised in regards to attachment avoidance:

a   Being single, separated, and divorced would be significant predictors of attachment avoidance, where individuals who are classified as single, separated, or divorced will score higher on attachment avoidance than those who are in a relationship.

b   Mindfulness and resilience would be significant predictors of attachment avoidance, where individuals with lower scores of mindfulness and resilience will have higher attachment avoidance.

c   Anxiety will be a significant predictor of attachment avoidance, where individuals with high scores of anxiety will have high attachment avoidance.

H_3: Resilience would mediate the relationship between being single and attachment anxiety.

3. Method

3.1. Participants

Participants were 27 male and 129 female university students ($N = 156$). Inclusion criteria required participants to be aged 18 years or above.

3.2. Measures

Demographic Questions. Participants were asked to provide information regarding their age, gender, and relationship status relevant to the study.

Depression Anxiety Stress Scale 21 (DASS-21). The DASS-21 is a short form of the original 42-item self-report measure assessing depression, anxiety, and stress. For the purpose of the current study, the depression and stress scales were not used, as anxiety was the only variable of interest. A total anxiety score was given by summing participant's scores, with greater scores indicating higher greater levels of anxiety.

Experiences in Close Relationship Scale—Short Form (ECR-S). The ECR-S [12] assesses romantic adult relationships in general, independent from participants' current relationship status. Items measure two underlying and continuous dimensions of adult attachment: attachment anxiety and attachment avoidance.

Freiburg Mindfulness Inventory (FMI-14). The FMI-14 [20] is a 14-item scale measuring experiences of mindfulness over a seven-day period. Possible scores range from 14 to 56, with higher scores indicative of greater levels of mindfulness.

The Connor Davidson-Resilience Scale (CD-RISC). The CD-RISC [22] is a 25-item scale measuring stress coping ability over a month long period. Possible scores range from 25 to 125, with higher scores indicating greater levels of resilience.

4. Results

Assumptions for Hierarchical Multiple Regression Analyses. Mean and standard deviations for each variable are shown in **Table 1**. Prior to the main analysis, a bivariate correlation was conducted to measure the linear association between the predictor and criterion variables. As seen in **Table 2**, Anxiety was significantly positively correlated with the relationship status single and married, and also with attachment anxiety and attachment avoidance. Mindfulness was significantly negatively correlated with attachment anxiety and anxiety. Resilience was significantly negatively correlated with the relationship status single, attachment anxiety, anxiety, and positively correlated with the relationship status married and mindfulness.

Main Analysis

Two hierarchical multiple regressions were conducted to examine the predictive ability of relationship status (single, defacto, married, separated, and divorced), anxiety, mindfulness, and resilience on adult attachment. As relationship status, anxiety, mindfulness and resilience were all significantly correlated with attachment anxiety, these predictor variables were all included in the first hierarchical multiple regression predicting attachment anxiety. However, as mindfulness and resilience did not significantly correlate with attachment avoidance, they were therefore excluded from the second hierarchical multiple regression predicting attachment avoidance.

Table 1. Number of participants, mean scores, and standard deviations for attachment anxiety, attachment avoidance, anxiety, mindfulness, and resilience.

	N	M	SD
Attachment Anxiety	156	22.31	6.602
Attachment Avoidance	156	20.02	4.279
Anxiety	156	4.93	4.762
Mindfulness	156	39.05	7.356
Resilience	156	69.06	13.692

Note: N = Number of Participants; M = Mean Score; SD = Standard Deviation.

Table 2. Hierarchical multiple regression analysis predicting attachment anxiety from relationship status, anxiety, mindfulness, and resilience.

Predictor	R	R^2 Change	B	SE B	β
Step 1	0.258*				
Single			3.587**	1.267	0.232
Separated			5.394	6.538	0.065
Divorced			-3.273	3.884	−0.068
Step 2	0.288	0.016			
Anxiety			0.183	0.111	0.132
Step 3	0.322	0.021			
Mindfulness			−0.134	.071	−0.149
Step 4	0.367*				
Resilience			−0.117*	.051	−0.243

*$p < 0.05$, **$p < 0.01$, ***$p < 0.001$.

A new categorical variable of "in a Relationship" was created in order to combine married and defacto into a single variable for comparison. Therefore, "in a Relationship" was excluded from the regression models to compare individuals who were in a relationship (married and defacto) to those who were not (single, separated, and divorced). Adjusted R^2 was used over R^2 as it provided a more accurate estimate of the true extent of the relationship between the predictor and criterion variables.

Relationship Status, Anxiety, Mindfulness, and Resilience as Predictors of Attachment Anxiety. On step one of the hierarchical multiple regression, relationship status accounted for a significant 4.8% of variance in attachment anxiety, $F(3, 152) = 3.603$, $p = 0.015$. On step two, anxiety was added and accounted for an additional non-significant 1.6% of variance in attachment anxiety, $\Delta F(1, 151) = 2.708$, $p = 0.102$. On step three, mindfulness was added and accounted for an additional non-significant 2.1% of variance in attachment anxiety, $\Delta F(1, 149) = 3.598$, $p = 0.060$. On step four, resilience was added and accounted for an additional significant 3.1% of variance in attachment anxiety $\Delta F(1, 149) = 5.346$, $p = 0.022$. In combination, relationship status, anxiety, mindfulness, and resilience accounted for 10% of variance in attachment anxiety, adjusted $R^2 = 0.100$, $F(6, 149) = 3.872$, $p = 0.001$. By Cohen's (1988) conventions, a combined effect of this magnitude can be considered "medium" ($f^2 = 0.15$). As can be seen in the standardised beta coefficients, relationship status and resilience were the strongest predictors of attachment anxiety, where individuals who were single had higher scores on attachment anxiety than individuals who were in a relationship, and those who scored lower on resilience also scored higher on attachment anxiety.

Relationship Status and Anxiety as Predictors of Attachment Avoidance. On step one, relationship status accounted for a significant 11.4% of the variance in attachment avoidance, adjusted $R^2 = 0.114$, $F(3, 152) = 7.637$, $p = < 0.001$. On step two, anxiety was added to the regression equation and accounted for an additional significant 5.9% of variance in attachment avoidance, $\Delta R^2 = 0.059$, $\Delta F(1, 151) = 11.042$, $p = 0.001$. In combination, relationship status and anxiety accounted for 16.9% of variance in attachment avoidance, adjusted $R^2 = 0.169$, $F(4, 151) = 8.867$, $p = < 0.001$. By Cohen's [23] conventions, a combined effect of this magnitude can be considered "medium" ($f^2 = 0.23$). As can be seen from the standardised beta coefficients in **Table 3**, relationship status was the greatest predictor of attachment avoidance, where individuals who were single had higher scores of attachment avoidance compared to individuals who were in a relationship. Additionally, divorce was the only relationship' status that significantly predicted attachment anxiety. Furthermore, individuals who scored higher on anxiety also scored higher on attachment avoidance.

Resilience as a Mediator between being Single and Attachment Anxiety. The four criteria stated by Baron and Kenny (1986) [24] were used to determine whether resilience mediated the relationship between being single and attachment anxiety. Thus, linear and hierarchical multiple regression analysis, and a Sobel test [25] were performed to test the third hypothesis that resilience mediated the relationship between being single and attach-

Table 3. Hierarchical multiple regression analysis predicting attachment avoidance from relationship status and anxiety.

Predictor	R	R^2 Change	B	SE B	β
Step 1	0.362**				
Single			3.710***	0.792	0.370
Separated			4.939	4.089	0.092
Divorced			4.939*	2.429	0.159
Step 2	0.436**	0.190			
Anxiety			0.225**	0.068	0.251

Note: N = 156; CI = confidence interval. $^*p < 0.05$; $^{**}p < 0.01$; $^{***}p < 0.001$.

ment anxiety. In the simple regression analysis, being single accounted for a significant 5.1% of the variability in attachment anxiety, adjusted $R^2 = 0.051$, $F(1, 154) = 9.379$, $p = 0.003$. Examination of the coefficients indicated being single predicted higher attachment anxiety ($B = 3.707$, $SE = 1.210$, $\beta = 0.240$, $p = 0.003$), with 95% confidence the true score is not zero.

The second criteria was also met where being single accounted for a significant 4.7% of the variability in resilience, adjusted $R^2 = 0.047$, $F(1, 154) = 8.652$, $p = 0.004$. Examination of the coefficients indicated that being single predicted lower scores of resilience ($B = -7.400$, $SE = 2.516$, $\beta = -0.231$, $p = 0.004$), with 95% confidence the true score is not zero.

The third criteria was also met where resilience accounted for a significant 8.4% of variability in attachment anxiety, adjusted $R^2 = 0.084$, $F(1, 154) = 15.291$, $p < 0.001$. Examination of the coefficients indicated that lower resilience predicted higher attachment anxiety, ($B = -0.145$, $SE = 0.037$, $\beta = -0.301$, $p < 0.001$), with 95% confidence the true score is not zero.

In addition, a hierarchical multiple regression analysis was conducted to determine if the fourth criteria stated by Baron and Kenny (1986) [24] was satisfied. As can be seen in **Figure 1**, the standardised regression coefficient between being single and attachment anxiety decreased when resilience was added to the model (a shift of $\beta = 0.240$ to $\beta = 0.180$). Resilience was found to reduce the significance of the standardised regression coefficient between being single and attachment anxiety (a shift of $p = 0.003$ to $p = 0.022$), indicating a full mediation of being single by mindfulness in prediction of attachment anxiety. **Figure 1** shows the mediating relationship of resilience between being single and attachment anxiety. As the addition of resilience weakened the strength of the predictive relationship between being single and attachment anxiety, a Sobel test [25], was conducted to determine whether this observed change was significant. This analysis showed the change in the predictive value of being single was significant. $Z = 2.35$, $p = 0.01$, indicating that the relationship between being single and attachment anxiety was mediated by resilience.

5. Discussion

The purpose of the current study was to investigate the relationship between adult attachment, relationship status, anxiety, mindfulness, and resilience in romantic relationships. In particular, this study aimed to determine whether relationship status, anxiety, mindfulness, and resilience significantly predicted scores of attachment anxiety and avoidance as measured by the ECR-S. The results indicated that the 12-item Experiences in Close Relationship Scale—Short Form [12] provided a reliable and valid measure of adult attachment within romantic relationships. To the researchers knowledge this is the first study to utilise the short form of the original Experiences in Close Relationship Scale [11] since its establishment, and therefore provides replicability and support of the ECR-S within a non-clinical and student population.

The main findings of this study showed that in regards to the first aspect of hypothesis one, which predicted attachment anxiety from relationship status, being single was the only relationship status that significantly predicted attachment anxiety. This is consistent with previous research by Noftle and Shaver (2006) [15] who found that within a sample of single individuals, relationship status was a significant predictor of attachment anxiety, where individuals who were not in a romantic relationship scored significantly higher on attachment anxiety. Furthermore, these findings are also in support of the increased anxiety reported by single individuals [7].

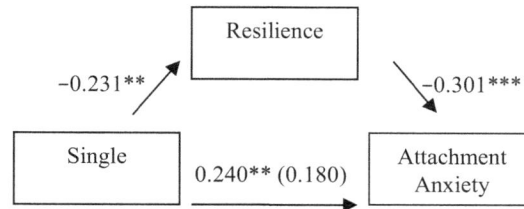

Figure 1. The relationship between being single and attachment anxiety, with resilience as a mediator. Note: Values represent the standardised β weights. β in the parenthesis indicates the changed value after resilience was added to the regression model. $^{*}p < 0.05$, $^{**}p < 0.01$, $^{***}p < 0.001$.

Additionally, resilience was also found to significantly predict attachment anxiety. This relationship supports the research by Caldwell and Shaver (2012) [21] who investigated the resilience-attachment relationship. However, in contrast to resilience, mindfulness was not found to be a significant predictor of attachment anxiety. This finding is inconsistent with research by Barnes *et al.* (2007) [17] that have associated mindfulness to positive relationship functioning.

In regards to attachment avoidance, being single or divorced were both found to be significant predictors, however, this relationship changed to only divorced being significant when the variable of anxiety was added into the regression equation. These findings that individuals who were either single or divorced significantly predicted attachment avoidance were consistent with previous research by Noftle and Shaver (2006) [15].

Mindfulness and resilience were not found to significantly predict attachment avoidance, as the main analyses could not be examined as both mindfulness and resilience did not significantly correlate with attachment avoidance. This was not anticipated as previous research as shown a negative relationship between attachment avoidance and mindfulness [18] and ego-resiliency (Caldwell & Shaver, 2012) [21]. It is possible that this occurred due to different sampling and methodological issues in the present study compared to previous research.

Additionally, anxiety was found to be a significant predictor of attachment avoidance. These results are in support of previous research such as Schachner *et al.* [7], who found that attachment avoidance predicted higher levels of anxiety. Although the current study was interested in whether anxiety predicted attachment avoidance, the results are still in favour of Schachner's and Colleagues anxiety-attachment relationship.

Finally, the results showed that resilience fully mediated the relationship between being single and attachment anxiety. As previously mentioned, the standardised regression coefficient between being single and attachment anxiety decreased when resilience was added into the model. Additionally, resilience was found to reduce the significance of the standardised regression coefficient between being single and attachment anxiety. These results suggest that although individuals who are single are predictive of attachment anxiety, if they also possess high levels of resilience, then this in turn can decrease their levels of attachment anxiety. This is a substantially important contribution to the field of adult attachment, considering that single individuals tend to report increased, depression, anxiety, and sexual displeasure [7]. To the researchers knowledge this is the first study to investigate whether resilience significantly mediates the relationship between being single and attachment anxiety. Therefore, the obtained results provide promising preliminary findings for future research on adult attachment, relationship status, and resilience.

A limitation must be considered when interpreting the results of this study. It is possible that the "single" category did not only include individuals who were single but also those who were "single again" as a result of separation, divorce, or widowhood. It is therefore likely that participants who classified themselves as "single" were in fact not true members of the single category. This is important to address for future research on romantic attachments, as experiences of individuals who have always been single may differ from those who find themselves single again after previously being married or in a long-term committed relationship.

The results obtained in this study further expand upon previous literature within adult attachment, in addition to establishing a platform for future research focusing on adult attachment and resilience. Not only has the current study highlighted the importance of investigating the different types of relationship status (single, defacto, married, separated, and divorced) in regards to adult attachment, but the findings also provide preliminary support for the significant predictive value of resilience in regards to attachment anxiety. As such, this study raised awareness and created dialogue of a promising arena of adult attachment that has very minimal research currently available. As resilience was found to be a significant predictor of attachment anxiety, in conjunction with significantly decreasing the relationship between being single and attachment anxiety, investigating resilience within romantic relationships is therefore a fundamental avenue in need of further research. In particular, an area that may warrant further investigation is the introduction of attachment-based resilience interventions within romantic relationships. Such interventions may address the consequences and issues concerning individuals who experience attachment anxiety, in conjunction with how resilience can enhance the quality of an individual's romantic relationship.

In conclusion, this study established a number of new and important relationships to the field of adult attachment that deserve further attention and replicability in order to fully ascertain the influence of the predictive factors that constitute a successful, healthy, and "loved up" relationship.

References

[1]   Collins, W.A., Welsh, D.P. and Furman, W. (2009) Adolescent Romantic Relationships. *Annual Review of Psychology*, **60**, 631-652. http://dx.doi.org/10.1146/annurev.psych.60.110707.163459

[2]   Mikulincer, B. and Shaver, P.R. (2007) Attachment in Adulthood: Structure, Dynamics, and Change. Guilford Press.

[3]   Plessis, K.D., Clarke, D. and Woolley, C.C. (2007) Secure Attachment Conceptualisations: The Influence of General and Specific Relational Models on Conflict Beliefs and Conflict Resolution Styles. *Interpersona: An International Journal on Personal Relationships*, **1**, 25-44. http://dx.doi.org/10.5964/ijpr.v1i1.3

[4]   Assad, K.K., Donnellan, M.B. and Conger, R.D. (2007) Optimism: An Enduring Resource for Romantic Relationships. *Journal of Personality and Social Psychology*, **93**, 285-297. http://dx.doi.org/10.1037/0022-3514.93.2.285

[5]   Wachs, K. and Cordova, J.V. (2007) Mindful Relating: Exploring Mindfulness and Emotion Repertoires in Intimate Relationships. *Journal of Marital Family Therapy*, **33**, 464-481. http://dx.doi.org/10.1111/j.1752-0606.2007.00032.x

[6]   Amato, P.R. (2000) The Consequences of Divorce for Adults and Children. *Journal of Marriage and Family*, **62**, 1269-1287. http://dx.doi.org/10.1111/j.1741-3737.2000.01269.x

[7]   Schachner, D.A., Shaver, P.R. and Gillath, O. (2008) Attachment Style and Long-Term Singlehood. *Personal Relationships*, **15**, 479-491. http://dx.doi.org/10.1111/j.1475-6811.2008.00211.x

[8]   Bowlby, J. (1973) Attachment and Loss. Basic Books, New York.

[9]   Daniel, S.I. (2006) Adult Attachment Patterns and Individual Psychotherapy: A Review. *Clinical Psychology Review*, **26**, 968-984. http://dx.doi.org/10.1016/j.cpr.2006.02.001

[10]   Bartholomew, K. and Horowitz, L.M. (1991) Attachment Styles among Young Adults: A Test of a Four-Category Model. *Journal of Personality and Social Psychology*, **61**, 226-244. http://dx.doi.org/10.1037/0022-3514.61.2.226

[11]   Brennan, K.A., Clark, C.L. and Shaver, P.R. (1998) Self-Report Measurement of Adult Attachment: An Integrative Overview. In: Simpson, J.A. and Rholes, W.S., Eds., *Attachment Theory and Close Relationships*, Guilford Press, New York, 46-76.

[12]   Wei, M., Russell, D.W., Mallinckrodt, B. and Vogel, D.L. (2007) The Experiences in Close Relationship Scale (ECR) —Short Form: Reliability, Validity, and Factor Structure. *Journal of Personality Assessment*, **88**, 187-204. http://dx.doi.org/10.1080/00223890701268041

[13]   Adamczyk, K. and Bookwala, J. (2013) Adult Attachment and Single vs. Partnered Relationship Status in Polish University Students. *Psychological Topics*, **22**, 481-500. Retrieved from Adult Attachment and Single vs. Partnered Relationship Status in Polish University Students—ProQuest.

[14]   Collins, N.L. and Read, S.J. (1990) Adult Attachment, Working Models, and Relationship Quality in Dating Couples. *Journal of Personality and Social Psychology*, **58**, 644-663. http://dx.doi.org/10.1037/0022-3514.58.4.644

[15]   Noftle and Shaver (2006).

[16]   Whisman, M.A. (2007) Marital Distress and DSM-IV Psychiatric Disorders in a Population-Based National Survey. *Journal of Abnormal Psychology*, **116**, 638-643. http://dx.doi.org/10.1037/0021-843X.116.3.638

[17]   Barnes Brown, Krusemark, Campbell and Roggee (2007).

[18]   Leigh, J. and Anderson, V.N. (2013) Secure Attachment and Autonomy Orientation May Foster Mindfulness. *Contemporary Buddhism: An Interdisciplinary Journal*, **14**, 265-283. http://dx.doi.org/10.1080/14639947.2013.832082

[19]   Baer, R.A., Smith, G.T., Hopkins, J., Krietemeyer, J. and Toney, L. (2006) Using Self-Report Assessment Methods to Explore Facets of Mindfulness. *Assessment*, **13**, 27-45. http://dx.doi.org/10.1177/1073191105283504

[20]   Walach, H., Buchheld, N., Buttenmuller, V., Kleinknecht, N. and Schmidt, S. (2006) Measuring Mindfulness—The

Freiburg Mindfulness Inventory (FMI). *Personality and Individual Differences*, **40**, 1543-1555. http://dx.doi.org/10.1016/j.paid.2005.11.025

[21] Caldwell and Shaver (2012).

[22] Connor, K.M. and Davidson, J.R. (2003) Development of a New Resilience Scale: The Connor-Davidson Resilience Scale (CD-RISC). *Depression and Anxiety*, **18**, 76-82. http://dx.doi.org/10.1002/da.10113

[23] Cohen, J. (1998) Statistical Power Analysis for the Behavioural Sciences. Lawrence Erlbaum Associates, Hillsdale.

[24] Baron and Kenny (1986).

[25] Sobel, M.E. (1982) Asymptotic Confidence Intervals for Indirect Effects in Structural Equation Models. In: Leinhardt, S., Ed., *Sociological Methodology*, American Sociological Association, Washington DC, 290-312.

9

The Cost-Effectiveness of Short-Term Psychodynamic Psychotherapy and Solution-Focused Therapy in the Treatment of Depressive and Anxiety Disorders during a Three-Year Follow-Up

Timo Maljanen[1], Tommi Härkänen[2], Esa Virtala[2], Olavi Lindfors[2], Päivi Tillman[1], Paul Knekt[2,3]

[1]Social Insurance Institution, Helsinki, Finland
[2]National Institute for Health and Welfare, Helsinki, Finland
[3]Biomedicum Helsinki, Helsinki, Finland
Email: timo.maljanen@kela.fi

Abstract

Background: Various psychotherapies are used extensively in treating different mental disorders, but still relatively little is known about the long-term health and cost effects of different therapies. The aim of this study is to compare the cost-effectiveness of short-term psychodynamic psychotherapy (SPP) and solution-focused therapy (SFT) in the treatment of depressive and anxiety disorders during a three-year follow-up. Methods: A total of 198 outpatients suffering from mood or anxiety disorder were randomized to SPP or SFT. Symptoms were assessed using the Beck Depression Inventory, the Hamilton Depression Rating Scale, the Symptom Check List Anxiety Scale, the Hamilton Anxiety Rating Scale, and the Symptom Check List Global Severity Index. Both direct and indirect costs due to mental health problems were measured. Results: The symptoms of depression and anxiety were reduced statistically significantly according to all 5 psychiatric outcome measures during the first 7 months, after which only minor changes were observed. The differences between the two groups were small and not statistically significant. The direct costs were about equal in both groups but the indirect costs were somewhat higher in the SPP group, although not statistically significantly. The costs of auxiliary treatments were much higher than the cost of SPP or SFT. Conclusions: With regard to cost-effectiveness, there is little difference between SPP and SFT.

Keywords

Depression, Anxiety, Psychotherapy, Cost Analysis

1. Introduction

Numerous studies have demonstrated that short-term psychotherapies are effective in the treatment of mood and anxiety disorders, and in meta-analyses no significant differences in the effectiveness of different types of short-term psychotherapies have been observed [1] [2]. However, as mood and anxiety disorders are frequently recurrent, the results of these studies must be interpreted with some caution, for the follow-up periods have in most studies been relatively short. Besides that, more attention should have been paid to monitoring the use of auxiliary psychiatric treatments, which may have a crucial effect both on symptoms and costs, especially in the long run [3]. The effects of auxiliary treatments are usually taken into account in economic evaluations, but although the need for economic evaluations of psychotherapies has been recognized for years, the number of such evaluations has remained modest, and especially studies with longer follow-up periods are rare. In addition to the paucity of existing research, cost-effectiveness comparisons are complicated by the fact that there is remarkable heterogeneity in the study designs due to differences in control treatments, patient inclusion criteria and outcome measures, for example. Before any firm conclusions about the cost-effectiveness of different therapies can be made, more information is needed about the costs and effects of different therapies. The aim of this study is to enlarge our knowledge in this respect by producing a comprehensive view of the various direct and indirect costs arising when patients have been treated either with short-term psychodynamic psychotherapy (SPP) or solution-focused therapy (SFT), as well as to assess changes in symptoms utilizing several health outcome indicators during a 3-year follow-up period. The cost-effectiveness of short-term therapies has been evaluated in a handful of studies [4] [5], but to our knowledge this is the first cost-effectiveness study where these two therapies are compared over a follow-up period covering several years.

2. Population and Methods

This cost-effectiveness study is a part of the Helsinki Psychotherapy Study [6]. The study follows the Helsinki Declaration and was approved by Helsinki University Central Hospital's ethics council. Patients gave written informed consent at the beginning of the study. The study population and methods used in the study are summarized only briefly here as they have been described in detail elsewhere [3] [6]-[8].

2.1. Patients and Settings

A total of 459 eligible and willing outpatients from the Helsinki region were referred for the Helsinki Psychotherapy Study from 1994 to 2000. Eligible patients were 20 - 45 years of age and had a longstanding (>1 year) disorder causing work dysfunction. The patients had to meet DSM-IV criteria [9] for anxiety or mood disorders. For the criteria of exclusion, see Knekt *et al.* [6]. Of the eligible patients, 133 refused to participate, and the remaining 326 patients were randomly assigned to short-term psychodynamic psychotherapy (SPP) (101 patients), solution-focused therapy (SFT) (97 patients), and long-term psychodynamic psychotherapy (LPP) (128 patients). The LPP group was not included in this study because the three-year follow-up was deemed to be too short to cover the long-run effects of LPP, *i.e.*, how symptoms and costs develop after the end of therapy. After assignment to treatment groups 3 SPP patients and 4 SFT patients refused to participate. Of the patients starting the assigned therapy, 21 (10 assigned to SPP and 11 to SFT) discontinued the treatment prematurely.

2.2. Treatments

2.2.1. Therapies

SPP is a brief, focal, transference based therapeutic approach which helps patients by exploring and working through specific intrapsychic and interpersonal conflicts. It is based on approaches described by Malan [10] and Sifneos [11]. SPP was scheduled for 20 treatment sessions, each lasting about 45 minutes with a frequency of one session per week. The SPP sessions were carried out, on average, over a period of 5.7 months (SD = 1.3).

SFT is a brief, resource oriented, goal focused therapeutic approach which helps clients change by constructing solutions [12]. It is based on an approach developed by de Shazer *et al*. [13]. The frequency of SFT sessions was flexible, usually one 60 to 90 minute session every two or three weeks for a maximum of up to 12 sessions over no more than 8 months. The mean duration of SFT was 7.5 months (SD = 3.0).

2.2.2. Therapists
SPP was provided by 12 therapists and SFT by 6 therapists. All therapists had received standard training in their respective forms of therapy. The mean number of years of experience in the therapy provided was 9 for both therapy forms. SPP was conducted in accordance with clinical practice, where the therapists might modify their interventions according to the patient's needs within the respective framework. None of the SPP therapists had received any training in SFT and vice versa. SFT was manualized and adherence monitoring was performed.

2.3. Assessment

2.3.1. Effectiveness
Effectiveness was measured by changes in psychiatric symptoms. Symptoms of depression were assessed with the Beck Depression Inventory (BDI) [14] and the Hamilton Depression Rating Scale (HDRS) [15]. Symptoms of anxiety were assessed with the Symptom Check List Anxiety Scale (SCL-90-ANX) [16] and the Hamilton Anxiety Rating Scale (HARS) [17]. Overall psychological distress was measured using the Symptom Check List Global Severity Index (SCL-90-GSI) [16]. Assessments based on self-administered questionnaires (BDI, SCL-90-ANX and SCL-90-GSI) were carried out at baseline and at 3, 7, 9, 12, 18, 24, and 36 months after baseline, while assessments based on interviews (HDRS and HARS) were performed at baseline and at follow-up points of 7, 12 and 36 months.

2.3.2. Costs
Altogether four different total cost components were estimated in this study. The most important of the four were the direct costs due to the treatment of mental disorders, which included costs accruing from 1) protocol-based and additional SPP and SFT sessions, 2) other psychotherapy sessions, 3) outpatient visits due to mental disorders, 4) psychotropic medication (prescription-only medicines), 5) inpatient care due to mental disorders, and 6) travel costs due to therapy visits. The indirect costs caused by mental disorders included 1) the value of lost productivity due to absenteeism from work because of psychiatric problems or 2) therapy visits, 3) the value of household work neglected because of psychiatric problems, 4) the value of leisure time lost due to therapy visits, and 5) the value of unpaid help received because of mental disorders. Direct costs due to non-mental disorders consisted of the cost of treatments (outpatient visits, inpatient care, and prescription-only medicines) for somatic disorders. Indirect costs due to non-mental disorders consisted of the value of lost productivity due to absenteeism from work and the value of household work neglected because of somatic problems.

Part of the cost data was readily available in monetary terms from patient registers covering all patients. Most of the cost items were estimated by multiplying the amount of services used by the corresponding unit costs. Information about the amounts of different services used was obtained either from patient level registers or from the patients themselves in five inquiries, which covered 0 - 7, 8 - 12, 13 - 18, 19 - 24 and 25 - 36 months' periods from the start of the therapy. All costs were included in the analysis in full regardless of the payer. All costs were converted to the 2010 price level by using official price indices. The costs were discounted by using a three percent yearly discount rate. Details of estimation of costs are described in Maljanen *et al*. [8].

2.3.3. Potential Confounding Factors
At baseline, demographic characteristics (age, sex, marital status, and education) and previous psychiatric treatments (medication, psychotherapy and hospitalization) were assessed by questionnaire, and suitability for psychotherapy [18], as well as factors related to psychiatric history (age at onset of first psychiatric disorder, childhood separation experiences), by interview.

2.4. Statistical Methods

2.4.1. Effectiveness
The effectiveness of the two therapies was studied in a design with repeated measurements of the outcome vari-

ables as "intention-to-treat" (ITT) analyses [6] [19]. The primary analyses were based on the assumption of ignorable dropouts, and in secondary analyses missing values were replaced by multiple imputation (MI) [20] [21]. The statistical analyses were based on linear mixed models, model-adjusted means and mean differences calculated using predictive margins [22] [23]. See Maljanen *et al.* for details [8].

The regression model for the effectiveness outcome assessed by repeated measurements included the main effects of time, treatment group, difference between theoretical and realized date of measurement, and first order interaction of time and treatment group [6]. Adjustment for the potential confounders was not found necessary.

2.4.2. Costs

The analyses of costs were based on comparisons of the arithmetic means of different cumulative cost items. Our earlier study [8] as well as many other studies have shown that due to the extremely high costs of some patients the distributions of cost variables are very skewed, and therefore the statistical analyses were performed using a non-parametric bootstrap approach [24]. In the cost analyses some of the missing values of cost variables were imputed using single-value imputation [8]. Potential confounding factors were not found in case of the cost outcomes, and thus the treatment group was the sole covariate in the model.

2.4.3. Cost-Effectiveness

The cost-effectiveness of the therapies was compared with the incremental cost-effectiveness ratio (ICER) [25], which is the difference in the mean costs of the two therapies divided by the difference of their mean effectiveness, *i.e.* $\left(\overline{C}_{SPP} - \overline{C}_{SFT} \right) / \left(\overline{E}_{SPP} - \overline{E}_{SFT} \right)$, where $\overline{C}_{SPP}$ stands for the mean costs and $\overline{E}_{SPP}$ for the mean effectiveness of SPP, and $\overline{C}_{SFT}$ and $\overline{E}_{SFT}$ respectively for SFT.

The effectiveness of the therapies was estimated by calculating the changes taken place in BDI, HDRS, SCL-90-ANX, HARS and SCL-90-GSI during the three-year follow-up period. The calculation was based on the area under the curve (AUC), a frequently used tool in clinical trials with repeated measurements, which is the mean value of the clinical indicator during the follow-up period [26]. Changes in symptoms over the whole three-year follow-up period were estimated by subtracting the AUC value of each psychiatric measure from the baseline value of that measure. These estimates of the overall symptom changes are marked with the symbol B-AUC. The confidence intervals of differences in average costs and the ICERs were calculated using the bootstrap method [24] [27]. Both effectiveness and costs were discounted by using a three percent yearly discount rate.

The principles used in calculating ICERs were the same as those used in our earlier study with a one-year follow-up period [8]. As these methods have been described in detail in an earlier article, only the main points are taken up here.

In the cost-effectiveness analyses, missing data were handled with MI. The effect of missing data was assessed using multi-dimensional sensitivity analyses [28]. The proportion of missing AUC values, and hence also that of missing B-AUC values, was larger (23% - 42%) than the proportion of missing health outcome values of the single measurement points, because a missing value at any of the measurement points of a patient causes a missing value in the AUC value of such a patient.

The results of the cost-effectiveness analyses are presented using cost-effectiveness planes with bootstrap iterations. Depending on how the iteration points are spread out across the four quadrants one is able to draw conclusions about the uncertainty associated with the cost-effectiveness results.

2.4.4. Sensitivity Analysis

In the sensitivity analyses different methods of handling the problem of missing observations were utilized [29]. Due to the uncertainties associated with different imputation methods, analyses based solely on non-missing observations were also performed. Also unit costs whose values were uncertain were changed to test the robustness of the results of the basic analyses.

All statistical analyses were performed using SAS software version 9.2 [30].

3. Results

3.1. Baseline Characteristics

The majority of the patients were females in their thirties who were employed or students and suffering from mood disorders (**Table 1**). Relatively few had received psychiatric treatment despite the fact that more than half

Table 1. Baseline characteristics of the 198 patients intended to treat by treatment group.

Characteristic	Treatment group	
	Short-term psychodynamic Psychotherapy [n = 101]	Solution-focused Therapy [n = 97]
Socioeconomic variables		
Age (years)	32.1 (7.0)[a]	33.6 (7.2)[a]
Males (%)	25.7	25.8
Full time employed or student (%)	61.4	65.2
Living alone (%)	48.5	56.7
University degree (%)	19.8	28.9
Psychiatric background		
Primary psychiatric disorder at age < 22 years (%)	57.6	66.0
Recurrent episodes of major depressive disorder (%)	68.3	60.0
Duration of disorder over 5 years (%)	33.0	36.5
Attempted suicide (SSI) (%)	7.1	9.4
Previous psychiatric treatment		
Psychotherapy (%)	18.8	20.0
Psychotropic medication (%)	21.8	27.8
Hospitalization (%)	0.0	2.1
Psychiatric diagnosis		
Mood disorder (%)	78.2	86.6
Anxiety disorder (%)	49.5	46.4
Personality disorder (%)	24.8	18.6
Psychiatric co-morbidity (%)	48.5	45.4

[a]Mean (SD).

had experienced recurrent episodes of major depression and a relatively early onset of psychiatric disorder. There were no statistically significant differences between the treatment groups with respect to demographic characteristics or the patients' baseline clinical status.

3.2. Effectiveness

During the period when the patients were receiving study therapy, *i.e.*, during the first 7 months of the follow-up, the scores of the two outcome measures assessing the symptoms of depression (BDI and HDRS) as well as the scores of the two outcome measures assessing the symptoms of anxiety (SCL-90-ANX and HARS) declined statistically significantly in both therapy groups (**Table 2**). A very similar development was observed in the overall psychological distress measured by SCL-90-GSI (data not shown). From there to the end of the three-year follow-up period the mean scores of all symptom indicators remained quite stable in both groups. There were no statistically significant differences between the therapy groups at any point of the follow-up for any of the outcome measures. Hence also the differences in the overall symptom changes (B-AUC values) were small and not statistically significant.

3.3. Costs

After the single-value imputation of missing cost values, the share of non-missing observations varied, depending on the service used, from 75% (cost of psychiatric outpatient care in the SFT group) to 100% (costs of study therapy visits and psychotropic medication in both groups). Complete cost data, *i.e.*, information about all cost items at every measurement point, were obtained from 79 SPP patients (78%) and from 72 SFT patients (74%). The mean total direct costs of patients with complete cost data were 4867 euros in the SPP group, being only marginally higher (by 29 euros, or 0.6%) than the costs in the SFT group (**Table 3**). If the total direct costs are

Table 2. Mean health outcome scores (s.e.) and mean score differences (95% confidence interval) between treatment groups by follow-up: ITT, Model 1.

Outcome variable	Time (months)	Mean scores[a] (s.e.)					
		Short-term psychodynamic Psychotherapy [n = 101]		Solution-focused therapy [n = 97]		Mean score difference[b] (95% confidence interval)	
BDI	0	17.9	(0.79)	18.2	(0.81)	0.0	
	3	12.8[*]	(0.84)	12.4[*]	(0.89)	+0.7	(−1.3, +2.8)
	7	10.3[*]	(0.88)	10.4[*]	(0.90)	+0.2	(−2.0, +2.5)
	9	9.6	(0.88)	10.7	(0.92)	−0.8	(−3.1, +1.5)
	12	9.6	(0.97)	10.6	(1.02)	−0.7	(−3.2, +1.9)
	18	8.7	(0.99)	10.1	(1.05)	−1.0	(−3.7, +1.8)
	24	9.5	(1.03)	10.0	(1.14)	−0.1	(−3.0, +2.8)
	36	10.3	(0.95)	9.8	(1.03)	−0.9	(−1.8, +3.5)
	Total change B-AUC[c] (= Baseline-AUC)	8.0		7.7		0.3	(−2.3, +2.6)
SCL-ANX-90	0	1.26	(0.07)	1.27	(0.07)	0.00	
	3	1.02[*]	(0.07)	1.03[*]	(0.07)	−0.01	(−0.16, +0.15)
	7	0.86[*]	(0.08)	0.94	(0.08)	−0.07	(−0.26, +0.12)
	9	0.82	(0.07)	0.87	(0.08)	−0.04	(−0.21, +0.14)
	12	0.82	(0.07)	0.90	(0.08)	−0.07	(−0.25, +0.11)
	18	0.74	(0.07)	0.86	(0.07)	−0.10	(−0.29, +0.09)
	24	0.83	(0.08)	0.94	(0.09)	−0.09	(−0.29, +0.12)
	36	0.82	(0.07)	0.82	(0.017)	+0.01	(−0.19, +0.21)
	Total change B-AUC[c] (= Baseline-AUC)	0.43		0.38		0.06	(−0.12, +0.23)
HDRS	0	15.4	(0.48)	15.8	(0.49)	0.0	
	7	10.7[*]	(0.60)	11.3[*]	(0.61)	−0.4	(−2.0, +1.1)
	12	10.5	(0.65)	11.4	(0.68)	−0.7	(−2.5, +1.0)
	36	10.8	(0.62)	10.7	(0.66)	+0.1	(−1.6, +1.9)
	Total change B-AUC[c] (= Baseline-AUC)	4.7		4.7		0.1	(−1.5, +1.6)
HARS	0	15.0	(0.52)	14.9	(0.53)	0.0	
	7	10.2[*]	(0.56)	10.8[*]	(0.57)	−0.5	(−2.0, +0.9)
	12	9.8	(0.59)	10.7	(0.62)	−0.9	(−2.5, +0.7)
	36	9.6	(0.55)	10.2	(0.59)	−0.7	(−2.2, +0.9)
	Total change B-AUC[c] (= Baseline-AUC)	5.1		4.4		0.7	(−0.8, +2.3)

[a]Basic model. [b]Basic model adjusted for the baseline level of the outcome measure considered. [c]According to 500 bootstrap iterations. [*]A statistically significant improvement from previous measurement point.

calculated by summing up the mean costs of the different cost items shown in **Table 3** the difference between the two groups turns out to be somewhat greater, with the total costs of the SPP group increasing to 5795 euros and the costs of the SFT group to 5306 euros. This difference was due to the fact that the patients in the SPP group used various auxiliary health care services more than or at least as much as the patients in the SFT group. During the three-year follow-up period the costs of all auxiliary health care services were in both groups much higher than the costs of study therapy: 247% and 98% higher, respectively, in the SPP and SFT groups. An overwhelming majority of patients in both groups, 83% in the SPP group and 82% in the SFT group, received some auxiliary treatments for their symptoms during the three-year follow-up period.

The largest cost item in both groups was auxiliary psychotherapy, which accounted for nearly 50% of all di-

Table 3. Direct costs (euros) and resource use (in cursive and in parentheses) due to mental disorders in short-term psychodynamic psychotherapy and solution-focused therapy group during the three-year follow-up period: Analysis based on non-missing observations of the single-value imputation data [n = number of patients with data at every measurement point].

Resource	Short-term psychodynamic Psychotherapy (SPP)		Solution-focused Therapy (SFT)		Difference of means (SPP-SFT)	95% confidence intervals for mean cost differences[a]
	Mean	10% - 90% quantiles (max)	Mean	10% - 90% quantiles (max)		
Study therapy	1297	920 - 1644 (1874)	1779	564 - 2255 (2818)	−482	−652, −323
(*number of visits*)		(18.0) [n=101]		(9.4) [n = 97]		
Other psychotherapy	2790	0 - 11 972 (28 723)	2448	0 - 8447 (36 621)	+342	−792, +1762
(*number of visits*)		(32.9) [n = 98]		(28.1) [n = 89]		
Psychiatric outpatient care[b]	873	0 - 2339 (9639)	598	0 - 1838 (6968)	+275	−88, +573
(*number of visits*)		(8.8) [n = 80]		(5.6) [n = 73]		
Psychotropic medication	368	0 - 1090 (3540)	373	0 - 1405 (4228)	−5	−193, +182
(*number of psychotropic medication days*)		(270.8) [n = 101]		(297.4) [n = 97]		
Psychiatric hospitalisation	368	0 - 0 (20 995)	0	0 - 0 (0)	+368	+32, +920
(*number of hospital days*)		(1.5) [n = 99]		(0) [n = 96]		
Travel to psychotherapy[c]	99	0 - 290 (803)	108	0 - 237 (3652)	−9	−104, +61
		[n = 97]		[n = 89]		
Total direct costs[d]	**4867**	1268 - 13,559 (30,937)	**4838**	1800 - 11,238 (21,982)	**+29**	−1344, +1213
		[n = 79]		[n = 72]		

[a]According to 500 bootstrap iterations. [b]Health centre, occupational health care, mental health clinic, hospital outpatient clinic, private physician, etc. [c]Information about the number of psychotherapy visits resulting in travel costs is not available. [d]Total direct costs or the difference in total direct costs do not equal the sum of individual cost items because due to the varying number of missing observations the mean calculations of total costs and different cost items are partly based on different sets of patient data.

rect costs in both groups. The relatively high cost of other psychotherapy was explained by the fact that in both therapy groups there were some patients who had had numerous psychotherapy sessions not included in the study protocol.

In both groups the mean direct costs were highest at the beginning of the three-year follow-up period when patients were receiving study therapy. In the first year of the follow-up the mean costs of patients in the SFT group were higher than the mean costs of the SPP group because SFT itself cost more than SPP. During the first year the costs showed a steep declining trend in both groups, the reason being that the number of patients receiving study therapy continued to diminish. In the last two years of the follow-up the mean costs showed a growing trend in both therapy groups and, unlike in the first year, the costs of the SPP group were consistently higher (**Figure 1**).

The mean indirect costs due to mental disorders were, like the direct costs, higher in the SPP group (**Table 4**). The reasons for this cost difference of 4128 euros was that both the value of lost productivity due to absenteeism from work because of sickness and the value of unpaid help received because of mental health problems were clearly higher in the SPP group. The share of these two cost items of all indirect costs was about 80% in the SPP group and 70% in the SFT group. Also the value of lost leisure time due to therapy visits and the value of neglected household work were considerable. No statistically significant differences between the two groups were observed in any cost item. It is worth noticing that the indirect costs were in both groups higher than the direct costs.

During the three-year follow-up, mean direct costs due to non-mental disorders were about the same in both groups: 1838 euros in the SPP group and 1570 euros in the SFT group. This difference was not statistically significant. In both therapy groups nearly 80% of these costs were caused by outpatient visits to physicians. Also the mean indirect costs due to non-mental disorders were similar in the two therapy groups: 3957 euros in the SPP group and 4066 euros in the SFT group. In both groups the indirect costs were mainly due to lost productivity.

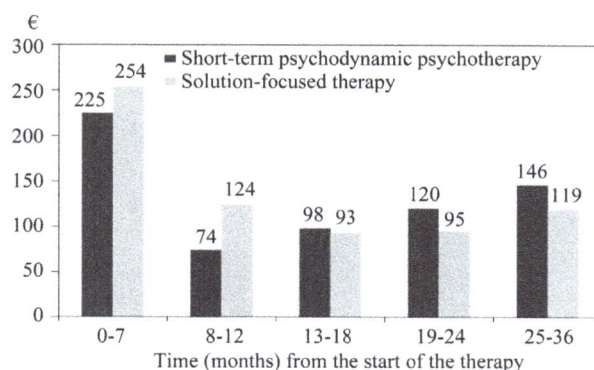

Figure 1. The mean monthly direct costs (euros) due to mental disorders in short-term psychodynamic psychotherapy and solution-focused therapy group during the three-year follow-up period.

Table 4. Indirect costs (euros) due to mental disorders in short-term psychodynamic psychotherapy and solution-focused therapy group during the three-year follow-up period: Analysis based on non-missing observations of the single-value imputation data [n = number of patients with data at every measurement point].

Resource	Short-term psychodynamic Psychotherapy (SPP)		Solution-focused Therapy (SFT)		Difference of means (SPP-SFT)	95% confidence intervals for mean cost differences[a]
	Mean	10% - 90% quantiles (max)	Mean	10% - 90% quantiles (max)		
Productivity lost due to sickness	6132	0 - 10 955 (118 459) [n = 73]	3526	0 - 8184 (39 173) [n = 61]	+2606	−846, +6220
Productivity lost due to therapy visits	31	0 - 0 (799) [n = 98]	61	0 - 270 (1162) [n = 84]	−30	−74, +16
Neglected household work due to sickness	850	0 - 1899 (13 163) [n = 65]	1148	0 - 2855 (13 242) [n = 55]	−298	−724, +460
Leisure time lost due to therapy visits	967	246 - 3007 (7920) [n = 98]	674	60 - 1729 (6667) [n = 89]	+293	−56, +593
Informal help	1700	0 - 0 (59 191) [n = 63]	959	0 - 4679 (9085) [n = 57]	+741	−525, +1985
Total indirect costs[b]	**10 525**	358 - 35,799 (122,546) [n = 59]	**6397**	179 - 17,087 (53,679) [n = 54]	**+4128**	−1420, +6602

[a]According to 500 bootstrap iterations. [b]Total indirect costs or the difference in total indirect costs do not equal the sum of individual cost items because due to the varying number of missing observations the mean calculations of total costs and different cost items are partly based on different sets of patient data.

3.4. Cost-Effectiveness

According to all five health outcome indicators the effectiveness of SPP seemed to be slightly better than that of SFT. The differences were, however, very small and as a result of this there is a lot of uncertainty in the ICERs. Due to this considerable uncertainty no point estimates or confidence intervals for this ratio were calculated. Instead, uncertainty associated with our results was analysed by running 500 ICER bootstrap iterations for each of the four health outcome measures assessing symptoms of depression or anxiety and direct costs (**Figure 2**). Because the cost outcome of these four analyses was the same, the locations of the iteration points with respect to the horizontal line were the same in all four **Figures 2(a)-(d)** excluding the variation caused by bootstrap iterations and imputation of missing values. Regardless of the outcome measure studied the iteration points are concentrated heavily around the origin and spread quite evenly among all four quadrants. Thus this cost-effective-

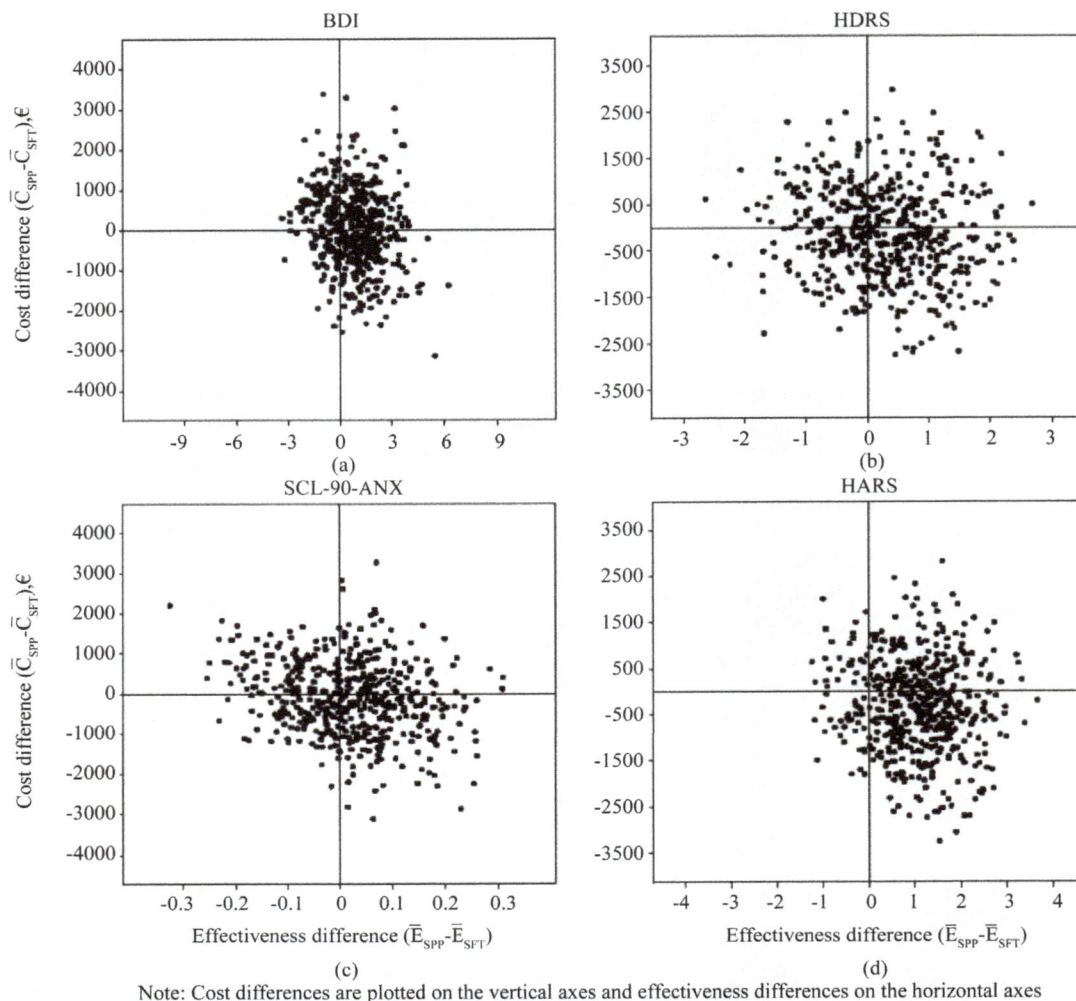

Figure 2. The incremental cost-effectiveness planes with 500 bootstrap iterations comparing short-term psychodynamic psychotherapy and solution-focused therapy: direct costs due to mental disorders as cost variable and BDI, HDRS, SCL-90-ANX and HARS as effectiveness variable.

ness analysis confirms our earlier findings that the differences between SPP and SFT are small both in terms of effectiveness and costs.

3.5. Sensitivity Analysis

In the sensitivity analyses we tested different imputation methods and changed the unit cost of those resources whose unit costs were known to be uncertain. The results for effectiveness, measured by all five health outcome measures, remained very similar to the basic results regardless of the imputation methods: during the first seven months the symptoms declined rapidly, but after that there were only small changes in the mean scores and no statistically significant differences between the two therapy groups at any measurement point. This stability of results is explained by the fact that the proportion of missing observations was reasonably small for all effectiveness measures.

With the economic outcome measures, the sensitivity analyses changed the results of the basic analysis more, but, again, the fundamental result remained the same: both direct and indirect costs due to mental disorders were greater in the group having received SPP. The sensitivity analyses changed the basic results mainly in the respect that the aggregate level of costs changed but the relationship between the two groups did not. This observation applies also to the costs arising from non-mental disorders. Independent of unit costs used or imputation method applied the differences in direct and indirect costs due to non-mental disorders were small between the two groups.

4. Discussion

Our study showed that symptoms of depression and anxiety were reduced substantially and by about the same amount in both therapy groups. The results thus confirm earlier findings indicating that both SPP and SFT are effective therapeutic approaches in the treatment of mental disorders [4] [31]. Differences in the direct health care costs due to mental disorders also were relatively small and not statistically significant either. As differences in the effectiveness means were very small the ICERs were extremely unstable and therefore no point estimates or confidence intervals for this ratio were estimated. Cost-effectiveness analysis in combination with the bootstrap method could, however, be used to handle the uncertainty associated with our results. The 500 bootstrap cost-effectiveness iterations made for each of the five health outcome measures supported the finding that SPP and SFT are quite similar with regard to their cost-effectiveness as the iteration points are situated quite evenly around the origin.

During the three-year follow-up period the mean total direct health care costs due to mental disorders were only marginally higher in the SPP group than in the SFT group. This difference was, however, not statistically significant, because the costs of individual patients varied considerably in both therapy groups. This difference in the total costs was due to fact that patients in the SPP group used auxiliary mental health care services more or at least as much as patients in the SFT group. Among the different cost items the greatest differences were, however, observed in the costs of study therapy, which were 482 euros (37%) higher in the SFT group, and this difference was also statistically significant. The reason for the observed difference in the cost of therapy sessions was that the price of one SFT visit was fixed at 188 euros (at 2010 prices) whereas the average price of one SPP visit was 71 euros. The higher price of an SFT visit was explained by the fact that the durations of SFT sessions were longer (1 - 1.5 hours vs. 45 minutes) and SFT therapists could consult with other SFT therapists if they considered it necessary. Both SPP and SFT therapists worked in the private sector, and so the price of a visit can be used as a proxy for the cost of one visit. Thus, although the realized number of study therapy visits by patients in the SPP group was, as planned in the protocol, nearly twice as high (18.0 vs. 9.4) as the number of visits by patients in the SFT group, the therapy costs were still clearly smaller in the SPP group.

An important finding in our study was that in the three-year follow-up period a great majority of patients in both therapy groups needed other treatments besides SPP or SFT for their symptoms. Studies with relatively short follow-up periods, too, have indicated that many patients need other treatments in addition to brief therapy [5] [32]. This study, with a follow-up period of three years, highlights very clearly that the need for additional treatments may be substantial especially in the long run, for the costs of all auxiliary treatments were observed to be much higher than the costs of SPP or SFT. Most of the cost of auxiliary treatments in both groups was due to the costs arising from the use of other psychotherapies received after the end of SPP or SFT. This indicates that in the long run short-term psychotherapies are quite seldom sufficient treatments for persons suffering from mood or anxiety disorders.

The total indirect costs due to mental disorders were in the SPP group as much as 4128 euros (65%) higher than the indirect costs of the SFT group. This great difference was due to the fact that the value of productivity lost and the value of informal help received because of mental disorders were much greater in the SPP group. Indirect costs were in both therapy groups clearly higher than direct costs. The mean indirect costs were, however, even more than the direct costs affected by the very high costs accrued by some individual patients. In the SPP group there were three patients with extremely high indirect costs which were due to productivity loss and informal help. If these patients had been excluded from the analysis, the mean indirect costs of the two therapy groups would have been quite similar.

The mean annual direct costs due to non-mental disorders during the three-year follow-up period were estimated to be 613 euros in the SPP group and 523 euros in the SFT group. This is much less than the corresponding average amount in the general Finnish population of same age (approximately 1100 euros in 2006) [33]. Although one must be very careful when comparing figures from different types of data (as was the case here), the differences in the above figures are so great that our finding does not seem to support the frequently expressed view that persons with depressive or anxiety disorders also have many other health problems and that their health care costs due to non-mental disorders are higher than those of persons without such disorders [34]. Possible explanations for our low estimates may be that the patients had relatively high educational attainment and that patients with severe organic diseases were excluded from our study. One further explanation could be that the reference figures [33] were partly based on registers where a certain share of mental health care expenditures, for instance, might be reported as somatic health care expenditures.

There are certain methodological considerations about our study that need to be addressed as well. First, compared to most clinical psychotherapy studies the sample size of our study (n = 198) can be regarded as relatively large, as sample sizes below 100 are very common [4] [31]. Second, in our study psychiatric symptoms were assessed using five different psychiatric measures which all yielded very similar results. This consistency of results together with the frequently repeated measurements increases the reliability of our results.

Third, the follow-up period of our study, three years, is considerably longer than what is usually the case with psychotherapy studies because in most studies the follow-up period is one year or less. Especially with mental health problems, which are often long-lasting and where relapses are frequent, a one-year follow-up period may be too short to capture the health or economic effects of the treatments compared.

In this study we tried to collect cost information about all the medication used in the treatment of mood and anxiety disorders. Some of the estimates on the direct costs of SPP and SFT can be regarded as highly reliable because part of the cost data was obtained directly from registers containing patient-level information about every patient. Part of the cost data was, however, based on information received from patients and with these cost items there is some uncertainty because of missing observations. In the sensitivity analyses different methods of handling missing observations were used and regardless of the way the missing observations were handled our results remained rather robust.

The missing observations were, however, a bigger problem in the case of indirect costs, as the estimation of indirect costs depended completely on information given by the patients. An additional weakness related to the estimation of indirect costs was that the estimation was partly based on questions to which it may have been difficult to give exact answers (e.g., for how long the respondent has been unable to study due to mental disorders or how much informal help the respondent has received). Also, considerable uncertainty attaches to the methods of valuing different indirect cost items, and there is no unanimity about how the valuation ought to be carried out. Regardless of these problems, the estimation of indirect costs is, however, considered to augment our understanding of the costs related to the treatment of depressive and anxiety disorders, especially because relatively few cost-effectiveness studies in the field of mental health have attempted to estimate indirect cost [35].

To our knowledge, this is the first economic long-term evaluation study comparing the costs and effects of SPP and SFT. According to our results, symptoms of depression and anxiety were reduced to a very similar extent in both therapy groups and there were no significant differences in costs between the two groups. Thus our results suggest that these two therapies are comparable in terms of cost-effectiveness, and this observation was confirmed by bootstrap iterations. More research with extensive data both about the effects and costs of the therapies compared, a sufficiently long follow-up period and rigorous economic evaluation are needed before any definite conclusions about the cost-effectiveness of these therapies, or short-term therapies in general, can be made.

Finding out the most cost-effective treatments for mood and anxiety disorders can be regarded as exceptionally important for the prevalence of these disorders is high, they cause considerable human suffering and lead to remarkable disability resulting in notable indirect costs, and there are various treatment options with probably very different health and cost effects. Thus the benefits to be gained by identifying the most cost-effective treatments for these disorders may be substantial and clearly surpass those obtainable with most other disorders.

Acknowledgements

The Helsinki Psychotherapy Study Group [7] was responsible for collection of the data. Financial support for the study received from: The Academy of Finland (Grant No. 138876) and the Social Insurance Institution of Finland.

References

[1]   Cuijpers, P., van Straten, A., Andersson, G. and van Oppen, P. (2008) Psychotherapy for Depression in Adults: A Meta-Analysis of Comparative Outcome Studies. *Journal of Consulting and Clinical Psychology*, **76**, 909-922.
        http://dx.doi.org/10.1037/a0013075

[2]   Cape, J., Whittington, C., Buszewicz, M., Wallace, P. and Underwood, L. (2010) Brief Psychological Therapies for Anxiety and Depression in Primary Care: Meta-Analysis and Meta-Regression. *BMC Medicine*, **8**, 38. http://dx.doi.org/10.1186/1741-7015-8-38

[3]   Knekt, P., Lindfors, O., Renlund, C., Sares-Jäske, L., Laaksonen, M.A. and Virtala, E. (2011) Use of Auxiliary Psychiatric Treatment during a 5-Year Follow-Up among Patients Receiving Short- or Long-Term Psychotherapy. *Journal of Affective Disorders*, **135**, 221-230. http://dx.doi.org/10.1016/j.jad.2011.07.024

[4]   Abbass, A.A., Hancock, J.T., Henderson, J. and Kisely, S.R. (2006) Short-Term Psychodynamic Psychotherapies for Common Mental Disorders. *Cochrane Database of Systematic Reviews*, Issue 4.

[5]   Bosmans, J., Schreuders, B., van Marwijk, H., Smit, J., van Oppen, P. and van Tulder, M. (2012) Cost-Effectiveness of Problem-Solving Treatment in Comparison with Usual Care for Primary Care Patients with Mental Health Problems: ARandomized Trial. *BMC Family Practice*, **13**, 98. http://dx.doi.org/10.1186/1471-2296-13-98

[6]   Knekt, P., Lindfors, O., Härkänen, T., Välikoski, M., Virtala, E., Laaksonen, M.A., Marttunen, M., Kaipainen, M., Renlund, C. and the Helsinki Psychotherapy Study·Group (2008) Randomized Trial on the Effectiveness of Long- and Short-Term Psychodynamic Psychotherapy and Solution-Focused Therapy on Psychiatric Symptoms during a 3-Year Follow-Up. *Psychological Medicine*, **38**, 689-703. http://dx.doi.org/10.1017/S003329170700164X

[7]   Knekt, P. and Lindfors, O. (2004) A Randomized Trial of the Effect of Four Forms of Psychotherapy on Depressive and Anxiety Disorders: Design, Methods, and Results on the Effectiveness of Short-Term Psychodynamic Psychotherapy and Solution-Focused Therapy during a One-Year Follow-Up. Social Insurance Institution, Helsinki, 15-112. http://www.ktl.fi/tto/hps/pdf/effectiveness.pdf.

[8]   Maljanen, T., Paltta, P., Härkänen, T., Virtala, E., Lindfors, O., Laaksonen, M.A., Knekt, P. and the Helsinki Psychotherapy Study Group (2012) The Cost-Effectiveness of Short-Term Psychodynamic Psychotherapy and Solution-Focused Therapy in the Treatment of Depressive and Anxiety Disorders during a One-Year Follow-Up. *Journal of Mental Health Policy and Economics*, **15**, 13-23.

[9]   American Psychiatric Association (1994) Diagnostic and Statistical Manual of Mental Disorders: DSM-IV. American Psychiatric Association, Washington DC.

[10] Malan, D.H. (1976) The Frontier of Brief Psychotherapy: An Example of the Convergence of Research and Clinical Practice. Plenum Medical Books, New York. http://dx.doi.org/10.1007/978-1-4684-2220-7

[11] Sifneos, P.E. (1978) Short-Term Anxiety Provoking Psychotherapy. In: Davanloo, H., Ed., *Short-Term Dynamic Psychotherapy*, Spectrum, New York, 35-42.

[12] Johnson, L.D. and Miller, S.D. (1994) Modification of Depression Risk Factors: A Solution-Focused Approach. *Psychotherapy: Theory, Research, Practice, Training*, **31**, 244-253. http://dx.doi.org/10.1037/h0090220

[13] deShazer, S., Berg, I.K., Lipchik, E., Nunnally, E., Molnar, A., Gingerich, W. and Weiner-Davies, M. (1986) Brief Therapy: Focused Solution Development. *Family Process*, **25**, 207-221. http://dx.doi.org/10.1111/j.1545-5300.1986.00207.x

[14] Beck, A.T., Ward, C.H., Mendelson, M., Mock, J. and Erbaugh, J. (1961) An Inventory for Measuring Depression. *Archives of General Psychiatry*, **4**, 561-571. http://dx.doi.org/10.1001/archpsyc.1961.01710120031004

[15] Hamilton, M. (1960) A Rating Scale for Depression. *Journal of Neurology, Neurosurgery and Psychiatry*, **23**, 56-61. http://dx.doi.org/10.1136/jnnp.23.1.56

[16] Derogatis, L.R., Lipman, R.S. and Covi, L. (1973) SCL-90: An Outpatient Psychiatric Rating Scale—Preliminary Report. *Psychopharmacology Bulletin*, **9**, 13-28.

[17] Hamilton, M. (1959) The Assessment of Anxiety States by Rating. *British Journal of Medical Psychology*, **32**, 50-55. http://dx.doi.org/10.1111/j.2044-8341.1959.tb00467.x

[18] Laaksonen, M.A., Lindfors, O., Knekt, P. and Aalberg, V. (2012) Suitability for Psychotherapy Scale (SPS) and Its Reliability, Validity and Prediction. *British Journal of Clinical Psychology*, **51**, 351-375. http://dx.doi.org/10.1111/j.2044-8260.2012.02033.x

[19] Härkänen, T., Knekt, P., Virtala, E. and Lindfors, O. (2005) A Case Study in Comparing Therapies Involving Informative Drop-Out, Non-Ignorable Non-Compliance and Repeated Measurements. *Statistics in Medicine*, **24**, 3773-3787. http://dx.doi.org/10.1002/sim.2409

[20] Rubin, D.B. (1987) Multiple Imputation for Nonresponse in Surveys. John Wiley, New York. http://dx.doi.org/10.1002/9780470316696

[21] Schafer, J.L. (1999) Multiple Imputation: A Primer. *Statistical Methods in Medical Research*, **8**, 3-15. http://dx.doi.org/10.1191/096228099671525676

[22] Lee, J. (1981) Covariance Adjustment of Rates Based on the Multiple Logistic Regression Model. *Journal of Chronic Diseases*, **34**, 415-426.http://dx.doi.org/10.1016/0021-9681(81)90040-0

[23] Graubard, B.I. and Korn, E.L. (1999) Predictive Margins with Survey Data. *Biometrics*, **55**, 652-659. http://dx.doi.org/10.1111/j.0006-341X.1999.00652.x

[24] Efron, B. (1982) TheJackknife, the Bootstrap and Other Resampling Plans. CBMS-NSF Regional Conference Series in Applied Mathematics, Monograph 38, SIAM. http://dx.doi.org/10.1137/1.9781611970319

[25] Drummond, M., Sculpher, M., Torrance, G., O'Brien, B. and Stoddart, G.L. (2005) Methods for the Economic Evaluation of Health Care Programmes. 3rd Edition, Oxford University Press, Oxford.

[26] Pruessner, J., Kirschbaum, C., Meinlschmid, G. and Hellhammer, D. (2003) Two Formulas for Computation of the Area under the Curve Represent Measures of Total Hormone Concentration versus Time-Dependent Change. *Psychoneuroendocrinology*, **28**, 916-931.http://dx.doi.org/10.1016/S0306-4530(02)00108-7

[27] Briggs, A.H. (2001) Handling Uncertainty in Economic Evaluation and Presenting the Results. In: Drummond, M. and McGuire, A., Eds., *Economic Evaluation in Health Care. Merging Theory with Practice*, Oxford University Press, Oxford, 172-214.

[28] Manning, W.G., Fryback, D.G. and Weinstein, M.C. (1996) Reflecting Uncertainty in Cost-Effectiveness Analysis. In: Gold, M.R., Siegel, J.E., Russell, L.B. and Weinstein, M.C., Eds., *Cost-Effectiveness in Health and Medicine*, Oxford University Press, Oxford, 247-275.

[29] Armitage, P. (2001) Theory and Practice in Medical Statistics. *Statistics in Medicine*, **20**, 2537-2548. http://dx.doi.org/10.1002/sim.727

[30] SAS Institute Inc. (2008) SAS/STAT® 9.2 User's Guide. SAS Institute Inc., Cary.

[31] Gingerich, W.J. and Eisengart, S. (2000) Solution-Focused Brief Therapy: A Review of the Outcome Research. *Family Process*, **39**, 477-498. http://dx.doi.org/10.1111/j.1545-5300.2000.39408.x

[32] Guthrie, E., Moorey, J., Margison, F., Barker, H., Palmer, S., McGrath, G., Tomenson, B. and Creed, F. (1999) Cost-Effectiveness of Brief Psychodynamic-Interpersonal Therapy in High Utilizers of Psychiatric Services. *Archives of General Psychiatry*, **56**, 519-526. http://dx.doi.org/10.1001/archpsyc.56.6.519

[33] Hujanen, T., Peltola, M., Häkkinen, U. and Pekurinen, M. (2008) Men's and Women's Health Care Expenditures by Age Groups in 2006 [in Finnish]. Stakesintyöpapereita 37/2008, Stakes, Helsinki.

[34] Simon, G., Ormel, J., VonKorff, M. and Barlow, W. (1995) Health Care Costs Associated with Depressive and Anxiety Disorders in Primary Care. *American Journal of Psychiatry*, **152**, 352-357.

[35] Konnopka, A., Leichsenring, F., Leibing, E. and König, H. (2009) Cost-of-Illness Studies and Cost-Effectiveness Analyses in Anxiety Disorders: A Systematic Review. *Journal of Affective Disorders*, **114**, 14-31. http://dx.doi.org/10.1016/j.jad.2008.07.014

10

Paroxetine Increased the Serum Estrogen in Postmenopausal Women with Depressive and Anxiety Symptoms

Borong Zhou*#, Shuangyan Xie#, Jiajia Hu#, Xiaofang Sun, Haitao Guan, Yanhua Deng

Department of Neurology, Key Laboratory of Reproduction and Genetics of Guangdong Higher Education Institutes, The Third Affiliated Hospital of Guangzhou Medical University, Guangzhou, China
Email: zhoubr8@aliyun.com

Abstract

Objective: Both of selective serotonin reuptake inhibitors (SSRIs) and estrogen can modulate emotion and cognition function in post-menopause women, moreover SSRIs can influence estrogen system in rats and aquatic wildlife but most of them for reproductive ability. The aim of this study was to investigate the possible relationship between SSRI, estrogen, and emotion and cognition in post-menopause women with anxiety and depressive symptoms .Methods: A double-blind, randomized controlled trials of Paroxetine, an SSRI (n = 44), versus placebo (n = 38) for 6 months in post-menopausal women with anxiety and depressive symptoms. For screening anxiety, depression and mild cognitive impairment (MCI), we use the Hamilton Anxiety Rating Scale (HAM-A), the Hamilton Depression Rating Scale (HAM-D) and the Chinese Version of the Montreal cognitive assessment (MoCA-CV). And sex hormones were measured by ELASE method which is serum estradiol (E2), follicle stimulating hormone (FSH) and luteinizing hormone (LH). Results: Paroxetine increased serum E2 and decreased LH, FSH significantly ($P < 0.05$). Meanwhile, HAM-A and HAM-D scores declined and MoCA-CV score raised by Paroxetine ($P < 0.05$). We also found that a negative association between E2 and scores of HAM-A and HAM-D at pre-treatment and post-treatment of Paroxetine (HAM-A: R = −0.27, R = −0.24; HAM-D: R = −0.65, R = −0.37), while a positive correlation between E2 and MoCA-CV scores (R = 0.52, R = 0.47). Conclusions: This founding suggests that SSRI can increase serum estrogen levels and the change of estrogen may be one of mechanism in SSRI's improve emotion and cognitive function in post-menopausal women.

Keywords

Paroxetine, Estrogen, Anxiety or Depressive Symptom, Cognition, Post-Menopausal Women

---

*Corresponding author.
#All authors made substantial contributions to the study and this manuscript. None was compensated for manuscript preparation.

1. Introduction

Mood disorder, especially depression, and dementia are commonly in comorbidity occurring in the aged population (Korczyn et al., 2009). Moreover, both of the diseases affect much more women than men (Korczyn et al., 2009). Many literatures have reported that, a hypoestrogenic state, such as premenstrual, postpartum, menopausal period, has been proposed to negatively affect emotional stability and cognitive function, especially in post-menopausal women (Shumaker et al. 2003). In the post-menopausal period, 18% of women had at least one psychiatric disorder with depression being the most common (16%) followed by general anxiety or panic (6%) and alcohol abuse (1%) (Colenda et al. 2010). Furthermore, the frequency of a psychiatric disorder is associated with poorer cognitive functioning among older women (Colenda et al. 2010). It also supported by another study which reported that the percent of women aged 48 to 50 suffering cognition disorder increase to 40% (Amyaloysi et al., 2006) (menopausal average age is 51). Thus, the hypoestrogenic state may be an important factor causing affective and cognitive disorder in post-menopausal women.

In consequence, several studies have analyzed that the role of estrogen in modulation of depression and cognitive impairment in elder women. First, estrogen produces antidepressant-like actions by themselves and facilitate the clinically used antidepressant (Estrada-Camarena et al., 2010) and in post-menopausal women (Zanardi et al., 2007). Second, randomized control trials, while clearly not entirely consistent, nevertheless have shown that performance on 47% of memory measures was better in postmenopausal women who received estrogen replacement therapy (ERT) (Zec et al., 2002). In another observational study reported by Tang et al., ERT was also associated with significantly reduced risk for Alzheimer disease (AD) in a sample of 1124 women enrolled in the Manhattan Study of Aging (Tang et al., 1996). Thus, a reduced risk of AD, improve cognitive functioning and depressive symptoms are found in postmenopausal women who use 17β-estradiol.

Overall, hypoestrogenic state resulting in affective and cognitive disorder while ERT improving depression and cognitive impairment suggest that estrogen play an important role in modulating affection and cognition in postmenopausal women.

Though estrogen have shown a positive effect, current guidelines do not recommend hormone therapy to improve depression and cognitive disorder not only because of no consistent association (Potyk, 2005) between estrogen therapy and cognitive function but also because HRT's disadvantages emerged from the large randomized controlled trial—the Women health initiative (WHI)—that found no benefit for prevention for cardiovascular diseases (Writing Group for the WHI Investigators, 2002) and, particularly, an increase in breast cancer incidence associated with hormone replacement therapy (HRT) (Million Women Study Collaborators, 2003). Thus, in last few years, interest in nonhormonal alternatives for treatment of depressive symptom in post-menopausal women has increased, in particular, the use of SSRI for treatment of mood disorders.

SSRIs has become favored treatment for female patients with depression, especially in late-life women with cognitive impairment. First, SSRIs are more effective and result in fewer adverse drug reactions in women than other antidepressions such as tricyclic antidepressants (TCAs) (Uher et al., 2009a). Second, in SSRIs treatment, women show a superior response to SSRIs comparing with men (Trivedi et al., 2006). In retrospective analysis of 235 men and 400 women randomly assigned to receive the SSRI sertraline or the TCA imipramine, women responded preferentially to Sertraline and men show a better response to imipramine (Kornstein et al., 2000). Third, in post-menopausal depressive women with mild cognitive impairment (MCI), SSRI, Paroxtine, treatment has been reported to improve performance in cognitive tasks and increase serum level of brain derived neurotrophic factor (BDNF) (Cubeddu et al., 2010; Wroolie et al., 2006; Fales et al. 2009). However, little is known what mechanism in gender preference of SSRIs in female.

It is mentioned above that estrogen played an important role in modulating affection and cognition in postmenopausal women, while, SSRIs also improve affective and cognitive disorder in late-life women. Thanks to the recent findings on the interaction between SSRIs and estrogen system on animal studies, such as rats (Taylor et al., 2004) and aquatic animals (Foran et al., 2004). Thus, we hypothesis that estrogen system may be one of mechanism of SSRIs involved in improving affection and cognition in postmenopausal women.

In the present study, we aimed to 1) clarify a possible relationship between Paroxetine which is one of SSRIs with the highest activity, and serum estrogen levels in a group of postmenopausal women with mood disorder undergoing treatment with Paroxetine for 6 months, 2) to evaluate the long-term modifications in cognition function as well as anxiety and depressive symptoms during treatment using Hamilton Anxiety Rating Scale-14 items (HAM-A), the Chinese version of the 17-item Hamilton Depression Rating Scale (HAM-D), Montreal cognitive assessment (MoCA-CV).

2. Materials and Methods

2.1. Participants

A total of 88 postmenopausal women with anxiety and depression were enrolled in the study from 2011 to 2012, including 6 patients lost to follow up, and 82 patients completed all sessions. All subjects had experienced their last menstrual period $\geq$ 12 months previously, therefore, they were postmenopausal according to the Stages of Reproductive Aging Workshop criteria (Soules et al., 2001). Moreover, they all met the standard anxiety and depression diagnosis in the ICD-10 (Cooper, 1989). None of them had taken psychoactive drugs or hormonal therapies for at least 6 months before the beginning of the protocol; and they had no mood or behavior disease before the onset of the menopausal transition. Subjects were randomized into two groups: experiment group intervened by Paroxetine (E-group, 44 cases) and control group treated with oryzanol (C-group, 38 cases). This study was approved by the institutional review board of the Third Affiliated Hospital of Guangzhou Medical College (Guangzhou, China) and written informed consent was obtained from every participant.

Protocol: In pre-therapy and post-treatment, HAM-A, HAM-D and MoCA-CV assessments were administered to determine the status of anxiety, depression and cognition before blood sample collection measuring sex hormone.

Treatment: The treatment in E-group consisted of 10 mg daily of Paroxetine (Glaxo Smith Kline) for the first week and the subsequent dose of 20 mg/day (quaque nocte) for the rest of time of 6 months. While the C-group were treated with Oryzanol at 20 mg three times per day for 6 months. 0.8 mg of Alprozolam per day (quaque nocte) was prescribed for both of the groups in the first month and then the dose of Alprozolam was gradually reduced to stop using.

2.2. Neuropsychological Scale Assessment

Participants were selected for the anxiety-depression status using the standard anxiety and depression diagnoses in the ICD-10 (Cooper, 1989). The criteria include: 1) Score of HAM-A $\geq$ 14 (Hamilton, 1959) and score of HAM-D $\geq$ 17 (Zheng et al., 1988); 2) experience of major anxiety symptoms for at least 3 months or major depression symptoms for at least 2 weeks; and 3) decline in functioning at work and home. Of these patients, 39 had mixed anxiety were diagnosed with depression disease (MADD, ICD-10 code F41.2), 28 suffered from anxiety only (ICD-10 code F41.8) and 15 suffered from depression only (ICD-10 code F32.0). Cognitive function was evaluated by MoCA-CV (Wong et al., 2009; Zhang et al., 2008).

2.3. Sex Hormones Evaluated by ELASA

After overnight fasting, a blood sample was drawn from the cubital vein of each participant between 7:00 and 8:00 AM. Serum estradiol, follicle stimulating hormone, luteinizing hormone and progesterone levels were measured with ELISA kit, similarly to these described previously (Zhou et al., 2012; Welt et al., 2003). The assay sensitivity for E2, FSH and LH is 0.1 pg/ml, 0.1 mIU/ml, and 0.1 mIU/ml. The intra-assay coefficients of variation (CVs) for E2, FSH, LH, and were 6.5%, 7.8%, and 6.12%. And the inter-assay CVs for E2, FSH, and LH were 6.5%, 7.8% and 6.12%.

2.4. Statistical Analysis

Statistical analysis was performed by using the SPSS16.0 statistical software package (standard version 16.0; SPSS, Chicago, IL). All data were recorded as mean $\pm$ standard deviation (x $\pm$ s).The demographic data were analyzed using Student's t-tests. In addition, we used one-way analyses of variance (ANOVA) to analyze the differences between pre-therapy and post-therapy in the two groups. To control for potential confounders, we employed repeated-measures analysis of covariance (ANCOVA) and multivariate regression analysis (logistic). We tested the effects of each variable on E2 level, including the severity of anxious/depressive symptoms (HAM-A or HAM-D scores), MoCA-CV scores, or demographic variables. A P-value of less than 0.05 was considered to indicate statistically significant differences.

3. Results

3.1. Baseline Characteristics

Baseline information of subjects was described in detail in **Table 1**. The age of patients range from 56 to 69 years old (mean, 61.89 ± 6.32 years), and there were no significant differences in demographic information, postmenopausal time, anxiety and depression course, HAM-A score, HAM-D score, MoCA-CV score and sex hormone levels before antidepressant treatment between the experiment group and the control group.

3.2. Estrogen Decreased, LH and FSH Has No Change in Natural State

To observe how the hypothalamic pituitary ovarian (HPO) axis work in natural state, we set the control group without intervened by Paroxetine to measure the sex hormones. In control group, estrogen declined to 37.54 ± 7.61pg/ml from 49.36 ± 12.75 pg/ml (**Figure 1(a)**), and there was no significantly change in LH and FSH (**Figures 1(b)** and **1(c)**).

3.3. Paroxetine Up-Regulated Estrogen, while Decreased LH and FSH

Women receiving Paroxetine for 6 months showed a significant increase in serum estrogen values with respect to pretreatment and control group values (57.24 ± 14.65 pg/ml at post-therapy vs 48.45 ± 10.25 pg/ml at the be-

Table 1. Demographics, neuropsychological test scores and hormone levels before treatment in the antidepressant treatment and control groups ($x \pm s$).

Groups	E-group (n = 44)	C-group (n = 38)	P value
Age (years)	61.96 ± 9.30	61.43 ± 8.41	0.88
Postmenopausal time (y)	5.40 ± 7.45	5.23 ± 6.80	0.83
Education (y)	8.96 ± 2.65	9.51 ± 3.47	0.65
Disease course (y)	2.26 ± 5.75	2.18 ± 4.12	0.85
HAM-A (scores)	21.42 ± 8.90	20.75 ± 7.32	0.68
HAM-D (scores)	23.89 ± 6.70	24.37 ± 8.14	0.67
MoCA-CA (scores)	24.08 ± 2.22	23.94 ± 2.68	0.68
E2 (pg/ml)	48.45 ± 10.25	49.36 ± 12.75	0.69
FSH (MIU/ml)	50.56 ± 16.78	49.80 ± 11.51	0.71
LH (MIU/ml)	24.18 ± 6.25	23.54 ± 6.58	0.74

E stands for experimental, and C stands for control.

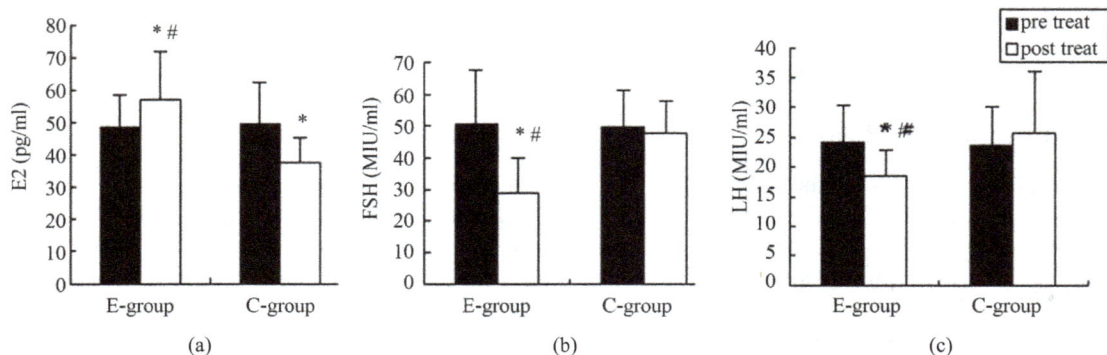

Figure 1. Paroxetine regulating on sex hormonal levels. The data are presented as mean ± SD. $^{*}P < 0.005$ versus pretreatment in the two groups; $^{#}P < 0.005$ versus post-treatment in control group.

ginning of therapy or 37.54 ± 7.61 pg/ml in control group, $P < 0.05$) (**Figure 1(a)**). And LH, FSH decreased significantly in the group treated by Paroxetine (LH from 24.18 ± 6.25 MIU/ml to 18.43 ± 4.55 MIU/ml, FSH from 50.56 ± 16.78 MIU/ml to 28.90 ± 11.34 MIU/ml) (**Figures 1(b)** and **1(c)**).

3.4. Paroxetine Relieved Anxiety and Depressive Symptom and Improve Cognitive Function

Similarly to estrogen levels, HAM-A score from 21.42 ± 8.90 to 9.78 ± 4.06, HAM-D score from 23.89 ± 6.70 to 11.54 ± 5.25 (**Figures 2(a)** and **2(b)**), declined significantly and MoCA-CV score raise to 26.92 ± 1.92 from 24.08 ± 2.22 by Paroxetine (**Figure 2(c)**). In control group, HAM-A score decreased, the HAM-D scores and MoCA-CV scores did not change (**Figures 2(a)**, **2(b)** and **2(c)**).

3.5. E2 Levels Was Significantly Associated with Scores of HAM-A, HAM-D and MoCA-CV at Pre-Treatment and Post-Treatment with Paroxetine

To gain further insight whether the estrogen is probably one of the mechanism of SSRI improve emotional and cognitive function in post-menopausal women, we analyses the correlation between estrogen and neuropsychological scale scores. E2 levels were significantly correlated with MoCA-CV scores at pre-($R = 0.52$, $P = 0.012$) and post-therapy of Paroxetine, ($R = 0.47$, $P = 0.015$), and negative correlated with HAM-D scores at pre ($R = -0.65$, $P = 0.0001$) and post-treatment ($R = -0.37$, $P = 0.036$) and HARDS-14 scores at pre ($R = -0.27$, $P = 0.043$) and post-treatment ($R = -0.24$, $P = 0.047$) (**Table 2**). The E2 levels was also associated with the rise in HAM-D scores ($R = 0.35$, $P = 0.038$) but this correlation did not happen in HARDS-14 scores ($R = 0.21$, $P = 0.052$) (**Table 2**).

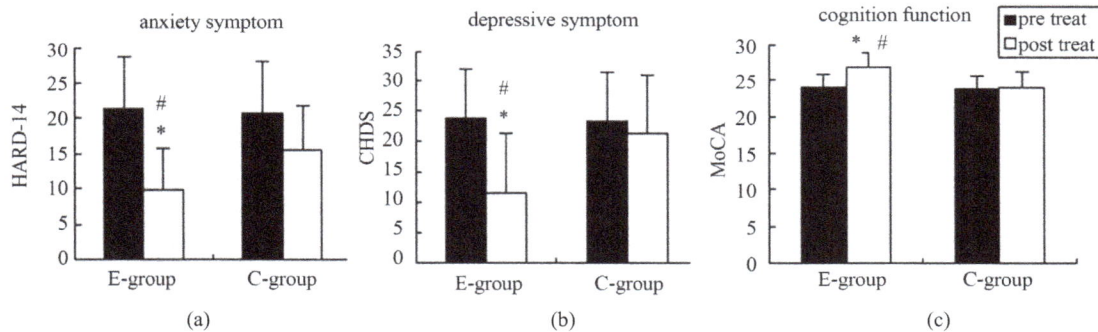

Figure 2. Paroxetine affecting clinical from the neuropsychological scale assessment. The data are presented as mean ± SD. $^*P < 0.005$ versus pretreatment in the two groups; $^\#P < 0.005$ versus post-treatment in control group.

Table 2. Correlation between E2 levels and MoCA-CA scores, HAM-A-14/HAM-D and demographic information pre- and post-therapy in the antidepressant treatment group.

E-group	E2 (pg/ml) pre-therapy		E2 (pg/ml) post-therapy	
Age	$R = 0.41$	$P = 0.028^*$	$R = 0.37$	$P = 0.06$
HAM-A-14 scores	$R = -0.27$	$P = 0.043^*$	$R = -0.24$	$P = 0.047^*$
HAM-D scores	$R = -0.65$	$P = 0.0001^*$	$R = -0.37$	$P = 0.036^*$
MoCA-CA scores	$R = 0.52$	$P = 0.047^*$	$P = 0.012$	$P = 0.015^*$
HAM-D scores	$R = -0.65$	$P = 0.0001^*$	$R = -0.37$	$P = 0.036^*$
Increased scores of HAM-A	\		$R = 0.21$	$P = 0.052^*$
Increased scores of HAM-D	\		$R = 0.35$	$P = 0.038^*$

$^*P < 0.05$.

4. Discussion

E2 increased, LH, FSH decreased significantly comparing pre therapy with post treatment of Paroxetine. And in the control group, E2 level fell, FSH and LH were not significantly altered.

Aging has dramatic effects on the reproductive system in women. The estrogen levels in the control group suggest that serum level estrogen decreased with the aging and no change of LH, FSH in control group even when estrogen decreased indicated that a loss of ovarian function and subsequent the loss of negative feedback on the hypothalamus and pituitary at low level of estrogen in their natural state (Hall, 2007). But when estrogen increased by Paroxetine, the LH and FSH declined demonstrating preservation of the negative feedback in HPO axis, which is consistent with the results of Shaw's study in 2011 (Shaw, 2011), that LH and FSH also decrease in 22 postmenopausal women by administering a controlled intravenous steroid infusion that mimics estradiol (E2) and progesterone (P) levels across the follicular phase.

In the condition of estrogen going down with aging in the post-menopausal women, by treating with Paroxetine the estrogen did not decrease, instead, it increased which reversed the estrogen decreasing trend. It strongly suggests that Paroxetine is able to affect the serum level of estrogen in postmenopausal women.

How SSRIs regulate estrogen system? To our knowledge, there have not been previous human researches but several animal studies which have shown that serotonergic agent can modify estrogen titers and vice versa (Maswood et al., 1999; Raap et al., 2000). Rats injected with Fluoxetine revealed that concentrations of 0.5 - 5 mg/kg may significantly alter circulating estrogen levels (Taylor et al., 2004). Moreover estradiol titers increased in Japanese medaka exposed to 0.1 and 0.5 mg/l Fluoxetine in water (Foran et al., 2004). The mechanism involved in the modulation of estradiol levels by Fluoxetine are unclear, but Rehavi et al. (2000) has speculated that in rats SSRIs may inhibit release of the luteinizing hormone (LH) which results in decreased ovarian release of estrogens in females. By contrast, in our experiment, estrogen increased and LH and FSH decreased after the treatment of Paroxetine, but we cannot exclude that the possibility of Paroxetine activating HPO axis to increase estrogen then followed by negative feedback in which LH and FSH went down. Moreover, in some cases SSRIs induce amenrrhea, hyperprolactinemia and galactorrhea, which have been also hypothesized that SSRIs may stimulate prolactin release directly via pre- or post-synaptic 5-HT receptors in the hypothalamus (Mondal et al., 2013), suggesting the existence of SSRIs effecting on hypothalamus.

Besides influencing HPO axis, attention can also be focused on data linking P450 and SSRI affecting estrogen synthesis and decomposition. For example, exposure to FLU has been shown to alter plasma estradiol levels and expression of the aromatase gene in the ovary of fish (Foran et al., 2004; Lister et al., 2009; Mennigen et al., 2010), the gen encoding cytochrome P450 enzyme aromatase in ovary catalyzing conversion of androgens into estrogens. Moreover, SSRIs have been also reported to influence a class of hepatic cytochrome P450 enzymes, responsible for metabolizing many endogenous and exogenous agents, including steroids (Brosen, 1995; Harvey et al., 1996). Thus, Paroxetine increases serum estrogen probably by modifying activity of cytochrome P450 enzymes in a manner that impacting the synthesis and decompose of estrogen.

Overall, SSRI's estrogenic effect has been confirmed, whose mechanism may be influencing HPO axis or estrogen's synthesis and composition. As we know, estrogen can regulate affective (Estrada-Camarena et al., 2010; Zanardi et al., 2007) and cognitive function (Zec et al., 2002; Tang et al., 1996) in postmenopausal women. However, there has been little information about estrogen involved in mechanism of SSRI improving affection and cognition in human. The current study is the first not only to show SSRI altering estrogen levels in human but also investigate the relations between the changes in estrogen and neuropsychological scale scores.

The Neuropsychological scale results showed a reduction in the score of HAM-A and HAM-D and an increase in MoCA-CV score in E-group comparing with C-group or pre-treatment. it indicates Paroxetine not only relieve anxiety and depressive symptoms but also improve cognitive function in post-menopausal women, which is consistent with previous reports (Paleacu et al., 2007; Savaskan et al., 2008). For example, Deanna M. Barch in 2012 found that both episodic memory and executive function demonstrated significant improvement among 166 adults with late-life depression during treatment with sertraline for 12 weeks (Barch et al., 2012).

Moreover, our results revealed that E2 levels were strongly correlated with HARDS-14 scores, HAM-D scores and MoCA-CV scores, which is also supported by previous evidence of a significant role of E2 on emotional disorder and cognitive function (Pae et al., 2008; Pan, 2010). Thus, this findings support our hypothesis that SSRI' altering estrogen levels may be one of mechanism in improve mood and cognitive disorder in the post-menopausal women.

Why SSRIs increasing estrogen can modulate our emotion and cognition? To answer this question, BDNF has to be firstly mentioned. The critical neurotrophin regulates many neuronal aspects including cell differentiation, cell survival, neurotransmission, and synaptic plasticity in the central nervous system (Numakawa et al., 2010), which may be involved in the pathophysiology of Alzheimer's disease and mental disorders (Numakawa et al., 2010). There is close relationship between BDNF and estrogen or SSRIs. On one hand, It was demonstrated that E2 action on calcineurin may, therefore, contribute to regulate the cAMP response element binding protein (CREB) signaling through which E2 increases the expression of BDNF that may underlie some of the effects of E2 on affective and cognitive function (Zhou et al., 2005). On the other, SSRIs indirectly up-regulate the CREB and BDNF which contribute to neural protection (Vinet et al., 2004). Moreover, Paroxetine increased plasm BDNF in post-menopausal women with major depression (Cubeddu et al., 2010) or climacteric symptoms (Yasui-Furukori et al., 2011). Thus, it suggests that the possibility that CREB-BDNF signaling is the common pathway for the effects of estrogen and SSRIs on brain function, such as modulating emotion and cognition. And the information was also provided that BDNF may be the reason of SSRI increasing estrogen to improve emotional and cognitive function.

5. Conclusion

As far as we know, the current study is the first one not only to evaluate the correlation between Paroxetine and estrogen in postmenopausal women, but also finding that the altered estrogen levels are significantly related to emotional and cognitive function. Since this is a preliminary study, further studies are needed to determine the extent of the relevance of the data obtained. For one hand, more researches should be conducted to investigate the concrete mechanism of Paroxetine increasing estrogen levels, via HPO axis or P450? (Our group has started to do). For the other hand, in fact, it would be very interesting to measure the serum BDNF in this study. If we had known the correlation between serum BDNF and estrogen by Paroxetine in this study, it would be more determined that BDNF may be the reason that altered estrogen by Paroxetine improves affective and cognitive function. Thus, studies investigating the effects of SSRIs altering estrogen on CREB-BDNF signaling are warranted.

Acknowledgements

This study was supported by a research grant from the Science Technology Planning Project (NO. 2011 B060300027) of Guangdong Province, China.

Conflict of Interest

The authors declare no conflict of interest.

References

Barch, D. M., D'Angelo, G., Pieper, C. et al. (2012) Cognitive Improvement Following Treatment in Late-Life Depression: Relationship to Vascular Risk and Age of Onset. *American Journal of Geriatric Psychiatry, 20*, 682-690. http://dx.doi.org/10.1097/JGP.0b013e318246b6cb

Brosen, K. (1995). Drug Interactions and the Cytochrome P450 System: The Role of Cytochrome P450 1A2. *Clinical Pharmacokinetics, 29*, 20-25. http://dx.doi.org/10.2165/00003088-199500291-00005

Colenda, C. C., Legault, C., Rapp, S. R. et al. (2010). Psychiatric Disorders and Cognitive Dysfunction among Older, Postmenopausal Women: Results from the Women's Health Initiative Memory Study. *American Journal of Geriatric Psychiatry, 18*, 177-186. http://dx.doi.org/10.1097/JGP.0b013e3181c65864

Cooper, J. E. (1989). An Overview of the Prospective ICD-10 Classification of Mental Disorders. *The British Journal of Psychiatry. Supplement, 4*, 21-23.

Cubeddu, A., Giannini, A., & Bucci, F. et al. (2010). Paroxetine Increases Brain-Derived Neurotrophic Factor in Postmenopausal Women. *Menopause: The Journal of The North American Menopause Society, 17*, 338-343. http://dx.doi.org/10.1097/gme.0b013e3181c29e44

Cubeddu, A., Giannini, A., Bucci, F. et al. (2010). Paroxetine Increases Brain-Derived Neurotrophic Factor in Postmenopausal Women. *Menopause, 17*, 338-343. http://dx.doi.org/10.1097/gme.0b013e3181c29e44

Estrada-Camarena, E., Lopez-Rubalcava, C., & Vega-Rivera, N. (2010). Antidepressant Effects of Estrogens: A Basic Approximation. *Behavioural Pharmacology, 21*, 451-464. http://dx.doi.org/10.1097/FBP.0b013e32833db7e9

Fales, C. L., Barch, D. M., Rundle, M. M. et al. (2009). Antidepressant Treatment Normalizes Hypoactivity in Dorsolateral Prefrontal Cortex during Emotional Interference Processing in Major Depression. *Journal of Affective Disorders, 112*, 206-211. http://dx.doi.org/10.1016/j.jad.2008.04.027

Foran, C. M., Weston, J., Slattery, M., Brooks, B. W., & Huggett, D. B. (2004). Reproductive Assessment of Japanese Medaka (*Oryzias latipes*) Following a Four-Week Fluoxetine (SSRI) Exposure. *Archives of Environmental Contamination and Toxicology, 46*, 511-517. http://dx.doi.org/10.1007/s00244-003-3042-5

Hall, J. E. (2007). Neuroendocrine Changes with Reproductive Aging in Women. *Seminars in Reproductive Medicine, 25*, 344-351. http://dx.doi.org/10.1055/s-2007-984740

Hamilton, M. (1959). The Assessment of Anxiety States by Rating. *British Journal of Medical Psychology, 32*, 50-55. http://dx.doi.org/10.1111/j.2044-8341.1959.tb00467.x

Harvey, A., & Preskorn, S. (1996). Cytochrome P450 Enzymes: Interpretation of Their Interactions with Selective Serotonin Reuptake Inhibitors. Part II. *Journal of Clinical Psychopharmacology, 16*, 345-355. http://dx.doi.org/10.1097/00004714-199610000-00002

Korczyn, A. D., & Halperin, I. (2009). Depression and Dementia. *Journal of the Neurological Sciences, 283*, 139-142. http://dx.doi.org/10.1016/j.jns.2009.02.346

Kornstein, S. G., Schatzberg, A. F., Thase, M. E., Yonkers, K. A., McCullough, J. P., Keitner, G. I. et al. (2000). Gender Differences in Treatment Response to Sertraline versus Imipramine in Chronic Depression. *American Journal of Psychiatry, 157*, 1445-1452. http://dx.doi.org/10.1176/appi.ajp.157.9.1445

Lister, A., Regan, C., Van Zwol, J., & Van Der Kraak, G. (2009). Inhibition of Egg Production in Zebrafish by Fluoxetine and Municipal Effluents: A Mechanistic Evaluation. *Aquatic Toxicology, 95*, 320-329. http://dx.doi.org/10.1016/j.aquatox.2009.04.011

Maswood, S., Truitt, W., Hotema, M., Caldarola-Pastuszka, M., & Uphouse, L. (1999). Estrous Cycle Modulation of Extracellular Serotonin in Mediobasal Hypothalamus: Role of the Serotonin Transporter and Terminal Autoreceptors. *Brain Research, 831*, 146-154. http://dx.doi.org/10.1016/S0006-8993(99)01439-0

Mennigen, J. A., Lado, W. E., Zamora, J. M., Duarte-Guterman, P., Langlois, V. S., Metcalfe, C. D. et al. (2010). Waterborne Fluoxetine Disrupts the Reproductive Axis in Sexually Mature Male Goldfish, *Carassius auratus. Aquatic Toxicology, 100*, 354-364. http://dx.doi.org/10.1016/j.aquatox.2010.08.016

Million Women Study Collaborators (2003). Breast Cancer and Hormone-Replacement Therapy in the Million Women Study. *Lancet, 362*, 419-427. http://dx.doi.org/10.1016/S0140-6736(03)14065-2

Mondal, S., Saha, I., Das, S., Ganguly, A., Das, D., & Tripathi, S. K. (2013). A New Logical Insight and Putative Mechanism behind Fluoxetine-Induced Amenorrhea, Hyperprolactinemia and Galactorrhea in a Case Series. *Therapeutic Advances in Psychopharmacology, 3*, 322-334. http://dx.doi.org/10.1177/2045125313490305

Numakawa, T., Suzuki, S., Kumamaru, E., Adachi, N., Richards, M., & Kunugi, H. (2010). BDNF Function and Intracellular Signaling in Neurons. *Histology and Histopathology, 25*, 237-258.

Numakawa, T., Yokomaku, D., Richards, M., Hori, H., Adachi, N., & Kunugi, H. (2010). Functional Interactions between Steroid Hormones and Neurotrophin BDNF. *World Journal of Biological Chemistry, 1*, 133-143. http://dx.doi.org/10.4331/wjbc.v1.i5.133

Pae, C. U., Mandelli, L., Han, C., Ham, B. J., Masand, P. S., Patkar, A. A. et al. (2008). Do Estradiol Levels Influence on the Cognitive Function during Antidepressant Treatments in Post-Menopausal Women with Major Depressive Disorder? A Comparison with Pre-Menopausal Women. *Neuro Endocrinology Letters, 29*, 500-506.

Paleacu, D., Shutzman, A., Giladi, N., Herman, T., Simon, E. S., & Hausdorff, J. M. (2007). Effects of Pharmacological Therapy on Gait and Cognitive Function in Depressed Patients. *Clinical Neuropharmacology, 30*, 63-71. http://dx.doi.org/10.1097/01.wnf.0000240949.41691.95

Pan, M., Li, Z., Yeung, V., & Xu, R. J. (2010). Dietary Supplementation of Soy Germ Phytoestrogens or Estradiol Improves Spatial Memory Performance and Increases Gene Expression of BDNF, TrkB Receptor and Synaptic Factors in Ovariectomized Rats. *Nutrition & Metabolism, 7*, 75-85. http://dx.doi.org/10.1186/1743-7075-7-75

Potyk, D. (2005). Treatments for Alzheimer Disease. *South Med J.* http://dx.doi.org/10.1097/01.SMJ.0000166671.86815.C1

Raap, D. K., DonCarlos, L., Garcia, F., Muma, N. A., Wolf, W. A., Battaglia, G. et al. (2000). Estrogen Desensitizes 5-HT$_{1A}$ Receptors and Reduces Levels of G$_z$, G$_{i1}$ and G$_{i3}$ Proteins in the Hypothalamus. *Neuropharmacology, 39*, 1823-1832. http://dx.doi.org/10.1016/S0028-3908(99)00264-6

Rehavi, M., Attali, G., Gil-Ad, I., & Weizman, A. (2000). Suppression of Serum Gonadal Steroids in Rats by Chronic Treatment with Dopamine and Serotonin Reuptake Inhibitors. *European Neuropsychopharmacology, 10*, 145-150. http://dx.doi.org/10.1016/S0924-977X(00)00066-3

Savaskan, E., Müller, S. E., Böhringer, A., Schulz, A., & Schächinger, H. (2008). Antidepressive Therapy with Escitalopram Improves Mood, Cognitive Symptoms, and Identity Memory for Angry Faces in Elderly Depressed Patients. *International Journal of Neuropsychopharmacology, 11,* 381-388. http://dx.doi.org/10.1017/S1461145707007997

Shaw, N. D., Srouji, S. S., Histed, S. N., & Hall, J. E. (2011). Differential Effects of Aging on Estrogen Negative and Positive Feedback. *American Journal of Physiology-Endocrinology and Metabolism, 301,* E351-E355. http://dx.doi.org/10.1152/ajpendo.00150.2011

Shumaker, S. A., Legault, C., Rapp, S. R., Thal, L., Wallace, R. B., Ockene, J. K. et al. (2003). Estrogen plus Progestin and the Incidence of Dementia and Mild Cognitive Impairment in Postmenopausal Women: The Women's Health Initiative Memory Study: A Randomized Controlled Trial. *JAMA, 289,* 2651-2662. http://dx.doi.org/10.1001/jama.289.20.2651

Soules, M. R., Sherman, S., Parrott, E., Rebar, R., Santoro, N., Utian, W., & Woods, N. (2001). Executive Summary: Stages of Reproductive Aging Workshop (STRAW). *Climacteric, 4,* 267-272. http://dx.doi.org/10.1080/713605136

Tang, M. X., Jacobs, D., Stern, Y., Marder, K., Schofield, P., Gurland, B. et al. (1996). Effect of Oestrogen during Menopause on Risk and Age at Onset of Alzheimer's Disease. *The Lancet, 348,* 429-432. http://dx.doi.org/10.1016/S0140-6736(96)03356-9

Taylor, G. T., Farr, S., Klinga, K., & Weiss, J. (2004). Chronic Fluoxetine Suppresses Circulating Estrogen and the Enhanced Spatial Learning of Estrogen-Treated Ovariectomized Rats. *Psychoneuroendocrinology, 29,* 1241-1249. http://dx.doi.org/10.1016/j.psyneuen.2004.03.001

Trivedi, M. H., Rush, A. J., Wisniewski, S. R. et al. (2006). Evaluation of Outcomes with Citalopram for Depression Using Measurement Based Care in STAR*D: Implications for Clinical Practice. *American Journal of Psychiatry, 163,* 28-40. http://dx.doi.org/10.1176/appi.ajp.163.1.28

Uher, R., Maier, W., Hauser, J., Marušič, A., Schmael, C., Mors, O. et al. (2009a). Differential Efficacy of Escitalopram and Nortriptyline on Dimensional Measures of Depression. *British Journal of Psychiatry, 194,* 252-259. http://dx.doi.org/10.1192/bjp.bp.108.057554

Vinet, J., Carra, S., Blom, J. M. C., Brunello, N., Barden, N., & Tascedda, F. (2004). Chronic Treatment with Desipramine and Fluoxetine Modulate BDNF, CaMKKα and CaMKKβ mRNA Levels in the Hippocampus of Transgenic Mice Expressing Antisense RNA against the Glucocorticoid Receptor. *Neuropharmacology, 47,* 1062-1069. http://dx.doi.org/10.1016/j.neuropharm.2004.07.035

Welt, C. K., Pagan, Y. L., Smith, P. C., Rado, K. B., & Hall, J. E. (2003). Control of Follicle-Stimulating Hormone by Estradiol and the Inhibins: Critical Role of Estradiol at the Hypothalamus during the Luteal-Follicular Transition. *Journal of Clinical Endocrinology & Metabolism, 88,* 1766-1771. http://dx.doi.org/10.1210/jc.2002-021516

Wong, A., Xiong, Y. Y., Kwan, P. W., Chan, A. Y. Y., Lam, W. W. M., Wang, K. et al. (2009). The Validity, Reliability and Clinical Utility of the Hong Kong Montreal Cognitive Assessment (HK-MoCA-CV) in Patients with Cerebral Small Vessel Disease. *Dementia and Geriatric Cognitive Disorders, 28,* 81-87. http://dx.doi.org/10.1159/000232589

Writing Group for the WHI Investigators (2002). Risks and Benefits of Estrogen plus Progestin in Healthy Postmenopausal Women: Principal Results from the Women's Health Initiative Randomized Controlled Trial. *JAMA, 288,* 321-333. http://dx.doi.org/10.1001/jama.288.3.321

Wroolie, T. E., Williams, K. E., Keller, J., Zappert, L. N., Shelton, S. D., Kenna, H. A. et al. (2006). Mood and Neuropsychological Changes in Women with Midlife Depression Treated with Escitalopram. *Journal of Clinical Psychopharmacology, 26,* 361-366. http://dx.doi.org/10.1097/01.jcp.0000227699.26375.f8

Yasui-Furukori, N., Tsuchimine, S., Nakagami, T., Fujii, A., Sato, Y., Tomita, T. et al. (2011). Association between Plasma Paroxetine Concentration and Changes in Plasma Brain-Derived Neurotrophic Factor Levels in Patients with Major Depressive Disorder. *Human Psychopharmacology, 26,* 194-200.

Zanardi, R., Rossini, D., Magri, L., Malaguti, A., Colombo, C., & Smeraldi, E. (2007). Response to SSRIs and Role of the Hormonal Therapy in Post-Menopausal Depression. *European Neuropsychopharmacology, 17,* 400-405. http://dx.doi.org/10.1016/j.euroneuro.2006.11.001

Zec, R. F., & Trivendi, M. A. (2002). The Effects of Estrogen Replacement Therapy on Neuropsychological Function in Postmenopausal Women with and without Dementia: A Critical and Theoretical Review. *Neuropsychology Review, 12,* 65-109. http://dx.doi.org/10.1023/A:1016880127635

Zhang, L. X., & Liu, X. Q. (2008). The Preliminary Application of Montreal Cognitive Assessment of Chinese Version in the Older People in Guangzhou. *Chinese Journal of Gerontology, 28,* 1632-1634.

Zheng, Y. P., Zhao, J. P., Phillips, M., Liu, J. B., Cai, M. F., Sun, S. Q., & Huang, M. F. (1988). Validity and Reliability of the Chinese Hamilton Depression Rating Scale. *British Journal of Psychiatry, 152,* 660-664. http://dx.doi.org/10.1192/bjp.152.5.660

Zhou, B., Sun, X., Zhang, M., Deng, Y. H., & Hu, J. J. (2012). The Symptomatology of Climacteric Syndrome: Whether Associated with the Physical Factors Or Psychological Disorder in Perimenopausal/Postmen-Opausal Patients with An-

xiety-Depression Disorder. *Archives of Gynecology and Obstetrics, 285,* 1345-1352.
http://dx.doi.org/10.1007/s00404-011-2151-z

Zhou, J., Zhang, H. B., Cohen, R. S., & Pandey, S. C. (2005). Effects of Estrogen Treatment on Expression of Brain-Derived
Neurotrophic Factor and cAMP Response Element-Binding Protein Expression and Phosphorylation in Rat Amygdalold
and Hippocampal Structures. *Neuroendocrinology, 81,* 294-310. http://dx.doi.org/10.1159/000088448

Abbreviations

ICD-10: International Classification of Diseases-10;
E2: Estradiol;
FSH: Follicle Stimulating Hormone;
LH: Luteinizing Hormone;
SSRIs: Selective Serotonin Reuptake Inhibitors;
HAM-A: Hamilton Anxiety Rating Scale-14 Items;
HAM-D: The 17-Item Hamilton Depression Rating Scale;
MoCA-CV: Montreal Cognitive Assessment;
HRT: Hormone Replacement Therapy;
BDNF: Brain Derived Neurotrophic Factor;
HPO: Hypothalamic Pituitary Ovarian.

11

Prediction of Anxiety and Behavioural Disturbances by Temperamental Characters in Children

Peyman Hashemian

Psychiatry and Behavioral Sciences Research Center, Faculty of Medicine, Mashhad University of Medical Sciences, Ibn-e-Sina Hospital, Mashhad, Iran
Email: hashemianp@mums.ac.ir

Abstract

Background: Temperament is a predictive factor of child behaviour. Thomas and Chess evaluated relationship of temperamental factor with behavioural disturbance in social milo. *Method*: In this study, 500 children between 4 to 10 years old, who have been admitted for their behavioural disturbance and anxiety to Dr-Sheikh Children Hospital in Mashhad, Iran, have been chosen. The parents fill Malhotra questionnaire and Conner's questionnaire. Then subscales of questionnaires are compared together. *Result*: Power and energy (activity) are the only factors which are in relation with conduct behaviour, impulsivity, hyperactivity and anxiety. *Conclusion*: Among temperament factor only power and energy (activity) have relation with conduct behaviour, impulsivity, hyperactivity and anxiety. Focus of attention (distractibility) is associated with hyperactivity. Sociability has no relationship with hyperactivity.

Keywords

Temperamental Characters, Behavioural Disturbances, Anxiety, Children

1. Introduction

Temperament is a predictive factor for child behaviour. It is an essential agent for self-regulation and a part of future personality formation.

Berdan L.E. and colleagues in 2008 studied the relationship of temperament with behavioural disturbance and social growth [1]. Goodnight J.A. and his team in 2007 found the relationship between difficult temperaments with behavioural disturbance as well as sleep disturbance [2]. Eisenberg N. and crew in 2009 evaluated the impact of negative emotion on behavioural disturbance [3].

Bates J.E. and colleagues studied the type of temperament and parents on future behavioural disturbance [4]. Researches of De Pauw and Mervielde [5] as well as Bucky and Edwards [6] showed the effectiveness of temperamental character on future personality and psychiatric state. Chess and Thomas and their team evaluated temperamental characters and environmental effect on future behavioural disturbance [7]. Miti found the efficacy of temperamental and environmental factors on personality growth [8]. Mc Inerny and Chamberl in conducted a study on the effect of temperamental characters on future behavioural disturbances [9]. Camerone valuated the influence of temperamental characters of child and parents on future behavioural disturbances [10].

The Malhotra temperament measurement schedule assesses temperament of children [11]. The test-retest reliability of this schedule is 0.83 to 0.94 with satisfactory factorial and construct validity [11]. The Conners' Parent Rating Scale is used to assess childhood behavioural disturbances [12]. Subscales of Conners' Parent Rating Scale are conduct symptom, impulsivity, anxiety, and hyperactivity [12]. Temperamental characters include power and energy (activity), focus of attention (distractibility), excitability, sociability, and regularity [11]. Sociability consists of approaching behaviour and adaptability and threshold of response [11]. Excitability consists of mood state and persistency [11]. Power and energy (activity) consist of activity level and intensity of response [11].

2. Method

In this study, 500 children between 4 - 10 years old were selected with the average age of 7.09 years. 304 of which were boys and 196 were girls. These children were referred to sheikh children hospital in Mashhad, Iran in 2011 for their symptoms of behavioural disturbance and anxiety. They had no medical disorder. Their behavioural symptoms included hyperactivity, impulsivity (aggression) and conduct disorder.

Informed consents were taken from their parents. Parents filled out Malhotra temperament measurement schedule [11] and Conners' Parent Rating Scale [12]. Subscales of Conner's Parent Rating Scale (including conduct symptom, impulsivity, anxiety, and hyperactivity) were compared with temperamental characters (including power and energy (activity), focus of attention (distractibility), excitability, sociability, regularity).

Mann-Whitney, two-tailed t-tests were used to compare the two questionnaires, with SPSS software, version 20.

3. Result

In this study 500 children were selected, 304 of which were boys (60.8%) and 196 were girls (39.2%).

Table 1 shows that among temperamental characters, only power and energy (activity) had been associated with conduct symptom. This means the more active the child, the more conduct symptom he/she has. (P-value = 0.001).

As can be seen in **Table 2**, among temperamental characters, only power and energy (activity) and focus of attention (distractibility) were related with impulsivity. This shows the more active and distracted the child, the more impulsive behaviour he/she might be (P-value = 0.000 and 0.018).

As shown in **Table 3**, among temperamental character only power and energy (activity) was related with symptoms of anxiety. The more active the child, the more anxious he/she might be (P-value = 0.004).

Table 4 shows that among temperamental character only sociability had no relationship with hyperactivity but other characters including excitability, energy, focus of attention (distractibility), regularity had relationship with hyperactivity. It means the more irregular, distractive, active and excited the child, the more hyperactive

Table 1. Relationship between conduct symptom and temperamental characters.

	Regularity	Focus of Attention	Energy	Excitability	Sociability
Asymp. Sig. (2-tailed)	0.034	0.167	0.001	0.523	0.310

Table 2. Relationship between impulsivity and temperamental characters.

	Regularity	Focus of Attention	Energy	Excitability	Sociability
Asymp. Sig. (2-tailed)	0.065	0.018	0.000	0.091	0.276

Table 3. Relationship between anxiety and temperamental characters.

	Regularity	Focus of Attention	Energy	Excitability	Sociability
Asymp. Sig. (2-tailed)	0.108	0.726	0.004	0.891	0.315

Table 4. Relationship between hyperactivity and temperamental characters.

	Regularity	Focus of Attention	Energy	Excitability	Sociability
Asymp. Sig. (2-tailed)	0.010	0.000	0.000	0.001	0.770

he/she can be (P-value = 0.010, 0.000, 0.000, 0.001).

4. Discussion

In this study, relationship between temperamental characters and behavioural disturbances and anxiety were compared. Temperamental characters include regularity, focus of attention, power and energy (activity), excitability and sociability. Behavioural disturbances include conduct, impulsivity, hyperactivity symptoms.

We found out that among temperamental factors, only power and energy (activity) had significant relation with conduct behaviour, impulsivity, hyperactivity and anxiety. Regularity and focus of attention (distractibility) and excitability and energy had significant relationship with hyperactivity.

Sociability had no relationship with hyperactivity. Regularity and focus of attention (distractibility) and excitability and sociability had no relation with conduct symptoms. Regularity and excitability and sociability had no relation with impulsivity symptoms. Regularity and focus of attention (distractibility) and excitability and sociability had no relationship with anxiety. This study is compatible with study of Burdan [1], Gunter [13], Rothbart [14], Foley [15], Harris [16], and Lonigan [17]. The above references show that temperament affects behavioural disturbances (externalizing symptoms), emotion and socializing behaviour.

5. Conclusions

Among all temperamental characters, high power and energy, excitability, distractibility and irregularity can be predictive as below:

1—high power and energy (high activity) in children can be predictive of anxiety and behavioural disturbance such as hyperactivity, conduct.

2—excitability and low focus of attention (distractibility) and irregularity can be predictive of hyperactivity.

Limitation and Recommendation

This study was performed in one center. Multi-center study is suggested.

The present study can be used as a preliminary study for a future prospective cohort study for evaluation of correlation of temperamental characters with emotional and behavioural disturbances.

References

[1] Berdan, L.E., Keane, S.P. and Calkins, S.D. (2008) Temperament and Externalizing Behavior: Social Preference and Perceived Acceptance as Protective Factors. *Developmental Psychology*, **44**, 957-968. http://dx.doi.org/10.1037/0012-1649.44.4.957

[2] Goodnight, J.A., Bates, J.E., Staples, A.D., Pettit, G.S. and Dodge, K.A. (2007) Temperamental Resistance to Control Increases the Association between Sleep Problems and Externalizing Behavior Development. *Journal of Family Psychology*, **21**, 39-48. http://dx.doi.org/10.1037/0893-3200.21.1.39

[3] Eisenberg, N., Valiente, C., Spinrad, T.L., Cumberland, A., Liew, J., Reiser, M., Zhou, Q. and Losoya, S.H. (2009) Longitudinal Relations of Children's Effortful Control, Impulsivity, and Negative Emotionality to Their Externalizing, Internalizing, and Co-Occurring Behavior Problems. *Developmental Psychology*, **45**, 988-1008. http://dx.doi.org/10.1037/a0016213

[4] Bates, J.E., Pettit, G.S., Dodge, K.A. and Ridge, B. (1998) Temperamental Resistance to Control and Restrictive Parenting in the Development of Externalizing Behavior. *Developmental Psychology*, **34**, 982-995. http://dx.doi.org/10.1037/0012-1649.34.5.982

[5]   De Pauw, S.S. and Mervielde, I. (2010) Temperament, Personality and Developmental Psychopathology: A Review Based on the Conceptual Dimensions Underlying Childhood Traits. *Child Psychiatry & Human Development*, **41**, 313-329.

[6]   Bucky, S.F. and Edwards, D. (1974) The Recruit Temperament Survey (RTS) as It Discriminates between Psychoses, Neuroses, and Personality Disorders. *Journal of Clinical Psychology*, **30**, 195-199. http://dx.doi.org/10.1002/1097-4679(197404)30:2<195::AID-JCLP2270300223>3.0.CO;2-2

[7]   Chess, S., Thomas, A., Rutter, M., Birch, H.G. and Birch, H. (1963) Interaction of Temperament and Environment in the Production of Behavioral Disturbances in Children. *American Journal of Psychiatry*, **120**, 142-148. http://dx.doi.org/10.1176/ajp.120.2.142

[8]   Miti, G. (1973) Temperament of the Child and Environmental Influences in Personality Development. *Minerva Pediatrica*, **25**, 1300-1306.

[9]   McInerny, T. and Chamberlin, R.W. (1978) Is It Feasible to Identify Infants Who Are at Risk for Later Behavioral Problems? The Carey Temperament Questionnaire as a Prognostic Tool. *Clinical Pediatrics*, **17**, 233-238. http://dx.doi.org/10.1177/000992287801700305

[10]   Cameron, J.R. (1978) Parental Treatment, Children's Temperament, and the Risk of Childhood Behavioural Problems: 2. Initial Temperament, Parental Attitudes, and the Incidence and Form of Behavioral Problems. *American Journal of Orthopsychiatry*, **48**, 140-147. http://dx.doi.org/10.1111/j.1939-0025.1978.tb01295.x

[11]   Malhotra, S. and Randhawa, A. (1982) A Schedule for Measuring Temperament in Children. Preliminary Date on Developement and Standardization. *Indian Journal of clinical psychology*, **9**, 203-210.

[12]   Conners, C.K. (1985) The Conners' Rating Scales. Pro-ED, Austin.

[13]   Gunter, K.L. (2007) Emotional Understanding and Social Behavior in School-Age Children. Published Annually by the Department of Psychology University of North Carolina at Charlotte, *The Undergraduate Journal of Psychology*, **20**, 1-7.

[14]   Rothbart, M.K. (2000) Temperament in Children. University of Oregon Douglas Derryberry Oregon State University. *Presented as a State of the Art Lecture at the 26th International Congress of Psychology*, Stockholm, 1-9. www.bowdoin.edu/~sputnam/rothbart-temperament-questionnaires/cv/publications/pdf/2002_temp_%20in_children_rothbart-derryberry.pdf

[15]   Foley, M.A., McClowry, S.G. and Castellanos, F.X. (2008) The Relationship between Attention Deficit Hyperactivity Disorder and Child Temperament. *Journal of Applied Developmental Psychology*, **29**, 157-169. http://dx.doi.org/10.1016/j.appdev.2007.12.005

[16]   Harris, J.R. Socialization, Personality Development, and the Child's Environments. http://www.thelizlibrary.org/liz/harris.htm

[17]   Lonigan, C.J., Vasey, M.W., Phillips, B.M. and Hazen, R.A. (2004) Temperament, Anxiety, and the Processing of Threat-Relevant Stimuli. *Journal of Clinical Child & Adolescent Psychology*, **33**, 8-20. http://dx.doi.org/10.1207/S15374424JCCP3301_2

Effects of Neurokinin-1 Receptor Inhibition on Anxiety Behavior in Neonatal Rats Selectively Bred for an Infantile Affective Trait

Amanda L. Schott, Betty Zimmerberg[*]

Department of Psychology and Program in Neuroscience, Williams College, Williamstown, USA
Email: [*]bzimmerb@williams.edu

Abstract

Interest in understanding the etiology and developing new treatments for anxiety disorders in children and adolescents has led to recent studies of neurotransmitters not traditionally associated with neural pathways for fear and anxiety. The binding of the neurotransmitter substance P (SP) to its neurokinin-1 (NK1) receptor may be a crucial component in mediating the anxiety response. While previous studies using rodent models have documented the anxiolytic effects of SP antagonists, the role of individual differences in affective temperament has not yet been examined in studies of drug response. This study used intracerebroventricular injections of the NK1 antagonist Spantide II at concentrations of 10 and 100 pmol to examine the consequences of blocking the SP-NK1 pathway in high and low line rats selectively bred for high or low levels of ultrasonic distress calls after a brief maternal separation. Affective temperament was a significant factor in determining drug response. Spantide II resulted in a significant reduction of distress calls in subjects in the high anxiety line, while low line subjects with low anxiety were resistant to the drug. These data indicate that the SP-NK1 pathway could be an important therapeutic target for the treatment of various stress disorders, but drug response might be influenced by the individual's state anxiety or history of chronic stress.

Keywords

Anxiety, Substance P, Neurokinin Receptor, Spantide, Ultrasonic Vocalizations

---

[*]Corresponding author.

1. Introduction

Anxiety disorders are among the most prevalent mental health disorders, including social phobia, post-traumatic stress disorder, obsessive-compulsive disorder, and panic disorder. Globally, estimates of the prevalence of anxiety disorders range from 5.3% in African cultures to 10.4% in Euro/Anglo cultures [1]. Anxiety behaviors are affective reactions that use neural pathways that evolved for mammalian fear responses. Fear responses can be observed very early in life; for example, the normative response of separation anxiety appears in infants at around 18 months of age and can persist until about three years of age. Recently, attention has focused on better detection and developing new treatments for anxiety disorders in adolescents and children. In a national survey of American teenagers, anxiety symptoms were reported by 31.9% of the respondents, with 8.3% meeting anxiety diagnostic criteria of severe impairment and/or distress [2]. The median age for disorder onset was also earlier for anxiety disorders (6 years of age) than for other mental health illnesses. Anxiety disorders in childhood and adolescence are associated with a variety of negative outcomes, including psychosocial and school impairments and an increase in suicide risk [3].

The neurobiological bases of anxiety are complex, involving multiple neurotransmitters and neural circuits. One neurotransmitter system recently implicated in the activation of anxiety behaviors is the neuropeptide substance P (SP). Stressful stimuli can trigger the *in vivo* release of SP in brain areas that are known to play roles in mediating anxiety behavior, such as the amygdala, hippocampus, periaqueductal gray, nucleus accumbens, and lateral septum [4] [5]. The influences of SP are mediated by its binding to the neurokinin-1 (NK1) receptor, the distribution pattern of which mainly overlaps with the locations of SP release itself [5] [6]. Microinjections of SP into the dorsal periaqueductal gray (dPAG), a major output station for the defense reaction, have significant anxiogenic effects [7].

The demonstration of SP-related anxiogenesis prompted studies of the therapeutic value of blocking its NK-1 receptor in animal models of anxiety. In rodents, fear behaviors manifest physiologically as freezing, ultrasonic vocalizations, and a reluctance to explore new environments [8]. NK1 receptor "knockout" mouse mutants show reductions in both depressive and anxious behaviors [9]. In neonatal guinea pigs, the SP antagonist GR73632 was noted to reduce distress vocalizations induced by an SP agonist [10]. In adult male rats, Spantide, a specific NK-1 receptor antagonist, at a dose of 100 pmol, reduced freezing and escape responses after the dPAG was electrically stimulated [11]. Spantide was similarly reported to block the anxiogenic effects of SP amygdalar injections on plus maze and exploratory behavior of male rats as well as reducing freezing after dPAG stimulation, also at a dose of 100 pmol [12].

Though the effects of the SP-NK1 pathway on anxiety behavior has been demonstrated in rodents, no studies examined whether individual differences in baseline affective temperament might interact with the pharmacological effects of blocking the NK-1 receptor. In this study, we used a rodent model useful in examining this question, ultrasonic vocalizations (USVs) after a brief maternal separation, analogous to human separation anxiety. These USVs are regarded as an indicator of the affective state of the pup (e.g. the term "distress calls" [13]), since they are reduced after the administration of anti-anxiety agents such as the benzodiazepines and neurosteroids [14]-[16]. The selective breeding of rats based on their rates of infantile ultrasonic vocalizations (USVs) has resulted in two unique lines (high and low) whose neonates reliably emit distress calls at high and low rates following a brief maternal separation [17]. The USV line difference, selected for an infantile trait, persists into adulthood. For example, heart rate in a novel environment, an indicator of stress reactivity, is significantly higher in juvenile high line rats as compared to low line rats [18]. Adult high line rats also behave more fearfully and inhibited than low line rats do; for example, high line rats take significantly longer than low line rats to emerge from a cylinder into an open field, while low line rats enter significantly more central squares and total squares in an open field than high line rats do [19].

This study examined the effects of an NK1 receptor antagonist, Spantide II, on USV rates in 7-day-old high and low line week-old pups following brief separation from the dam. USVs are a corroborated behavioral indicator of anxiety in pups [20], and infantile vocalization behavior predicts scores on independent measures of anxiety in adulthood [21]. Spantide II, an analogue of substance P that blocks SP functioning via competitive binding at the NK1 receptor sites [22], is injected into the cerebral lateral ventricles [23]. The experiment sought to characterize individual differences in the SP-NK1 pathway as well as to determine whether an anxiolytic effect of this SP antagonist would be observable in neonatal rats.

2. Materials and Methods

2.1. Subjects

Subjects were 194N:NIH Norway infant rats bred from the 46th generation of high and low lines in the Williams College Animal Facility, Williamstown, MA. Pregnant females were housed in clear plastic breeding cages (44 cm × 22 cm × 20 cm) after successful mating with a same-line male, in a room with a 12-hour light-dark cycle with ad libitum access to food and water. All testing was performed during the light cycle. Experiments were performed in accordance with the National Institutes of Health Guide for Care and Use of Laboratory Animals and were approved by the Institutional Care and Use Committee. Births were noted on postnatal day 0. Litters smaller than 6 or larger than 10 pups were not used.

2.2. Behavioral Testing

On postnatal day 7, the entire litter was brought to the testing room in a transfer cage, which was placed on a heating pad set at 32°C for 20 minutes. There were four experimental injections conditions: non-injected control, vehicle control, and two dose conditions of Spantide II. Four male and four female subjects were randomly selected from the litter; in some cases the litter did not have all possible subjects but for each litter, only one male and one female pup were tested per injection condition. Subjects were randomly assigned to experimental conditions and testing was also performed in a random order for condition and sex. Subjects (n = 49) in the vehicle condition received 2 μl intracerebroventricular (ICV) injections of saline. Experimental subjects received ICV 2 μl injections of either 10 pmol (n = 47) or 100 pmol (n = 43) of Spantide II obtained from Sigma Aldrich Chemical Company (St. Louis, MO). ICV injections were made using a glass Hamilton syringe (Cole Parmer, Chicago. IL) and a 30 gauge needle sharpened and beveled to a 22° angle tip. The needle was inserted 2 mm into the lateral ventricle at 1 mm lateral and dorsal to bregma; at this age landmarks are easily visible through the skin covering the skull. Control subjects (n = 55) received the same handling but no injection.

Subjects were individually placed in a flat-bottomed glass dish, 190 mm × 100 mm, directly under a capacitance microphone with a mylar diaphragm (S-25 ultrasound bat detector, Ultra Sound Advice, London) suspended from a clamp. This system was set to detect signals at 45 ± 5 kHz, and produced an audible signal in earphones worn by the experimenter, who could then manually count ultrasounds using a software counting program (OD Log). Calls were recorded for two minutes. Testing was conducted in an adjacent room under dim lighting.

2.3. Data Analysis

The effects of line, condition, and sex on USV number were evaluated with a three-factor Analysis of Variance (ANOVA), followed by LSD post-hoc testing where appropriate (criterion of $p < 0.05$). All analyses were conducted using IBM SPSS Statistics Version 21 (IBM Corp., Armonk, NY).

3. Results

There was a significant interaction between line and condition on the number of USVs emitted, $F(3,178) = 10.439$, $p < 0.001$), as shown in **Figure 1**. This interaction is explained by the finding that the effect of condition was only significant in the high line subjects; no significant effects of the drug were apparent in low line subjects. Post-hoc testing revealed that high line subjects in the 10 pmol and 100 pmol drug conditions emitted significantly fewer USVs than non-injected control and vehicle control subjects (p's < 0.001). The two control groups did not differ from each other. Interestingly, high line subjects injected with 10 pmol Spantide II called marginally less than those injected with a 100 pmol solution of the drug ($p < 0.07$).

There was a significant main effect of condition on the number of USVs, $F(3,178) = 7.929$, $p < 0.001$, an artifact due to the effects on the high line subjects. There was also a significant main effect of line on the number of USVs, $F(1,178) = 371.275$, $p < 0.001$). Since the high line rats were bred specifically for high rates of USVs after brief maternal separation, the mean number of USVs was expected to be significantly higher; across conditions, low line subjects (N = 80) emitted a mean of 32 calls per two minutes, while high line (N = 114) produced a mean of 201 USVs. There was no main effect of sex, not any interaction of sex with any other factor.

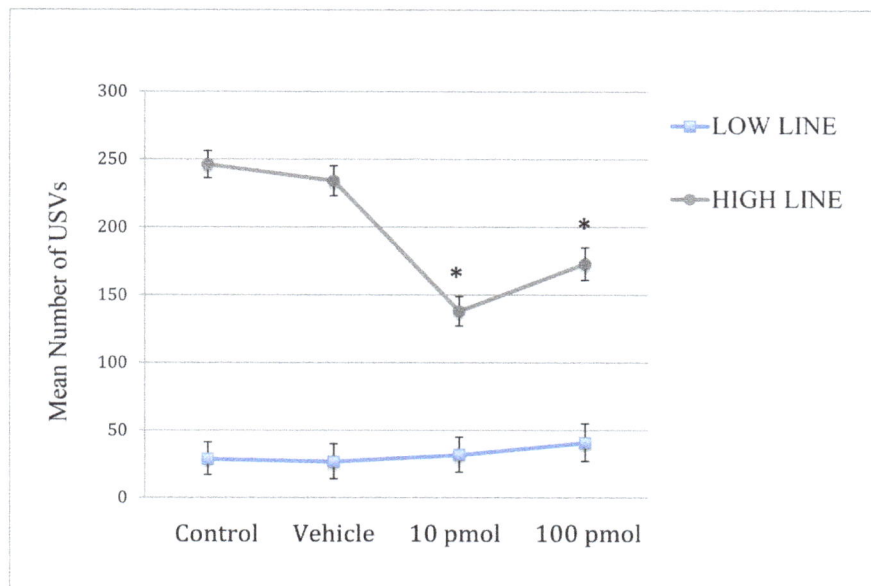

Figure 1. Mean USVs per two minutes (±SEM) for low and high line subjects injected with Spantide II at concentrations of 10 and 100 pmol, saline vehicle, or a no-injection control. *Significantly different from both control groups (p's < 0.001).

4. Discussion

A significant reduction of distress calls was observed in high line rats injected with either 10 pmol or 100 pmol Spantide II, as compared to control and vehicle groups. These results indicate that blocking NK1 receptors has an anxiolytic effect on subjects with high baseline anxiety levels. The failure of either dose of Spantide II to reduce USV rates in low line animals may be due to a line difference in density or subunit composition of NK1 receptors. Further investigation of the SP/NK1 system in this animal model might prove useful in determining this neurotransmitter system's role in stress and anxiety disorders.

The suggestion that the lower concentration (10 pmol) was more effective than the higher dose (100 pmol) of Spantide II parallels a similar finding in an earlier study in adult male rats. In that study, 10 pmol of Spantide II was more effective than 100 pmol in reversing the hippocampal excitability induced by infusions of SP [24]. In this study, the mean number of USV calls in the 10 pmol drug group decreased by 43% compared to the controls, and the USV rate for the 100 pmol group was reduced by 30%. The results also extend previous research on adult male rodents to neonatal subjects of both sexes. Although no sex effects were detected, it is possible that sex effects in response to NK1 antagonists would appear after puberty.

High line rats may be a useful model system for studying stress pathologies, since humans diagnosed with anxiety disorders exhibit above-average baseline stress responses. Highlighting the interaction between baseline affective temperament and drug response emphasizes the value of matching drug treatment with individual differences in affect. The high line also offers the advantage of high rates of anxiety behavior emitted without artificial induction. While previous experiments on NK1 antagonists have used electrical stimulation of brain areas involved in defensive responses [11] [12] or infusions of SP [10], the paradigm used in this study may better correspond to environmental stressors likely to be found in the course of normal daily activities. NK1 receptor antagonists may also be useful outside the realm of anxiety, as substance P has also been implicated in modulating depression in animal models and humans [10] [25].

5. Conclusion

The substance P/NK1 neurotransmitter system has been demonstrated to be active in regulating anxiety in neonatal rats, which might be clinically important in developing new medications for children with anxiety disorders. The anxiolytic effect of the SP antagonist Spantide II was also found to be dependent on the subject's affective state.

Acknowledgements

We thank the Groff Foundation for their support of this research. We thank Susan Brunelli and Myron Hofer for initiating the selective breeding of the high and low lines and their generosity in sharing this resource. We also thank Daniela Zarate for her technical support.

References

[1]   Baxter, A.J., Scott, K.M., Vos, T. and Whiteford, H.A. (2012) Global Prevalence of Anxiety Disorders: A Systematic Review and Meta-Regression. *Psychological Medicine*, **43**, 897-910. http://dx.doi.org/10.1017/S003329171200147X

[2]   Merikangas, K.R., He, J.P., Burstein, M., Swanson, S.A., Avenevoli, S., Cui, L., Benjet, C., Georgiades, K. and Swendsen, J. (2010) Lifetime Prevalence of Mental Disorders in U.S. Adolescents: Results from the National Comorbidity Survey Replication—Adolescent Supplement (NCS-A). *Journal of the American Academy of Child and Adolescent Psychiatry*, **49**, 980-989. http://dx.doi.org/10.1016/j.jaac.2010.05.017

[3]   Salum, G.A., Desousa, D.A., do Rosário, M.C., Pine, D.S. and Manfro, G.G. (2013) Pediatric Anxiety Disorders: From Neuroscience to Evidence-Based Clinical Practice. *Revista Brasileira de Psiquiatria*, **35**, S3-S21. http://dx.doi.org/10.1590/1516-4446-2013-S108

[4]   Ebner, K., Muigg, P., Singewald, G. and Singewald, N. (2008) Substance P in Stress and Anxiety: NK-1 Receptor Antagonism Interacts with Key Brain Areas of the Stress Circuitry. *Annals of the New York Academy of Sciences*, **1144**, 61-73. http://dx.doi.org/10.1196/annals.1418.018

[5]   Ebner, K. and Singewald, N. (2006) The Role of Substance P in Stress and Anxiety Responses. *Amino Acids*, **31**, 251-272. http://dx.doi.org/10.1007/s00726-006-0335-9

[6]   Mantyh, P.W. (2002) Neurobiology of Substance P and the NK1 Receptor. *Journal of Clinical Psychiatry*, **11**, 6-10.

[7]   De Araújo, J.E., Silva, R.C., Huston, J.P. and Brandão, M.L. (1999) Anxiogenic Effects of Substance P and Its 7-11 C Terminal, but Not the 1-7 N Terminal, Injected into the Dorsal Periaqueductal Gray. *Peptides*, **20**, 1437-1443. http://dx.doi.org/10.1016/S0196-9781(99)00154-0

[8]   Steimer, T. (2011) Animal Models of Anxiety Disorders in Rats and Mice: Some Conceptual Issues. *Dialogues in Clinical Neuroscience*, **13**, 495-506.

[9]   Bilkei-Gorzo, A. and Zimmer, A. (2005) Mutagenesis and Knockout Models: NK1 and Substance P. *Handbook of Experimental Pharmacology*, **169**, 143-162. http://dx.doi.org/10.1007/3-540-28082-0_5

[10] Kramer M.S., Cutler, N., Feighner, J., Shrivastava, R., Carman, J., Sramek, J.J., *et al.* (1998) Distinct Mechanism for Antidepressant Activity by Blockade of Central Substance P Receptors. *Science*, **281**, 1640-1645. http://dx.doi.org/10.1126/science.281.5383.1640

[11] Brenes, J.C., Broiz, A.C., Bassi, G.S., Schwarting, R.K.W. and Brandão, M.L. (2012) Involvement of Midbrain Tectum Neurokinin-Mediated Mechanisms in Fear and Anxiety. *Brazilian Journal of Medical and Biological Research*, **45**, 349-356. http://dx.doi.org/10.1590/S0100-879X2012007500030

[12] Carvalho, C., Santos, J.M., Bassi, G.S. and Brandão, M.L. (2013) Participation of NK1 Receptors of the Amygdala on the Processing of Different Types of Fear. *Neurobiology of Learning and Memory*, **102**, 20-27. http://dx.doi.org/10.1016/j.nlm.2013.03.004

[13] Allin, J.T. and Banks, E.M. (1972) Functional Aspects of Ultrasound Production by Infant Albino Rats (*Rattus norvegicus*). *Animal Behavior*, **20**, 175-185. http://dx.doi.org/10.1016/S0003-3472(72)80189-1

[14] Carden, S.E. and Hofer, M.A. (1990) Independence of Benzodiazepine and Opiate Action in the Suppression of Isolation Distress in Rat Pups. *Behavioral Neuroscience*, **104**, 160-166. http://dx.doi.org/10.1037/0735-7044.104.1.160

[15] Winslow, J.T. and Insel, T.R. (1991) The Infant Rat Separation Paradigm: A Novel Test for Novel Anxiolytics. *Trends in Pharmacological Sciences*, **12**, 402-404. http://dx.doi.org/10.1016/0165-6147(91)90616-Z

[16] Zimmerberg, B., Brunelli, S.A. and Hofer, M.A. (1994) Reduction of Rat Pup Ultrasonic Vocalizations by the Neuroactive Steroid Allopregnanolone. *Pharmacology, Biochemistry and Behavior*, **47**, 735-738. http://dx.doi.org/10.1016/0091-3057(94)90181-3

[17] Brunelli, S.A. (2005) Development and Evolution of Hidden Regulators: Selective Breeding for an Infantile Phenotype. *Developmental Psychobiology*, **47**, 243-252. http://dx.doi.org/10.1002/dev.20090

[18] Brunelli, S.A. and Hofer, M.A. (2007) Selective Breeding for Infant Rat Separation-Induced Ultrasonic Vocalizations: Developmental Precursors of Passive and Active Coping Styles. *Behavioural Brain Research*, **182**, 193-207. http://dx.doi.org/10.1016/j.bbr.2007.04.014

[19] Zimmerberg, B., Brunelli, S.A., Fluty, A.J. and Frye, C.A. (2005) Differences in Affective Behaviors and Hippocampal Allopregnanolone Levels in Adult Rats of Lines Selectively Bred for Infantile Vocalizations. *Behavioral Brain Re-

search, **159**, 301-311. http://dx.doi.org/10.1016/j.bbr.2004.11.009

[20] Schwarting, R.K.W. and Wöhr, M. (2012) On the Relationships between Ultrasonic Calling and Anxiety-Related Behavior in Rats. *Brazilian Journal of Medical and Biological Research*, **45**, 337-348. http://dx.doi.org/10.1590/S0100-879X2012007500038

[21] de Gomes, V., Hassan, W., Maisonnette, S., Johnson, L.R., Ramos, A. and Landeira-Fernandez, J. (2013) Behavioral Evaluation of Eight Rat Lines Selected for High and Low Anxiety-Related Responses. *Behavioural Brain Research*, **257**, 39-48. http://dx.doi.org/10.1016/j.bbr.2013.09.028

[22] Håkanson, R., Leander, S., Asano, N., Feng, D.M. and Folkers, K. (1990) Spantide II, a Novel Tachykinin Antagonist Having High Potency and Low Histamine-Releasing Effect. *Regulatory Peptides*, **31**, 75-82. http://dx.doi.org/10.1016/0167-0115(90)90197-5

[23] Glascock, J.J., Osman, E.Y., Coady, T.H., Rose, F.F., Shababi, M. and Lorson, C.L. (2011) Delivery of Therapeutic Agents through Intracerebroventricular (ICV) and Intravenous (IV) Injection in Mice. *Journal of Visualized Experiments*, **56**, 2968. http://dx.doi.org/10.3791/2968

[24] Liu, H., Mazarati, A.M., Katsumori, H., Sankar, R. and Wasterlain, C.G. (1999) Substance P Is Expressed in Hippocampal Principal Neurons during Status Epilepticus and Plays a Critical Role in the Maintenance of Status Epilepticus. *Proceedings of the National Academy of Sciences of the United States of America*, **96**, 5286-5291. http://dx.doi.org/10.1073/pnas.96.9.5286

[25] Bondy, B., Baghai, T.C., Minov, C., Schule, C., Schwarz, M.J., Zwanzger, P., *et al.* (2003) Substance P Serum Levels Are Increased in Major Depression: Preliminary Results. *Biological Psychiatry*, **53**, 538-542. http://dx.doi.org/10.1016/S0006-3223(02)01544-5

Prevalence of Depression and Anxiety Disorders in Peri-Natal Sudanese Women and Associated Risks Factors

Abdelgadir H. Osman[1*], Taissier Y. Hagar[2], Abdelaziz A. Osman[2], Hussein Suliaman[3]

[1]Department of Psychiatry, Faculty of Medicine University of Khartoum, Khartoum, Sudan
[2]Formerly Registrar in Sudan Medical Council, Currently Specialists in Saudi Arabia
[3]Khartoum Neuropsychiatric Centre, Khartoum, Sudan
Email: [*]abdelgadir1159@yahoo.com

Abstract

The purpose of this study was to estimate a point prevalence of depression and anxiety disorders among Sudanese peri-natal women attending ant-natal and postnatal clinics in the capital city of Sudan. Simultaneously, to examine the associated risks factors. Participants were 945 peri-natal women in two main women antenatal and post natal clinics in the Capital City of Sudan screened consecutively. They were divided into two groups. The first group was of, Four Hundreds eighty (480) women in their third trimester, and the second group consisted of Four Hundreds Sixty Five (465) women in the first 10 week of postnatal period. All participants were screened, using Beck Depression Inventory (BDI), Hospital Anxiety and Depression scale (HADS), and Personal information Questionnaire (PIQ) for collecting socio-demographic, personal, medical, social and family history data. Routine urine and blood results were recorded. Results: 59% of prenatal and 46% of postnatal women suffered from high levels of distress in the form of mixed anxiety and depressive symptoms. However, only 20.9% of peri-natal women suffered of moderate to severe depression. Over 90% of the depressed women were not formally diagnosed or received psychiatric help. Poor marital relationship, physical co-morbidity, positive family history and past psychiatric history of depression were the main significant risk factors associated with perinatal depression and anxiety. Conclusion: Contrary to the commonly held views that perinatal women are mainly plighted with depression as the main mental illness, this study confirms initial findings that, anxiety disorder is far more prevalent and more distressing to this vulnerable group. Moreover, psychiatric morbidities in both prenatal and postnatal periods attract high prevalence rates in low income countries. Maternal health policies in low income countries must incorporate routine screening for mental health status, basic support and interventions for mental illnesses in perinatal women. Depression and emotional disorders in perinatal women should be seen as important public health priority.

---

[*]Corresponding author.

Prevalence of Depression and Anxiety Disorders in Peri-Natal Sudanese Women...

113

Keywords

Prenatal, Postnatal, Peri-Natal, Depression, Anxiety, Psychiatric Morbidities, Risks Factors

1. Background

Symptoms of anxiety and depressive disorders in perinatal women have received considerable attention in high income countries over the last three decades. However, little attention and limited resources, if any, were directed to this group, in low income countries. Only a few prevalence studies were conducted in low income countries to examine the prevalence of the common mental disorders in perinatal women and especially so in Africa, Sudan included [1] [2].

Peri-natal depression has long been recognized to be associated with a number of risks factors such as genetic vulnerability, hormonal changes, major life events, psychosocial stressors and past and present medical complication [3]-[5]. High stress during pregnancy can increase susceptibility to maternal infections by mechanisms that inhibit components of the immune system, also lead to premature delivery and post natal complications [5]-[7]. Post natal depression however, has been associated with low infant body weight, higher infant physical morbidity including diarrhea, vitamin deficiencies weaker mother baby bond and risk of maternal suicide [8]-[12].

Despite all the high maternal and infant morbidity as a consequence to maternal mental health problems, yet the total number of all the prevalence studies that were conducted in Africa did not exceed a total of 11,000 cases, at a recent systemic review of prevalence of depression in perinatal women in Africa [1] [13] [14]. Most studies on perinatal women and mental health disorders have focused on depression and depressive disorders in this sensitive period, rightly so. However, little attention has been given to high rate and distressing symptoms of anxiety which has by itself significant consequences to both mother and baby's health. This can only be unraveled, by using appropriate tools to pick up this condition [15]-[17].

Prevalence findings for anxiety disorders in prenatal and postnatal women attracted rates between 10% - 20% which can either be purely anxiety disorder or mixed anxiety depressive symptoms with anxiety features predominating the psychiatric presentation. Therefore, both anxiety and depression warrant appropriate attention and investigation by researchers and women's mental health strategists [18] [19].

There is conflicting evidence as to whether or not symptoms of anxiety deserve separate attention in the perinatal period, as it might be seen as part of a depressive spectrum by some researchers [20].

Many recent researchers have investigated the initial reported risk factors by Kendal *et al.* in 1976, with anxiety during pregnancy, viz, poor quality of intimate relationship, previous episodes of depression and anxiety, perinatal obstetric complications, positive family history of depression, past history of depression and general low annual income [21] [22]. However, many studies consistently found that past psychiatric history of depression, strong family history of depressive disorder and poor quality of intimate relationship or violence were the strongest risk factors for perinatal depression and mostly so for post natal depression. However, some other risk factors such as presence of high anxiety symptoms during pregnancy as, predictor and risk factor for future development of post natal depression received less attention [23]. Likewise, health factors such as low hemoglobin levels, chronic physical co-morbidity, the number of already born children, job and employment status and presence or absence of family support received less attention in perinatal psychiatric studies [24].

2. Method

2.1. Subjects

Subjects were consecutively collected from two main antenatal clinics at Khartoum Teaching Hospital, and Omdurman antenatal clinic. These two clinics serve a large catchment areas of around 2 million population and overseen by obstetricians, midwives *and senior University consultant obstetricians. Inclusion criteria were designed to include all women who presented to the antenatal clinics in their 3rd trimester in the period between, 1st of June to 30th of September* 2009. Written informed consents to participate in the study in Arabic were obtained. The only exclusion criteria was language barrier for only a few women that didn't speak clear Arabic or

Sudanese dialect leading to clear communication barriers.

Total of 945 consecutive candidate satisfying inclusion criteria were interviewed by trained psychiatric registrars and clinical psychologists.

480 Prenatal women in their third trimester, and 465 postnatal women in the 2nd to 10th week of the postnatal period, had been interviewed in the specified research period.

Separate postnatal clinics exists, serving the same territory, therefore all postnatal women were interviewed at these clinics, as they arrived to see their midwives and health visitors for routine checkup. Most of postnatal women presented between the second and the 10th week of their post natal period (90% were between the 4th to 8th week post delivery).

2.2. Assessments

Six research psychologists and two psychiatrists received three days training on applying interview questionnaires. Most of inter-rater differences were ironed out during training. Then, a pilot phase was carried out in the first two weeks prior to commencement of the study phase which revealed 96.5% of inter-rater reliability for all instruments used for the study. Three instruments were used to collect relevant information.

The first questionnaire was Personal information Questionnaire (PIQ) used to obtain detailed social demographic information about candidates with special reference to, important personal, family, past and present psychiatric history and physical morbidities beside social stressors and circumstances. There was special section for recording hemoglobin and urine results obtained on the same day.

The second questionnaire was a standardized Hospital anxiety and Depression scale (HADS) to report on symptoms of anxiety and depression with this instrument, indicating distress level.

HADS is a self report scale, contains 14 items rated on 4-point Likert-type scale. HADS, has, subscales assess depression and anxiety. The seven-items for either depression or anxiety, yields a score of 0 - 21 that is interrupted with the following cut points: 0 - 7, normal; 8 - 10, mild mood disturbance; 11 - 14, moderate mood disturbance; and 12 - 21, severe mood disturbance [25].

However, a third questionnaire, Beck Depression Inventory (BDI), was used to validate the reported depressive symptoms and obtained by (HADS). The other reason for using BDI was to report on the degree and intensity of the depressive illness. BDI, it's also Likert-type scale, of 21 items, reports symptoms from 0 - 3 (0 meaning symptom not existing, 3, the symptom is sever). BDI, yields score from 0 - 63. The score for moderate depression is 18 - 23, whilst 23 and over indicate severe depression [26].

HADS scale has been validated to be a sensitive instrument to detect symptoms of anxiety and depression, compared with the widely used, Edinburgh Depression Inventory (EDI), which is only sensitive for depressive disorders in perinatal period. Both HADS and BDI instruments have been validated in the Sudanese culture.

The study protocol was approved by the Ethics and research Committee of the University. Written authorizations were obtained from relevant health authorities, beside individual patient's written informed consents.

2.3. Statistical Analysis

All information obtained was entered on the statistical package for social science (SPSS) version 15. Chi square and T-test were calculated for all subjects as per results.

3. Results

3.1. Social Demographic Characteristics

Table 1 gives important socio-demographic characteristics of our participants. 566 (59.9%) of the participants were under the age of 35, 492 (52.1%) finished school before university level while 59 (6.4%) were illiterate. 730 (77.3%) were housewives, that, had previously worked or never worked. 583 (61.7%) of the subjects reported low socio economic background as defined by comparative criteria for an average income in Sudanese community *i.e.* the total family income per year is less than 2500 dollars per year (as defined by Sudanese Social Security and Welfare office). 489 (51.1%) had, had no supporting hand from relatives or other sources to help with the running of the household apart from husbands. While 476 (49%) of the participants had a close relative such as a mother, or a sister, regularly giving them a hand for the household chores and with kids support. It is part of Sudanese culture to have a close relative or senior female relative moving in to live with the pregnant woman prior to giving birth and shortly afterwards to support the family. It is customary that such relative will offer sympathy, and support to the young mother. Most women were of multi-parity (had more than one previously born child), with an average of 2.3 children at the household.

3.2. Clinical Characteristics

Table 2 and **Table 3** show 496 (52.5%) of our perinatal women *i.e.* antenatal and post natal showed high levels of distress (either depression/anxiety, or mixed condition) as reflected by, HADS questionnaire with a threshold above 12 as a cutoff point which denoting clinical threshold from mild to moderate for both anxiety and depression whilst, 449 (47.5%) did not manifest with clinically significant symptoms of anxiety or depression. Prenatal women in particular showed high levels of distress and anxiety (59%) **Table 4**, but only 24% of them presented with clinically significant symptoms of depression as per Becks results, **Table 5** and **Table 6**.

Table 1. Demographics characteristics.

	Number	percentage %
25 - 35 years of age	566	59.9%
Undergraduates	492	52.1%
Illiterates	59	6.4%
Housewives	730	77.3%
Low socioeconomic background	583	61.7%
No helping hand at home apart from the husband	489	51.1%
Average no. of children	2.33	

Table 2. Risks factors leading to high symptoms of mixed anxiety and depression.

	Number of Children		Marital relationship			Past psychiatric		Family history of depression		Physical co-morbidity with pregnancy	
	0 - 4	5 - 10	Good	Average	Poor	Yes	No	Yes	No	Yes	No
Normal	162	34	208	14	1	13	205	13	203	23	174
Mild	185	17	219	4	0	23	202	12	217	21	161
Moderate	205	21	251	18	0	38	233	24	239	38	192
Severe	176	28	184	40	4	42	189	31	188	48	148
Total	728	100	862	76	5	116	829	80	847	130	675

$$X^2 = 50.99 \ DF = 30 \ P = 0.010 \ X^2 = 51.1 \ DF = 6. \ P = 0000 \ X^2 = 15.9, DF = 3, P = 0.001 \ X^2 = 13.8 \ DF = 3, P = 0.003$$

Table 3. Shows distribution of Psychiatric disorder in perinatal period.

	Number	Percentage
HADS	497	52.6%
Beck	198	20.9%

Table 4. Shows prevalence of mixed anxiety and depressive symptoms in prenatal and postnatal period using HADS.

	Prenatal		Postnatal	
	Number	Percentage	Number	Percentage
Normal	87	18.10%	139	30%
Mild	110	22.90%	112	24%
Moderate	149	31%	121	26%
severe	134	28%	93	20%
Total	480	100%	465	100%

Table 5. Positive risk factors for depression with BDI.

	Marital relationship			Past history of depression		Family history of psychiatric illness		Organic illness	
	Good	Average	Poor	Yes	No	Yes	No	Yes	No
Normal	394	18	0	29	384	28	383	42	329
Mild	306	26	0	48	334	27	303	46	226
Moderate	118	18	4	22	140	15	115	30	82
Severe	44	14	0	16	57	10	45	11	38
Total	862	76	4	115	829	89	846	129	675

$X^2 = 55.6$ DF = 6 P = 0.000 $X^2 = 26.9$, DF = 3, P = 0.000 $X^2 = 9.6$ DF = 3 P = 0.023 $X^2 = 17.4$ DF = 3 P = 0.001

Table 6. Shows prevalence of depressive symptoms in prenatal and postnatal period using BECK.

	Prenatal		Postnatal	
	Number	Percentage	Number	Percentage
Normal	182	37.9%	237	51%
Mild-borderline	183	38.10%	149	32%
moderate	81	17%	56	12%
severe	34	7%	23	5%
Total	480	100%	465	100%

3.3. Comparing Prenatal versus Postnatal Morbidities

When, both anxiety and depression were dichotomized to case and non case, taking 12 score as cut off points on the HADS for anxiety and depression, (which were previously validated in Sudanese culture), (**Table 4**), this, revealed that, 383 (59%) of prenatal women showed clinically significant results for both anxiety and depression. On the other hands, 214 (46%), as reflected in HADS, results for postnatal women (**Table 4**).

However, only 115 (24%) of prenatal women presented with clinically significant score for depression of a moderate and severe degree, and 79 (17%) of postnatal women attracted high score results for moderate to severe depression as manifested on the Beck Depression Inventory (BDI), **Table 6**.

3.4. Risk Factors and Associations (Table 7)

Poor marital relationship emerged as a major risk factor for developing both antenatal depression and anxiety as well as post natal, with p-value below 0.0001. Physical co-morbidity with pregnancy came as a second factor especially for a combination of anxiety and depression when it is taken as a spectrum with a p-value of 0.001 as reflected in the HADS test, **Table 7**. Other significant associations were past psychiatric history of depression and anxiety and positive family history for psychiatric illness with a p-value of 0.001, and 0.003 consecutively. Women who had more than 3 children showed higher symptoms for anxiety and depression with a p-value of 0.01, whilst, whether the mother was working or holding a job at the time of her pregnancy or shortly afterwards did not manifest as a major risk factor for depression or anxiety. Educational level whether illiterate or post graduate did not bear any correlation to probability of developing anxiety or depression, nor seen as a protective factor. On the other hand the three most significant factors for developing severe depression for, both pre-natal and postnatal women, were poor marital relationship, past psychiatric illness (both P values below 0.001), and family history of psychiatric illness **Table 7**.

4. Discussion

This study found high prevalence of both anxiety and depression for antenatal (59%) and post natal (46%) women more than previously thought. These disorders were assessed by the HADS test as it was previously noted by O'Hara *et al.* (1990). A diagnosis of depression is only one index of psychological distress which could be rather insensitive and may be more useful to identify psychological distress in the perinatal period with the

Table 7. Collated P values for all risks factors.

Risk Factors	P value against HADS	P value as Per BDI
Poor marital relationship	0.000	0.000
Urine general	0.000	0.009
Co-morbidity with pregnancy	0.001	0.001
Past history of psychiatric illness	0.001	0.000
Family history of psychiatric illness	0.003	0.023
Number of Children	0.010	0.010
Type of co-morbidity	0.020	0.001
Occupation	0.026	
Educational level	0.036	

use of an instrument capable of tapping a common core or psychological impairment. We believe that the HADS test is both sensitive and valid for tapping high levels of distress in perinatal period which reflects the higher result found in this study [27].

Most studies on perinatal psychiatric prevalence didn't take into account the strong co-morbidity between depressive mood and anxiety disorders. Therefore, one of the aims of the present study is to report on the prevalence of these two conditions together and, separate in perinatal periods. Moreover, this study examined a wide range of risk factors that had been noted by different researchers elsewhere.

Principal Findings

This study identified two categories of associated risk factors for perinatal emotional disorders (depression and anxiety), confirmed the widely known risks factors for depression that may occur at any period in a woman's life, such as associated perceived lack of social support or hostility from intimate husband, past psychiatric history of depression or anxiety and family history of depression or anxiety.

However, this study, revealed, a second category of risks factors that are relatively specific to peri-natal emotional disorders such as, physical co-morbidity in the prenatal period, anemia and presence of high psychological distress at the first and second trimester of pregnancy.

Most importantly, we reported, higher rates of psychiatric morbidity, than previously thought, in the form of general distress (stress, anxiety, and depression) at the prenatal period up (59%), and 46% for postnatal period, leading to detrimental health consequence for both the mother and her baby.

Moreover, we were able to discover that, most of this high rates of distress did not receive any formal recognition or treatment via the psychiatric system, (90% of cases) that were found to have moderate to severe mood disorders had not received any formal mental health treatment. Therefore, the distress was endured by the sufferer unrecognized or diagnosed and not treated or supported by mental health team in the developing countries, as was the case in Sudan. Many factors can be cited to this failure, of provisions and recognition for mental ill-health of peri-natal women, not least, due to, stigma associated with mental illness, but, also one can cite other factors, such, as, ignorance, and limitations of resources.

It's worth noting that, contrary to the widely believed vulnerability factor for depression, this study could not detect association of mental morbidity with type of employment or the lack of it, level of education a woman might have attained, or presence or absence of a family support extra to that of the partner. Although, the findings of this paper suggest that dimensional or categorical anxiety is a major risk factor for post natal depression. However, interpretation of the two conditions were hampered by methodological limitations such as, being, relatively small sample size, a cross sectional study, and, lacked adjustment for confounding factors.

Strengths and Weaknesses

This study examined a large number of cases, more that most studies conducted in developing countries, that is to say 945 candidate, and was able to tap on categorical findings of perinatal depression and anxiety.

Among the weaknesses of this study, the inherent problem of being a cross sectional study, one would want to see a longitudinal cohort findings after the initial assessment. Moreover a more structured and standardized assessment tool such as, SCID (Structured Clinical Interview Schedule) would have revealed more elaborate and specific psychiatric diagnosis than HADS and BDI would have allowed.

Declaration of Interest

None.

References

[1] Sawyer, A., Ayers, S. and Smith, H. (2010) Pre- and Postnatal Psychological Wellbeing in Africa: A Systematic Review. *Journal of Affective Disorders*, **123**, 17-29. http://dx.doi.org/10.1016/j.jad.2009.06.027

[2] O'Hara, M.W. and Swain, A.M. (1996) Rates and Risks of Postpartum Depression—A Meta-Analysis. *International Review of Psychiatry*, **8**, 37-54. http://dx.doi.org/10.3109/09540269609037816

[3] Eberhard-Gran, M., Eskild, A., Tambs, K., Samuelsen, S.O. and Opjordsmoen, S (2002) Depression in Postpartum and Non-Postpartum Women: Prevalence and Risk Factors. *Acta Psychiatrica Scandinavica*, **106**, 426-433http://dx.doi.org/10.1034/j.1600-0447.2002.02408.x

[4] O'Hara, M.W., Schlechte, J.A., Lewis, D.A. and Varner, M.W. (1991) Controlled Prospective Study of Postpartum Mood Disorders: Psychological, Environmental, and Hormonal Variables. *Journal of Abnormal Psychology*, **100**, 63-73. http://dx.doi.org/10.1037/0021-843X.100.1.63

[5] Faisal-Cury, A., Tedesco, J.J.A., Kahhale, S., Menezes, P.R. and Zugaib, M. (2004) Postpartum Depression: In Relation to Life Events and Patterns of Coping. *Archives of Women's Mental Health*, **7**, 123-131. http://dx.doi.org/10.1007/s00737-003-0038-0

[6] Fisher, J.R.W., Morrow, M.M., Nhu Ngoc, N.T. and Hoang Anhc, L.T. (2004) Prevalence, Nature, Severity and Correlates of Postpartum Depressive Symptoms in Vietnam. *BJOG*, **111**, 1353-1360. http://dx.doi.org/10.1111/j.1471-0528.2004.00394.x

[7] Gausia, K., Fisher, C., Ali, M. and Oosthuizen, J. (2009) Magnitude and Contributory Factors of Postnatal Depression: A Community-Based Cohort Study from a Rural Subdistrict of Bangladesh. *Psychological Medicine*, **39**, 999-1007. http://dx.doi.org/10.1017/S0033291708004455

[8] Patel, V., DeSouza, N. and Rodrigues, M. (2003) Postnatal Depression and Infant Growth and Development in Low-Income Countries: A Cohort Study from Goa, India. *Archives of Disease in Childhood*, **88**, 34-37. http://dx.doi.org/10.1136/adc.88.1.34

[9] Lack, M.M., Baqu, A.H., Zaman, K., McNary, S.W., Le, K., El Arifeen, S., *et al.* (2007) Depressive Symptoms among Rural Bangladeshi Mothers: Implications for Infant Development. *Journal of Child Psychology and Psychiatry*, **48**, 764-772. http://dx.doi.org/10.1111/j.1469-7610.2007.01752.x

[10] Evans, J., Heron, J., Patel, R.R. and Wiles, N. (2007) Depressive Symptoms during Pregnancy and Low Birth Weight at Term: Longitudinal Study. *The British Journal of Psychiatry*, **191**, 84-85. http://dx.doi.org/10.1192/bjp.bp.105.016568

[11] Orr, S.T., James, S.A. and Blackmore Prince, C. (2002) Maternal Prenatal Depressive Symptoms and Spontaneous Preterm Births among African-American Women in Baltimore, Maryland. *American Journal of Epidemiology*, **156**, 797-802. http://dx.doi.org/10.1093/aje/kwf131

[12] Murray, L., Cooper, P.J., Wilson, A., *et al.* (2003) Controlled Trial of the Short- and Long-Term Effect of Psychological Treatment of Post-Partum Depression: 2. Impact on the Mother-Child Relationship and Child Outcome. *British Journal of Psychiatry*, **182**, 420-427. http://dx.doi.org/10.1192/bjp.182.5.420

[13] Agoub, M., Moussaoui, D. and Battas, O. (2005) Prevalence of Postpartum Depression in a Moroccan Sample. *Archives of Women's Mental Health*, **8**, 37-43. http://dx.doi.org/10.1007/s00737-005-0069-9

[14] Mirza, I. and Jenkins, R. (2004) Risk Factors, Prevalence, and Treatment of Anxiety and Depressive Disorders in Pakistan: Systematic Review. *BMJ*, **328**, 794-797. http://dx.doi.org/10.1136/bmj.328.7443.794

[15] Eberhard-Gran, M., Tambs, K., Opjordsmoen, S., Skrondal, A. and Eskild, A. (2003) A Comparison of Anxiety and Depressive Symptomatology in Postpartum and Non-Postpartum Mothers. *Social Psychiatry and Psychiatric Epidemiology*, **38**, 551-556. http://dx.doi.org/10.1007/s00127-003-0679-3

[16] Klein, D.N., Lewinsohn, P.M., Rohde, P., Seeley, J.R. and Shankman, S.A. (2003) Family Study of Co-Morbidity between Major Depressive Disorder and Anxiety Disorders. *Psychological Medicine*, **33**, 703-714. http://dx.doi.org/10.1017/S0033291703007487

[17] Littleton, H.L., Breitkopf, C.R. and Berenson, A.B. (2007) Correlates of Anxiety Symptoms during Pregnancy and Association with Perinatal Outcomes: A Meta-Analysis. *American Journal of Obstetrics and Gynecology*, **196**, 424-432. http://dx.doi.org/10.1016/j.ajog.2007.03.042

[18] Meades, R. and Ayers, S. (2011) Anxiety Measures Validated in Perinatal Populations: A Systematic Review. *Journal of Affective Disorders*, **133**, 1-15.

[19] Lau, Y. and Keung, D.W. (2007) Correlates of Depressive Symptomatology during the Second Trimester of Pregnancy among Hong Kong Chinese. *Social Science & Medicine*, **64**, 1802-1811. http://dx.doi.org/10.1016/j.socscimed.2007.01.001

[20] Bolton, H.L., Hughes, P.M., Turton, P. and Sedgwick, P. (1998) Incidence and Demographic Correlates of Depressive Symptoms during Pregnancy in an Inner London Population. *Journal of Psychosomatic Obstetrics & Gynecology*, **19**, 202-209. http://dx.doi.org/10.3109/01674829809025698

[21] Husain, N., Bevc, I., Husain, M., Chaudhry, I.B., Atif, N. and Rahman, A. (2006) Prevalence and Social Correlates of Postnatal Depression in a Low Income Country. *Archives of Women's Mental Health*, **9**, 197-202.

[22] Abiodun, O.A., Adetoro, O.O. and Ogunbode, O.O. (1993) Psychiatric Morbidity in a Pregnant Population in Nigeria. *General Hospital Psychiatry*, **15**, 125-128. http://dx.doi.org/10.1016/0163-8343(93)90109-2

[23] Rahman, A., Iqbal, Z. and Harrington, R. (2003) Life Events, Social Support and Depression in Childbirth: Perspectives from a Rural Community in the Developing World. *Psychological Medicine*, **33**, 1161-1167. http://dx.doi.org/10.1017/S0033291703008286

[24] Kumar, R. and Robson, K. (1984) A Prospective Study of Emotional Disorders in Childbearing Women. *The British Journal of Psychiatry*, **144**, 35-47. http://dx.doi.org/10.1192/bjp.144.1.35

[25] Snaith, R.P. and Zigmond, A.S. (1994) The Hospital Anxiety and Depression Scale Manual. Nfer-Nelson, Windsor.

[26] Beck, A.T. (1993) Beck Depression Inventory Manual. Psychological Corporation, San Antonio.

[27] Bjelland, I., Dahl, A.A., Haug, T.T. and Neckelmann, D. (2002) The Validity of the Hospital Anxiety and Depression Scale. An Updated Literature Review. *Journal of Psychosomatic Research*, **52**, 69-77. http://dx.doi.org/10.1016/S0022-3999(01)00296-3

Antidepressant Prescribing Patterns for Depressive and Anxiety Disorders in a Singapore Hospital

Teck Hwee Soh[1], Leslie Lim[1*], Herng Nieng Chan[1], Yiong Huak Chan[2]

[1]Department of Psychiatry, Singapore General Hospital, Singapore
[2]National University Health System, Singapore
Email: *leslie.lim.e.c@sgh.com.sg

Abstract

Objective: Although antidepressants are the recommended first-line pharmacological treatments for depressive and anxiety disorders, their prescribing patterns have not been studied in Singapore. We investigate antidepressant prescription patterns for outpatients with depressive and anxiety disorders in a general hospital in Singapore. We hypothesize that intolerance to side effects and lack of efficacy may contribute to medication switching, and that initiation of antidepressant therapy is not easily tolerated. Methods: A retrospective review of the casenotes of outpatients was carried out between January 2013 and December 2013. A total of 206 patients were randomly selected. The study was approved by the hospital's institutional review board. Data analysis was carried out using SPSS version 18. Results: There were more females than males (ratio 1.7:1) with a mean age of 50.6 ± 15.2 years. Depressive disorder, comprising 50% of the sample, was the most frequent diagnosis followed by anxiety disorder (27.2%), mixed anxiety-depression (16%) and adjustment disorder (5.8%). Almost all patients (97.1%) were prescribed antidepressants, the most common being selective serotonin reuptake inhibitors (SSRI) (75.5%), followed by the noradrenaline and specific serotonin antidepressant (NaSSA) (13.5%) and tricyclic antidepressants (TCA) (8.5%). Patients prescribed SSRIs tended to be younger and better educated (p = 0.0005). More than half of the patients (52.1%) required antidepressant switching mainly due to lack of efficacy and intolerance of side effects. Combination therapy was prescribed for 17% of patients with SSRI-NaSSA, the most preferred combination. Nearly a quarter (23.8%) patients required augmentation therapy with atypical antipsychotics. Combination (p = 0.024) and augmentation (p = 0.033) were utilized more often for depression than for anxiety disorders. Conclusion: Antidepressant medications are commonly prescribed for depression and anxiety disorders. The main reasons for switching antidepressants were intolerance and lack of efficacy. That about half of the patients reported side effects necessitating medication change confirmed our hypothesis that an-

---

*Corresponding author.

tidepressant therapy was not easy to initiate. This has important implications for treatment adherence and outcome.

Keywords

Antidepressants, Anxiety Disorders, Depressive Disorders, Augmentation, Combination, Switching

---

1. Introduction

Antidepressant prescribing patterns have shown an increasing trend over the years [1] [2]. These medications are recommended first-line treatments for depressive and anxiety disorders [1] [3]. According to published evidence, it would appear that selective serotonin reuptake inhibitors have become the most commonly prescribed class of antidepressant drugs worldwide [1]-[5]. The clinician's decision on which antidepressant to prescribe is complex and multifactorial, with the ultimate choice affected by patient factors and psychosocial reasons [6]. Tolerability and efficacy of medications influence patient adherence and this in turn affects treatment outcomes. Should these agents be less than effective in achieving remission? Successful augmentation with lithium [7] buspirone [8], bupropion [9], and atypical antipsychotic agents [10] has been documented. Combination with mirtazapine has been supported on the basis of a randomized placebo control trial [11]. In cases of treatment resistant depression and anxiety disorders, a variety of therapeutic options have been proposed [12]-[14].

However, there is scant data on the usage of antidepressants in South East Asia. A multi-centered international study on antidepressant prescription patterns in East Asia in 2007 showed that selective serotonin reuptake inhibitors (SSRIs) were the most commonly prescribed antidepressants [15]. This finding was corroborated by other authors who also found that SSRIs formed the majority of prescriptions [16].

This study seeks to investigate the prescribing patterns of antidepressants for psychiatric outpatients with depressive and anxiety disorders in a general hospital psychiatric department in Singapore, with particular reference to switching, combination and augmentation therapy.

We hypothesize that side effect intolerance and lack of efficacy may contribute to switching before arriving at the final choice of antidepressant. Antidepressant class, whether singly or combined, details of augmentation strategy, and reasons for switching facilitate understanding as to why patients/ doctors prefer/reject one antidepressant over another. Such information is invaluable for the guidance of trainee psychiatrists in this country.

2. Methods

The study is a retrospective case record review of outpatients attending psychiatric clinics at the Department of Psychiatry in the Singapore General Hospital. This is the largest general hospital in the country and also serves as a teaching hospital for undergraduates and postgraduate students and residents.

The study sample included patients attending outpatient follow up between January 2013 and December 2013. A random sampling of one in 5 case records of patients was performed.

Patients with the following DSM-IV-TR conditions were included in the study: Depressive disorder with or without psychotic features, anxiety disorders, mixed anxiety-depressive disorder, adjustment disorder (with depressive mood, or anxious mood or mixed anxious and depressed mood). Patients who satisfied the aforementioned inclusion criteria but who had medical comorbidities or a diagnosis of personality disorder were included in the study. Those with any of the following conditions: primary psychotic disorder with secondary depression, bipolar disorder, schizoaffective disorder, other conditions with secondary depression/anxiety, substance induced conditions, organic brain conditions, and eating disorders were excluded.

The following data were collected, viz. socio-demographic characteristics, clinical diagnosis, antidepressants prescribed, and reasons for medication choices. The data collection forms were anonymized without identifiers. Any ambiguity was resolved by consensus among the investigators at meetings chaired by the second author, who is also a senior clinician in the department.

All department psychiatrists were notified of the study and written approval obtained from the prescribing doctors for investigators to study the case records of their patients. None of the treating psychiatrists was involved in data collection to avoid the possibility of bias, or conflict of interest. The study was approved by the hospital's Centralised Institutional Review Board (CIRB).

Statistical Analysis

Data was analyzed using the Statistical Package for Social Sciences (SPSS) version 18 (SPSS Inc, Chicago). Descriptive statistics were performed to tabulate the socio-demographic characteristics of the sample. Frequency data was analyzed using the Fisher exact probability test, while continuous variables were analyzed using Student's unpaired t-test. A p-value of less than 0.05 was considered significant.

3. Results

A total of 206 patients were randomly sampled from the pool of patients. The socio-demographic characteristics are presented in **Table 1**.

There were 131 females (63.6%). The majority ethnic group was Chinese (86.9%), with age range 20-88 years, and mean age 50.6 ± 15.2 years for the whole sample. Majority of the patients (70.9%) were married. Most had some form of education, with only 5.3% having no formal education. Almost half (46.1%) had tertiary education.

The clinical characteristics of the sample are presented in **Table 2**. The predominant diagnosis was depressive disorder in 50% of the sample, followed by anxiety disorder in about a quarter (27.2%). The rest of the patients were diagnosed with mixed anxiety-depressive disorder (16%) and adjustment disorder (5.8%).

The duration of illness for most of the patients was between 1 to 5 years (52.9%), while 11.7% were ill for more than 10 years and 6.8% for less than one year.

Previous medical or surgical history was reported by 68.4% of patients. The 3 most common medical comorbidities were cardiovascular, gastrointestinal and metabolic/endocrine conditions, respectively.

3.1. Prescription Pattern of Antidepressants

As shown in **Table 3**, almost all patients (97.1%) received antidepressant medication with SSRIs, the most commonly prescribed (75.5%), followed by NaSSA (13.5%) and TCAs (8.5%). Patients prescribed SSRIs upon initiation of treatment tended to be younger (p = 0.0005) and to have at least secondary level education (p = 0.00017). (Please refer to **Table 4**).

3.2. Switching

Switching to another antidepressant was carried out for more than half (52.1%) of the patients. The main reason for switching was lack of efficacy (36.7%), side effects (30.3%) and patients' preference (22.9%). The most common side effects reported were headache, gastrointestinal upset (nausea and abdominal discomfort) and dizziness. Patients who suffered from cardiovascular disorders were significantly less likely to experience switching (p = 0.006, OR = 3.3, 95% CI 1.4 to 7.8).

3.3. Combination Therapy

Combination therapy was prescribed for 17% of patients. Types of combinations are shown in **Table 5**. The SSRI-NaSSA combination was the most frequently preferred in about 37% patients, followed by the SSRI-TCA combination in 20%. The most cited reason for use of combination therapy was lack of efficacy in nearly half (49%) of patients, and to improve sleep in 17%. Combination therapy was prescribed more for patients with depression than for anxiety disorders (p = 0.024)

In contrast to other medical diagnoses, those with neurological conditions were more likely to have combination therapy (p = 0.029, OR = 4.0, 95% CI 1.2 to 13.7).

3.4. Augmentation Therapy

Augmentation therapy was prescribed for 23.8% (n = 49) of the patients. Atypical antipsychotics were the most preferred augmenting agent, followed by mood stabilizers and typical antipsychotic medication. The most popular choice of atypical antipsychotic in our study was risperidone, followed by quetiapine, with olanzapine, a distant third.

Table 1. Socio-demographic characteristics of sample.

Characteristic (n = 206)	Number	%
Gender		
Male	75	36.4%
Female	131	63.6%
Race		
Chinese	179	86.9%
Malay	12	5.8%
Indian	9	4.4%
Other	6	2.9%
Marital status		
Married	146	70.9%
Single	41	19.9%
Divorced	12	5.5%
Widowed	7	3.4%
Educational level		
No formal education	11	5.3%
Primary	34	16.5%
Secondary	66	32.1%
Tertiary	95	46.1%
Employment status		
Full time	124	60.2%
Part time	9	4.4%
Unemployed	73	35.4%

Table 2. Clinical characteristics of sample.

Characteristic (n = 206)	Number	%
Diagnosis		
Depressive disorder without psychotic features	97	47.1%
Depressive disorder with psychotic features	6	2.9%
Anxiety disorder	56	27.2%
Mixed anxiety-depressive disorder	33	16.0%
Adjustment disorder	12	5.8%
Others	2	1.0%
Duration of illness (years)		
<1	14	6.8%
1 - 5	109	52.9%
6 - 10	59	28.6%
>10	24	11.7%
History of suicide attempts		
Yes	15	7.3%
No	191	92.7%
Past medical history		
Yes	141	68.4%
No	65	31.6%

Table 3. Types of antidepressants prescribed on initiation of treatment.

Prescribed Antidepressants	No. (%)
SSRI	151 (75.5)
NaSSA	27 (13.5)
TCA	17 (8.5)
SNRI	2 (1.0)
RIMA	1 (0.5)
Others	7 (3.5)

*Some patients were on more than one antidepressant. TCA = tricyclic antidepressant; RIMA = reversible inhibitor of monoamine oxidase; SSRI = specific serotonin reuptake inhibitor; SNRI = serotonin noradrenaline reuptake inhibitor; NaSSA = noradrenaline specific serotonin antidepressant.

Table 4. Correlation of prescribing patterns of antidepressants to patient characteristics.

Characteristic	SSRI (n = 151)	TCA (n = 17)	Significance
Age (mean)	48.9	61.9	p = 0.0005
Gender			NS
Male	53 (35.1%)	6 (35.3%)	
Female	98 (64.9%)	11 (64.7%)	
Educational level			p = 0.00017
Up to secondary level	29 (19.2%)	11 (64.7%)	
Secondary and above	122 (80.8%)	6 (35.3%)	
Diagnosis*	N = 141	N = 16	NS
Depressive illness	76 (65.5%)	7 (43.7%)	
Anxiety disorder	40 (34.5%)	7 (43.7%)	
Mixed anxiety-depression	25 (17.7%)	2 (12.6%)	

SSRI = specific serotonin reuptake inhibitor; TCA = tricyclic antidepressant; *patients with other diagnoses were not included in the analysis.

Table 5. Types of Combination therapy.

Combinations	n = 35 (100%)
SSRI + NaSSA	13 (37.1%)
SSRI + TCA	7 (20.0%)
SSRI + trazodone	4 (11.5%)
SSRI + SNRI	1 (2.9%)
SSRI + SSRI	2 (5.7%)
SSRI + bupropion	2 (5.7%)
TCA + SNRI	2 (5.7%)
TCA + NaSSA	2 (5.7%)
Others	2 (5.7%)

TCA = tricyclic antidepressant; RIMA = reversible inhibitor of monoamine oxidase; SSRI = specific serotonin reuptake inhibitor; SNRI = serotonin noradrenaline reuptake inhibitor; NaSSA = noradrenaline specific serotonin antidepressant.

The main reasons for augmentation therapy were the presence of comorbid conditions (36.7%) and lack of efficacy (20.4%) of single agent therapy. Augmentation was prescribed more frequently for patients suffering from depression (p = 0.033) compared to other conditions (please refer to **Table 6**).

There were no associations between age and sex with switching, augmentation or combination therapy (in all cases p > 0.05).

4. Discussion

Compared to the general population, there was an over representation of Chinese patients in the study, which could be a reflection of the demographic characteristics of patients referred to the hospital, or living in the Tanjong Pagar constituency where the hospital is sited. According to the Singapore Elections Department, the num-

Table 6. Relationship between therapy and clinical characteristics.

Characteristic	Combination	Monotherapy	Significance
Diagnosis	%	%	p = 0.024
Depressive disorder	84.6	60.9	
Anxiety disorder	15.4	39.1	
Duration of illness			NS
<5 years	57.1	60.2	
>5 years	42.9	39.8	
	Augmentation	**No augmentation**	**Significance**
Diagnosis	%	%	p = 0.033
Depressive disorder	79.5	60	
Anxiety disorder	20.5	40	
Duration of illness			NS
<5 years	59.2	59.9	
>5 years	40.8	40.1	

ber of eligible voters within the constituency in 2014 was 137,464 persons [17]. Thus a generous estimate of the size of the hospital's catchment area, which includes non-voters, temporary residents, and non-citizens would be about 180,000 persons.

A greater preponderance of females in this sample is consistent with the higher prevalence of anxiety and depression in females in Singapore [18] [19].

Almost all patients in our study (97%) were offered treatment with an antidepressant, of which SSRIs were the most commonly prescribed. This is in keeping with the results of studies done in Asia [5] [17] [20], the United States [4] and Europe [21] which supported this finding.

SSRI usage has been previously associated with younger age, female gender and diagnosis of depression, compared to TCAs [22]. These findings were also reflected in our study, which suggested that those prescribed SSRIs tended to be better educated. There was no correlation with gender in our sample.

The use of "dual-action" antidepressants, for example NaSSAs and SNRIs, has been on the rise in recent years. Mirtazapine (NaSSA) and venlafaxine (SNRI) were the 2nd and 4th most commonly used antidepressants in this study. Some researchers have suggested that the treatment of depression with newer antidepressants that enhance both norepinephrine and serotonin neurotransmission may result in higher response and remission rates than SSRIs [23].

Treatment is not always effective, and some found that only one third of patients achieve full remission after their first antidepressant treatment in a naturalistic setting [24]. In our case, efficacy was assessed by the treating psychiatrist based on clinical examination of patients, as formal rating scales were not utilized in our clinics.

Our study revealed that more than half required switching. About a third cited side effects and another third efficacy issues. This is in keeping with our hypothesis that intolerance to side effects and a lack of efficacy contribute to switching before settling on the final choice of antidepressant. Whether our patients were more likely to experience side effects, or report side effects, compared to those from the West is open to question. It appears that a greater proportion in our study required switching compared to those from other countries. While it is possible that our patients are more prone to side effects, this observation was supported by Lin who suggested that Asians metabolize drugs in the CYP4502D6 system more slowly than patients of other ethnic groups, and hence it were more likely to develop side effects at lower doses compared to their Western counterparts [25]. In order to avoid side effects, we usually start with lower dosages, and thereafter titrate them upwards cautiously. Taking our most commonly prescribed SSRI, Fluvoxamine, as an example, we used starting dosages as low as 25 mg for anxiety disorder. Our average dose of this medication was 77.5 mg. This is below the recommended range of 100 - 300 mg for this drug in the European guidelines [26]. Whereas in the case of Fluoxetine, our average dose was 36 mg, within the recommended range of 20 - 40 mg [26].

There are many options available for switching, including use of a second SSRI, novel dual-acting antidepressants, selective norepinephrine or noradrenergic/dopaminergic agents, TCAs or mianserin [27]. However, in our hospital, mianserin is not available, although a drug similar in structure to mianserin viz. mirtazapine appears to be used as a drug of second choice.

The proportion of patients who were switched to another class of antidepressants for this study was 52.9%, which appears to be a higher rate compared to other studies. For example, researchers in France, based on a general practice database, showed that 16% of patients switched antidepressants, with 72% occurring within 3 months of treatment initiation [28]. Others reported switching for the purpose of optimizing treatment in about 40% of patients [29].

In our study, 17% of patients received combination therapy. Although our preferred combination was SSRI-NaSSA, with the exception of a few small studies demonstrating the efficacy of this method [30] [31], the literature is generally rather sparse in regards the use of this approach. Combinations involving other classes of antidepressants have been described [32]-[34] (although used less commonly in our hospital).

An interesting observation of our study was the combination of trazodone and SSRI. Although trazodone is an older antidepressant, it has been used more as a sedative hypnotic in recent times [35]. This could explain its relative lack of utility as a combination agent elsewhere. Some have found that the SSRI-trazodone combination could be useful in alleviating the sleep problems associated with SSRI monotherapy [36], which is in keeping with the fact that the second most common reason for combination was for improvement of sleep. The addition of buproprion or an SNRI to an SSRI were the popular options in other studies [9] [29], although less preferred in our department. This could be due to the relative infrequent use of Bupropion or of SNRIs in our hospital, a reflection of prescribing habits rather than availability.

This study shows that 23.8% of patients had augmentation therapy. This is similar to the 20% quoted in a study done in Korea [20]. In a multi-centre study in Spain, Garcia-Toro *et al.* found that about 19% patients [29] were prescribed augmentation therapy, with atypical antipsychotics being the more common choice (rather similar to our case).

The lack of association between age and sex with switching, combination or augmentation therapies would suggest that strategies to alleviate side effects or lack of efficacy were implemented regardless of demographic characteristics of the patient. Patients with cardiovascular conditions were significantly less likely to be switched to another antidepressant in the event of poor response or when they experienced side effects. For instance, there was no association between cardiovascular problems and the use of augmentation (p = 0.629), or combination therapy (p = 0.064). This would suggest that our psychiatrists tended to be more cautious with cardiac patients, preferring to wait for the initial antidepressant to take effect rather than try other medications or strategies to overcome efficacy problems.

In contrast, those with neurological comorbidities were more likely to receive combination therapy, as our clinicians probably felt that such strategies were not likely to worsen their patients' neurological status.

A retrospective study with a small sample size has its limitations, the most common problem being missing data or illegible entries in case records. As a naturalistic observational study with broad inclusion criteria, it has not been possible to control for clinical and socio-economical characteristics of the sample population, thus limiting inferences about cause-and-effect relationships. As we only analyzed outpatients receiving care from psychiatrists, our findings could neither be generalized to mild depressive patients, mainly managed by family physicians, nor the severely ill in the inpatient population.

5. Conclusion

Notwithstanding some limitations, this is the first study to examine antidepressant prescription patterns in a Singapore hospital. Our findings confirmed the hypothesis that antidepressant therapy was not easy for patients to tolerate. Side effects may seriously reduce treatment adherence and efficacy, hence necessitating strategies of switching, augmentation and combination prescriptions. Conversely, these options could also be selected for efficacy problems in the absence of side effects. This raises the need for further research to examine the extent of treatment non-adherence, and to correlate this with attitudes towards intake of psychiatric medications and their side effects.

Acknowledgements

The authors would like to thank Joyce Lim, a research assistant, for her help in data collection, and Dr Ng Kah Wee and Dr Cecilia Kwok for assistance rendered during the preparation of this manuscript.

References

[1] Abbing-Karahagopian, V., Huerta, C., Souverein, P.C., de Abajo, F., Leufkens, H.G.M., Slattery, J., *et al.* (2014) Antidepressant Prescribing in Five European Countries: Application of Common Definitions to Assess the Prevalence, Clinical Observations, and Methodological Implications. *European Journal of Clinical Pharmacology*, **70**, 49-57. http://dx.doi.org/10.1007/s00228-014-1676-z

[2] Exeter, D., Robinson, E. and Wheeler, A. (2009) Antidepressant Dispensing Trends in New Zealand between 2004 and 2007. *Australia and New Zealand Journal of Psychiatry*, **43**, 1131-1140. http://dx.doi.org/10.3109/00048670903279879

[3] National Institute for Clinical Excellence (2004) Management of Depression in Primary and Secondary Care. Clinical Guideline 23. National Institute for Clinical Excellence, London. http://www.nice.org.uk/pdf/CG023quickrefguide.pdf

[4] Ivanova, J.I., Bienfait-Beuzon, C., Birnbaum, H.G., Connolly, C., Emani, S. and Sheehy, M. (2011) Physicians' Decisions to Prescribe Antidepressant Therapy in Older Patients with Depression in a US Managed Care Plan. *Drugs and Aging*, **28**, 51-62. http://dx.doi.org/10.2165/11539900-000000000-00000

[5] Zhang, Y., Becker, T., Kösters, M. (2013) Preliminary Study of Patterns of Medication Use for Depression Treatment in China. *Asia-Pacific Psychiatry*, **5**, 231-236. http://dx.doi.org/10.1111/appy.12022

[6] Zimmerman, M., Posternak, M., Friedman, M., Attiullah, N., Baymiller, S., Boland, R., *et al.* (2004) Which Factors Influence Psychiatrists' Selection of Antidepressants? *The American Journal of Psychiatry*, **161**, 1285-1289. http://dx.doi.org/10.1176/appi.ajp.161.7.1285

[7] Bauer, M., Adli, M., Ricken, R., Severus, E. and Pilhatsch, M. (2014) Role of Lithium Augmentation in the Management of Major Depressive Disorder. *CNS Drugs*, **28**, 331-342. http://dx.doi.org/10.1007/s40263-014-0152-8

[8] Joffe, R.T. and Schuller, D.R. (1993) An Open Study of Buspirone Augmentation of Serotonin Reuptake Inhibitors in Refractory Depression. *The Journal of Clinical Psychiatry*, **54**, 269-271.

[9] Spier, S.A. (1998) Use of Bupropion with SRIs and Venlafaxine. *Depression and Anxiety*, **7**, 73-75. http://dx.doi.org/10.1002/(SICI)1520-6394(1998)7:2<73::AID-DA4>3.0.CO;2-6

[10] Shelton, R.C., Tollefson, G.D., Tohen, M., Stahl, S., Gannon, K.S., Jacobs, T.G., *et al.* (2001) A Novel Augmentation Strategy for Treating Resistant Major Depression. *The American Journal of Psychiatry*, **158**, 131-134. http://dx.doi.org/10.1176/appi.ajp.158.1.131

[11] Carpenter, L.L., Yasmin, S. and Price, L.H. (2002) A Double-Blind Placebo-Controlled Study of Antidepressant Augmentation with Mirtazapine. *Biological Psychiatry*, **51**, 183-188. http://dx.doi.org/10.1016/S0006-3223(01)01262-8

[12] Shelton, R.C., Osuntokun, O., Heinloth, A.N. and Corya, S.A. (2010) Therapeutic Options for Treatment-Resistant Depression. *CNS Drugs*, **24**, 131-161. http://dx.doi.org/10.2165/11530280-000000000-00000

[13] Ammar, G., Naja, W.J. and Pelissolo, A. (2014) Treatment-Resistant Anxiety Disorders: A Literature Review of Drug Therapy Strategies. *Encéphale*, **14**, pii: S0013-7006(14)00040-2.

[14] Spijker, J. and Nolen, W.A. (2010) An Algorithm for the Pharmacological Treatment of Depression. *Acta Psychiatrica Scandinavica*, **121**, 180-189. http://dx.doi.org/10.1111/j.1600-0447.2009.01492.x

[15] Elections Department, Singapore (2014) http://www.eld.gov.sg/elections_type_electoral.html

[16] Uchida, N., Chong, M.Y., Tan, C.H., Nagai, H., Tanaka, M., Lee, M.S., *et al.* (2007) International Study on Antidepressant Prescription Pattern at 20 Teaching Hospitals and Major Psychiatric Institutions in East Asia: Analysis of 1898 Cases from China, Japan, Korea, Singapore and Taiwan. *Psychiatry and Clinical Neurosciences*, **61**, 522-528. http://dx.doi.org/10.1111/j.1440-1819.2007.01702.x

[17] Sim, K., Lee, N.B., Chua, H.C., Mahendran, R., Fujii, S., Yang, S.Y., *et al.* (2007) Newer Antidepressant Drug Use in East Asian Psychiatric Treatment Settings: REAP (Research on East Asia Psychotropic Prescriptions) Study. *British Journal of Clinical Pharmacology*, **63**, 431-437. http://dx.doi.org/10.1111/j.1365-2125.2006.02780.x

[18] Lim, L., Ng, T.P., Chua, H.C., Chiam, P.C., Won, V., Lee, T., *et al.* (2005) Generalised Anxiety Disorder in Singapore: Prevalence, Co-Morbidity and Risk Factors in a Multi-Ethnic Population. *Social Psychiatry and Psychiatric Epidemiology*, **40**, 972-979. http://dx.doi.org/10.1007/s00127-005-0978-y

[19] Chua, H.C., Lim, L., Ng, T.P., Lee, T., Mahendran, R., Fones, C. and Kua, E.H. (2004) The Prevalence of Psychiatric Disorders in Singapore Adults. *Annals Academy of Medicine Singapore*, **33**, S102.

[20] Bae, K.Y., Kim, S.W., Kim, J.M., Shin, I.S., Yoon, J.S., Jung, S.W., *et al.* (2001) Antidepressant Prescribing Patterns in Korea: Results from the Clinical Research Center for Depression Study. *Psychiatry Investigation*, **8**, 234-244.

[21] Bauer, M., Monz, B.U., Montejo, A.L., Quail, D., Dantchev, N., Demyttenaere, K., *et al.* (2008) Prescribing Patterns of Antidepressants in Europe: Results from the Factors Influencing Depression Endpoints Research (FINDER) Study. *European Psychiatry*, **23**, 66-73. http://dx.doi.org/10.1016/j.eurpsy.2007.11.001

[22] Sclar, D.A., Robinson, L.M., Skaer, T.L. and Galin, R.S. (1998) What Factors Influence the Prescribing of Antidepressant Pharmacotherapy? An Assessment of Office-Based Encounters. *International Journal of Psychiatry in Medicine*, **28**, 407-419. http://dx.doi.org/10.2190/6VR0-XRCG-G1H3-N9Q0

[23] Papakostas, G.I., Thase, M.E., Fava, M., Nelson, J.C. and Shelton, R.C. (2007) Are Antidepressant Drugs That Combine Serotonergic and Noradrenergic Mechanisms of Action More Effective than the Selective Serotonin Reuptake Inhibitors in Treating Major Depressive Disorder? A Meta-Analysis of Studies of Newer Agents. *Biological Psychiatry*, **62**, 1217-1227. http://dx.doi.org/10.1016/j.biopsych.2007.03.027

[24] Rush, A.J., Trivedi, M.H., Wisniewski, S.R., Nierenberg, A.A., Stewart, J.W., Warden, D., *et al.* (2006) Acute and Longer-Term Outcomes in Depressed Outpatients Requiring One or Several Treatment Steps: A STAR*D Report. *American Journal of Psychiatry*, **163**, 1905-1917. http://dx.doi.org/10.1176/ajp.2006.163.11.1905

[25] Lin, K.M. (2001) Biological Differences in Depression and Anxiety across Races and Ethnic Groups. *Journal of Clinical Psychiatry*, **62**, 13-19.

[26] Bandelow, B., Zohar, J., Hollander, E., Kasper, S., Möller, H.J., *et al.* (2008) World Federation of Societies of Biological Psychiatry (WFSBP) Guidelines for the Pharmacological Treatment of Anxiety, Obsessive-Compulsive and Post-Traumatic Stress Disorders—First Revision. *World Journal of Biological Psychiatry*, **9**, 248-312. http://dx.doi.org/10.1080/15622970802465807

[27] Connolly, K.R. and Thase, M.E. (2001) If at First You Don't Succeed: A Review of the Evidence for Antidepressant Augmentation, Combination and Switching Strategies. *Drugs*, **71**, 43-64. http://dx.doi.org/10.2165/11587620-000000000-00000

[28] Saragoussi, D., Chollet, J., Bineau, S., Chalem, Y. and Milea, D. (2012) Antidepressant Switching Patterns in the Treatment of Major Depressive Disorder: A General Practice Research Database Study. *International Journal of Clinical Practice*, **66**, 1079-1087. http://dx.doi.org/10.1111/j.1742-1241.2012.03015.x

[29] Garcia-Toro, M., Medina, E., Galan, J.L., Gonzalez, M.A. and Maurino, J. (2012) Treatment Patterns in Major Depressive Disorder after an Inadequate Response to First Line Antidepressants. *BMC Psychiatry*, **12**, 143. http://dx.doi.org/10.1186/1471-244X-12-143

[30] Debonnel, G., Gobbi, G., Turcotte, J., Boucher, N., Hébert, C., De Montigny, C. and Blier, P. (2000) Effects of Mirtazapine, Paroxetine and Their Combination: A Double-Blind Study in Major Depression. *European Neuropsychopharmacology*, **10**, 252. http://dx.doi.org/10.1016/S0924-977X(00)80213-8

[31] Anttila, S.A. and Leinonen, E.V. (2001) A Review of the Pharmacological and Clinical Profile of Mirtazapine. *CNS Drug Reviews*, **7**, 249-264. http://dx.doi.org/10.1111/j.1527-3458.2001.tb00198.x

[32] Horgan, D., Dodd, S. and Berk, M. (2007) A Survey of Combination Antidepressant Use in Australia. *Australasian Psychiatry*, **15**, 26-29. http://dx.doi.org/10.1080/10398560601109855

[33] Shelton, R.C. (2003) The Use of Antidepressants in Novel Combination Therapies. *Journal of Clinical Psychiatry*, **64**, 14-18.

[34] Lam, R.W., Wan, D.C., Cohen, N.L. and Kennedy, S.H. (2002) Combining Antidepressants for Treatment Resistant Depression: A Review. *Journal of Clinical Psychiatry*, **63**, 685-693. http://dx.doi.org/10.4088/JCP.v63n0805

[35] Schatzberg, A.F. (1987) Trazodone: A 5-Year Review of Antidepressant Efficacy. *Psychopathology*, **20**, 48-56. http://dx.doi.org/10.1159/000284523

[36] Fagiolini, A., Comandini, A., Catena Dell'Osso, M. and Kasper, S. (2012) Rediscovering Trazodone for the Treatment of Major Depressive Disorder. *CNS Drugs*, **26**, 1033-1049. http://dx.doi.org/10.1007/s40263-012-0010-5

Predictors of Comorbid Psychological Symptoms among Patients with Social Anxiety Disorder after Cognitive-Behavioral Therapy

Sei Ogawa[1], Risa Imai[1], Masaki Kondo[1], Toshi A. Furukawa[2], Tatsuo Akechi[1]

[1]Department of Psychiatry and Cognitive-Behavioral Medicine, Nagoya City University Graduate School of Medical Sciences, Nagoya, Japan
[2]Department of Health Promotion and Human Behavior, Kyoto University Graduate School of Medicine/School of Public Health, Kyoto, Japan
Email: seiogawa1964@nifty.com

Abstract

Aim: The present study aimed to examine the predictors of comorbid psychological symptoms in social anxiety disorder (SAD) after cognitive-behavioral therapy (CBT). **Methods:** One hundred fourteen SAD patients completed manualized group CBT. We examined associations between the personality dimensions of NEO Five Factor Index (NEO-FFI) and the subscales of Symptom Checklist-90 Revised (SCL-90-R) in SAD patients after CBT using multiple regression analysis. **Results:** High levels of conscientiousness at baseline predicted symptom reduction on 4 SCL-90-R scales, including somatization, obsessive-compulsive, anxiety and global severity index in patients with SAD after CBT. And high levels of agreeableness predicted symptom reduction on 2 SCL-90-R scales, including Hostility and Paranoid Ideation. High levels of openness predicted psychoticism. **Conclusion:** The present study suggested that high levels of three NEO-FFI dimensions (openness, agreeableness, conscientiousness) might predict comorbid psychological symptoms reduction in SAD patients after CBT. For the purpose of improving comorbid psychological symptoms with SAD patients, it might be useful to pay more attention to these dimensions of NEO-FFI at baseline.

Keywords

Social Anxiety Disorder, Cognitive-Behavioral Therapy, Comorbid Psychological Symptoms

1. Introduction

Social anxiety disorder (SAD) is one of the most common psychiatric disorders with lifetime prevalence of 12% [1]. Epidemiological studies have established that psychiatric comorbidity is frequent in SAD patients [1]. SAD patients with other psychiatric disorders are associated with increased symptom severity [2].

The efficacy of cognitive-behavioral therapy (CBT) encompassing exposure therapy and cognitive restructuring has been established for SAD [3]. There is now evidence indicating that CBT for a targeted anxiety disorder yields positive benefits upon comorbid disorders [4] [5]. Predictors of less effective treatment may save patients' time by avoiding ineffective treatments, which may be sometimes associated with economic burden [6]. However, few studies have addressed predictors of outcomes in comorbid psychological symptoms after CBT for SAD.

Some studies suggest that personality mediates part of comorbidity [7] [8]. Whether personality characteristics have an impact on CBT outcome is also an important question. In CBT for SAD, however, research to identify predictive personality characteristics has been limited.

The purpose of the present study is to examine the predictive personality characteristics of comorbid psychiatric symptoms in CBT for SAD.

2. Materials and Methods

2.1. Participants

One hundred forty-four SAD patients attended the group CBT program. All of the patients met the following entry criteria: 1) principal Axis I diagnosis of SAD according to the DSM-IV criteria, as assessed by the Structured Clinical Interview for DSM-IV(SCID) [9]; 2) absence of current psychosis, bipolar disorder and substance-use disorder. The patients provided their written informed consent after receiving full explanation of the study's purpose and procedures. The study was performed in accordance with the Declaration of Helsinki and the study's protocol was approved by the Ethics Committee of our institute.

2.2. Treatment

The group CBT for SAD at our department was originally based on the programme developed by Andrews *et al.* [10]. The program consists of the following components: 1) psychoeducation; 2) behavioral experiments; 3) attention training; 4) cognitive restructuring; and 5) *in vivo* graded exposures. The program is run in 16 2-h weekly sessions by two therapists.

2.3. Measures

At pre- and post-treatment the Symptom Checklist-90 Revised (SCL-90-R) and the Liebowitz Social Anxiety Scale (LSAS) were assessed. The NEO Five Factor Index (NEO-FFI) was assessed at pre-treatment.

The SCL-90-R is a widely used and self-reported assessment tool for general psychopathology [11]. It contains 90 items, subdivided into nine subscales of somatization, obsessive-compulsive, interpersonal sensitivity, depression, anxiety, hostility, phobic anxiety, paranoid ideation, psychosis and global severity index (GSI). Each item is scored between 0 (not at all) and 5 (extremely), and the average of the relevant items was taken to be the subscale score [11].

The NEO-FFI is a 60-item self-reported questionnaire designed to measure the five major personality dimensions of neuroticism, extraversion, conscientiousness, openness and agreeableness [12]. There are 12 items per dimension and the items are answered on a 5-point scale ranging from 0 (strongly disagree) to 4 (strongly agree) [12].

The LSAS is the most frequently used clinician-administered instrument for assessment of social anxiety disorder [13]. It is a 24-item scale that provides separate scores for fear (0 - 3 indicate none, mild, moderate, and severe, respectively) and avoidance (0 - 3 indicate never, occasionally, often, and usually, respectively) of social interaction and performance situations [13].

2.4. Statistical Analysis

All the data were examined using SPSS 18.0 for Windows [14]. First, we used an independent samples t-test or

χ^2 test to compare the demographic and clinical data among the patients who completed the program and those who did not. Second, to examine the predictors of the indices of psychological comorbidity, we performed step-wise multiple linear regression analysis using age, sex, onset, total score of LSAS at baseline, subscales of SCL-90-R at baseline and five personality dimensions of NEO-FFI, involving neuroticism, extraversion, conscientiousness, openness and agreeableness as independent variables and subscales of SCL-90-R at endpoint as dependent variables. All the statistical tests were two-tailed, and $p \leq 0.05$ was considered statistically significant.

3. Results

3.1. Patients Characteristics

Thirty patients (26.3%) out of the 144 who started the treatment dropped out prematurely from the CBT program and 114 patients were included in the current analysis. The reasons for dropouts were mainly the increased anxiety and the difficulties in this therapy to pursue. In baseline demographic and clinical characteristics, no statistically significant differences were seen among the subgroups (**Table 1**).

3.2. Predictors of the Comorbid Psychiatric Symptoms

In regression analysis (**Table 2**), high levels of Conscientiousness of NEO-FFI at baseline predicted symptom reduction on 4 SCL-90-R scales, including somatization, obsessive-compulsive, anxiety, and GSI at endpoint. And high levels of agreeableness predicted symptom reduction on 2 SCL-90-R scales, including hostility and paranoid ideation. High levels of openness predicted psychoticism. In demographic variables, sex (female) predicted symptom reduction on interpersonal sensitivity. Neuroticism, extraversion, and LSAS at baseline predicted nothing significantly.

4. Discussion

The present study suggests that high levels of three dimensions of NEO-FFI (openness, agreeableness, conscientiousness) at baseline may predict comorbid psychological symptoms reduction in patients with SAD after CBT. Especially high levels of conscientiousness may predict symptom reduction on somatization, obsessive-compulsive, anxiety and GSI at endpoint.

Although number of studies has examined the role of particular variables in predicting response to treatment for SAD, the results were inconsistent and inconclusive [15]. From the point of view of group therapy, our findings concerning openness and conscientiousness are consistent with those of Ogrodniczuk *et al.* (2003), who found openness and conscientiousness were directly associated with favorable outcome in group psychotherapy for psychiatric outpatients [16].

High openness patients are more likely benefit from group psychotherapy by being able to embrace the novel experience that psychotherapy offers [16]. High agreeableness is related favorable outcome in psychotherapy because high agreeableness patients are trusting, sympathetic, and cooperative [16]. High conscientiousness

Table 1. Baseline characteristics and mean clinical scores.

	Completer (N = 114)	Dropout (N = 30)	*P* value
Mean age (SD)	33.4 (10.5)	30.7 (10.8)	0.23
Sex (Male, %)	50%	46.7%	0.75
Mean age of onset (SD)	18.9 (7.8)	16.7 (5.9)	0.10
LSAS (SD)	75.3 (25.8)	77.1 (22.5)	0.70
NEO-FFI Neuroticism (SD)	31.6 (8.4)	29.6 (8.2)	0.24
NEO-FFI Extraversion (SD)	21.5 (8.2)	22.3 (6.5)	0.60
NEO-FFI Openness (SD)	28.8 (7.1)	28.7 (4.5)	0.86
NEO-FFI Agreeableness (SD)	30.9 (6.2)	29.9 (5.6)	0.37
NEO-FFI Conscientiousness (SD)	25.3 (7.3)	22.1 (8.0)	0.06

Note: LSAS, Liebowitz social anxiety scale; NEO-FFI, NEO five factor index ; SD, Standard deviation.

Table 2. Predictors at baseline for comorbid psychological symptoms after CBT (N = 114).

	SOM	O-C	I-S	DEP	ANX	HOS	PHOB	PAR	PSY	GSI
Baseline	0.64**	0.73**	0.59**	0.61**	0.54**	0.51**	0.69**	0.46**	0.56**	0.63**
Sex	a	a	0.17*	a	a	a	a	a	a	a
Age	a	a	a	a	a	a	a	a	a	a
Onset	a	a	a	a	a	a	a	a	a	a
LSAS	a	a	a	a	a	a	a	a	a	a
Neuroticism	a	a	a	a	a	a	a	a	a	a
Extraversion	a	a	a	a	a	a	a	a	a	a
Openness	a	a	a	a	a	a	a	a	−0.17*	a
Agreeableness	a	a	a	a	a	−0.28**	a	−0.25**	a	a
Conscientiousness	−0.15*	−0.16*	a	a	−0.16*	a	a	a	a	−0.15*
Adjusted R-square	0.41	0.57	0.40	0.36	0.31	0.42	0.47	0.32	0.31	0.42

Note: Table shows the standardized Beta coefficients (*$P < 0.05$, **$P < 0.01$). a Entered into analysis but not selected in the multiple regression model through application of a stepwise method. Appendices: SOM, Somatization; O-C, Obsessive-compulsive; I-S, Interpersonal sensitivity; DEP, Depression; ANX, Anxiety; HOS, Hostility; PHOB, Phobic anxiety; PAR, Paranoid ideation; PSY, Psychosis; GSI, Global Severity Index; LSAS, Liebowitz Social Anxiety Scale.

patients are also more likely to benefit from psychotherapy because they work hard, tolerate discomfort, and delay gratification of impulses and desires [16].

For the purpose of improving comorbid symptoms with SAD patients, it might be useful to pay more attention to some dimensions of NEO-FFI, especially conscientiousness.

The present study has some limitations. First, we lacked follow-up data and could not refer to long-term effect of CBT for comorbid psychological symptoms. Second, this study did not include several predictors like expectancy regarding therapy or therapist [15]. Future studies should be conducted as follow-up study and place more focus on other predictors like patient expectancy.

5. Conclusion

The present study suggests that high levels of openness, agreeableness, and conscientiousness of NEO-FFI personality dimensions may predict some comorbid psychological symptoms reduction in SAD patients after CBT.

Acknowledgements

This study was supported by Grant-in-Aid from the Ministry of Health, Labour and Welfare, Japan.

Conflict of Interest

The authors do not have any conflict of interest to report regarding this study.

References

[1]   Kessler, R.C., Chiu, W.T., Demler, O., Merikangas, K.R. and Walters, E.E. (2005) Prevalence, Severity, and Comorbidity of 12-Month DSM-IV Disorders in the National Comorbidity Survey Replication. *Archives of General Psychiatry*, **62**, 617-627. http://dx.doi.org/10.1001/archpsyc.62.6.617

[2]   Schneier, F.R., Johnson, J., Hornig, C.D., Liebowitz, M.R. and Weissman, M.M. (1992) Social Phobia. Comorbidity and Morbidity in an Epidemiologic Sample. *Archives of General Psychiatry*, **49**, 282-288. http://dx.doi.org/10.1001/archpsyc.1992.01820040034004

[3]   Acarturk, C., Cuijpers, P., van Straten, A. and de Graaf, R. (2009) Psychological Treatment of Social Anxiety Disorder: A Meta-analysis. *Psychological Medicine*, **39**, 241-254. http://dx.doi.org/10.1017/S0033291708003590

[4]   Craske, M.G., Farchione, T.J., Allen, L.B., Barrios, V., Stoyanova, M. and Rose, R. (2007) Cognitive Behavioral

Therapy for Panic Disorder and Comorbidity: More of the Same or Less of More? *Behaviour Research and Therapy*, **45**, 1095-1109. http://dx.doi.org/10.1016/j.brat.2006.09.006

[5]   Tsao, J.C., Lewin, M.R. and Craske, M.G. (1998) The Effects of Cognitive-Behavior Therapy for Panic Disorder on Comorbid Conditions. *Journal of Anxiety Disorders*, **12**, 357-371. http://dx.doi.org/10.1016/S0887-6185(98)00020-6

[6]   Mululo, S.C.C., Menezes, G.B.D., Vigne, P. and Fontenelle, L.F. (2012) A Review on Predictors of Treatment Outcome in Social Anxiety Disorder. *Revista Brasileira de Psiquiatria*, **34**, 92-100. http://dx.doi.org/10.1590/S1516-44462012000100016

[7]   Battaglia, M., Przybeck, T.R., Bellodi, L. and Cloninger, C.R. (1996) Temperament Dimensions Explain the Comorbidity of Psychiatric Disorders. *Comprehensive Psychiatry*, **37**, 292-298. http://dx.doi.org/10.1016/S0010-440X(96)90008-5

[8]   Bienvenu, O.J., Brown, C., Samuels, J.F., Liang, K.Y., Costa, P.T., Eaton, W.W. and Nestadt, G. (2001) Normal Personality Traits and Comorbidity among Phobic, Panic and Major Depressive Disorders. *Psychiatry Research*, **102**, 73-85. http://dx.doi.org/10.1016/S0165-1781(01)00228-1

[9]   First, M.B. (1997) Structured Clinical Interview for DSM-IV Axis I Disorders : SCID-I : Clinician Version: Administration Booklet. American Psychiatric Press, Washington DC.

[10]   Andrews, G., Creamer, M., Crino, R., Hunt, C., Lampe, L. and Page, A. (2003) The Treatment of Anxiety Disorders: Clinician Guides and Patient Manuals. 2nd Edition, Cambridge University Press, Cambridge and New York.

[11]   Derogatis, L.R. (1992) SCL-90-R: Administration, Scoring & Procedures Manual-II, for the R (Revised) Version and Other Instruments of the Psychopathology Rating Scale Series. 2nd Edition, Clinical Psychometric Research, Inc., Towson.

[12]   Costa, P.T. and McCrae, R.R. (1992) Revised Neo Personality Inventory (NEO PI-R) and Neo Five-Factor Inventory (NEO-FFI). Psychological Assessment Resources, Inc., Odessa.

[13]   Fresco, D.M., Coles, M.E., Heimberg, R.G., Liebowitz, M.R., Hami, S., Stein, M.B. and Goetz, D. (2001) The Liebowitz Social Anxiety Scale: A Comparison of the Psychometric Properties of Self-Report and Clinician-Administered Formats. *Psychological Medicine*, **31**, 1025-1035. http://dx.doi.org/10.1017/S0033291701004056

[14]   SPSS (2009) SPSS for Windows (Version 18.0).

[15]   Rodebaugh, T.L., Holaway, R.M. and Heimberg, R.G. (2004) The Treatment of Social Anxiety Disorder. *Clinical Psychology Review*, **24**, 883-908. http://dx.doi.org/10.1016/j.cpr.2004.07.007

[16]   Ogrodniczuk, J.S., Piper, W.E., Joyce, A.S., McCallum, M. and Rosie, J.S. (2003) NEO-Five Factor Personality Traits as Predictors of Response to Two Forms of Group Psychotherapy. *International Journal of Group Psychotherapy*, **53**, 417-442. http://dx.doi.org/10.1521/ijgp.53.4.417.42832

16

Effect of Exercise on Mental Health in the Physical Dimension, Anxiety and Mental Disorder, Social Dysfunction and Depression

Morteza Alibakhshi Kenari

Martyr Beheshti University of Medical Sciences and Health Services, Tehran, Iran
Email: Morteza.alibakhshikenari@gmail.com

Abstract

In the last twenty years, a lot of attention to issues of psychology and psychotherapy are associated with physical activity. Due to the increasing rate of mental disorders in country, this study attempts to compare the health of athletes and non-athletes in Beheshti University. Mental Health in schools will also compare. In this study, the health measured using the General Health Questionnaire GHQ-28 has performed. University students participated in this study of 260 patients who were randomly selected to represent the school. Statistical methods are used for the analysis and comparison of two sample t-test. The results show that the significant differences of symptoms of physical, anxiety, sleep disorder, social dysfunction and depression in the two groups were observed between athletes and non-athletes. The college student mental health and physical education than other students in four scales were much more favorable situation.

Keywords

Exercise; Physical Dimension; Anxiety and Sleep Disorders; Depression; Mental Health; Impaired Social Functioning

1. Introduction

In recent years much attention has been psychological and psychotherapy, because people today are more than anything suffering from mental health problems. Now in the world, especially in developing countries, about 150 million people suffer from some form of mental disorder. These figures are somewhat higher population growth and changes in lifestyle and family breakdown and economic problems involved. One of the ways that psychologists have identified a role for the reduction and treatment in mental health is exercise (McGannon & Poon, 2005). In other words, the researchers found a strong link between exercise and mental health and mental disorder there. Since our country is a developing country and the future of the students and mothers of tomorrow and the search for identity and age may be due to various reasons such as being away from family and feel more responsibility and career and marriage and other issues have been under a lot of stress and trauma are at risk. It is important to note. Obviously neglecting their health status may be irreparable damage to the family that they formed under the direct supervision and follow it to the community (Humphreys, 2003).

2. Health and Mental Tension

The World Health Organization defines mental health state of complete physical, mental and social be called (WHO, 2007). Some psychologists believe that the ability and flexibility to adapt to the environment and the judge denied and fair and reasonable in the face of mental health and psychological criteria (Knechtle, 2004). And treatment of mental illness as well as social and family life and enable compatibility of environmental. It should be noted that those with no mental disorder but its necessarily mentally healthy people to account, just as those who have no mental disease but are not considered to be healthy (Pereira, 2007).

Stress is a condition in which the emotions and expressions of the human body comes into tension and heaviness. To say to the stress of the human capacity for doing work that requires mental focus as well as the weakening of the human forces that began to fatigue.

3. The Role of Exercise in Mental Health Care

Studies on the effect of exercise on mental health in children have found that play an important role in maintaining the health of sick children's physical activity (Matsudo, 2006). According to a study conducted in 1991 also found that aerobic exercise is an important factor in reducing the effects of stress (Samad, 2004). In addition, it was found most effective exercise in elderly hospitalized and non-hospitalized alleviate symptoms of anxiety, depression, mood and stress reactions , as well as aerobic exercise is important for stress reduction (Brunner & Suddarth, 2004). In 1990 it was found exercise improves mood and mental health and increased self-esteem and self-respect, Bornak and colleagues (1995) found that intense exercise can have many benefits on mood and behavior and reduce stress and increase self-esteem and aerobic exercise may improve the self-esteem of dust.

4. Materials and Methods

This research is a descriptive search. Beheshti University student population with a bachelor's or master's in school year 2013 were enrolled in MQT form. The number of participants is 260 persons who comprise 80 individual athletes and 180 non-athletes. These were in addition to several sports teams of the members of the group selected College of Engineering and Physical education and art and literature and science and theology and psychology and social science has been formed, which were randomly selected.

The instrument used in this research questionnaire is 28 questions, {GHq28} is a standard tool designed by Goldberg and Hiller. This questionnaire was formed of 28 questions to ask first eight physical symptoms and eight second question anxiety and eight third question of social dysfunction and Eight quarters of the symptoms of depression and sleep disturbances were assessed. To compare the mental health of athletes and non-athletes of all indices t test for independent groups was used. All statistical calculations were performed using computer SPSS software.

5. Results and Findings

After statistical analysis and hypothesis testing, research findings revealed significant differences in mental health status than non-athlete student athlete "as shown in table". The problem in all dimensions: physical symptoms of anxiety and sleep disorder symptoms, social functioning and depressive symptoms compared to non-athletes were better {$p < 0/05$} "as shown in **Table 1**".

Considering the above table mental health scores of athletes is very better than non-athletes "as shown in **Table 2**".

According to information found in each of the four scale athletes are a more favorable situation as shown in **Figure 1**.

Table 1. Scores on mental health subjects.

ATHLETES		NON-ATHLETES	
mean	Standard deviation	mean	Standard deviation
19.81	11.94	24.94	15.26

Table 2. Scores on the four scales the mental health in the participants.

Depression		Impairment in social functioning		Anxiety and sleep disorders		Physical		
Standard deviation	mean	Standard deviation	mean	Standard deviation	mean	Standard deviation	mean	Index
3.38	4.14	4.01	5.58	3.43	5.13	2.38	4.3	ATHLETES
3.41	5.18	4.84	7.01	3.81	6.5	399	6.31	NON-ATHLETES

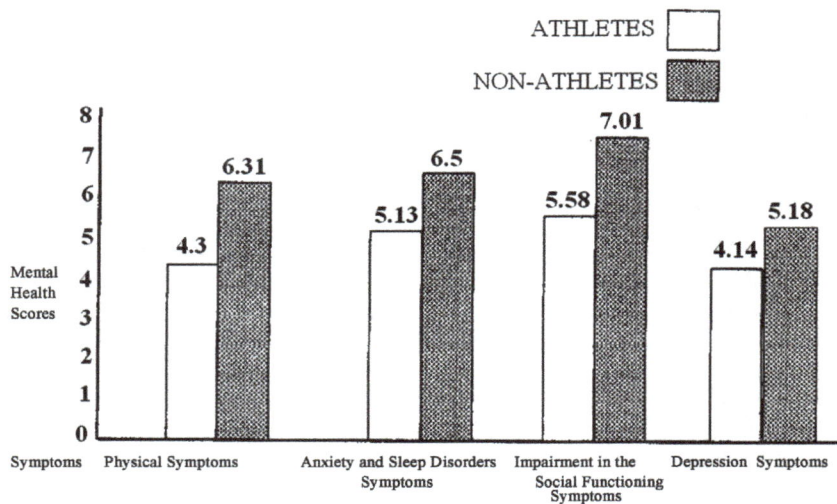

Figure 1. Comparison of four scales in the student-athletes and non-athletes.

In this study, four mental health scales were calculated separately for the eight colleges as shown in **Figure 2**.

So that diagram 2 is shown the Students School of Physical Sciences and Engineering and Theology and social sciences, art and psychology of better mental health. The results of the four mental health scales were also segregated schools. Charts tree showing physical signs to separate colleges as shown in **Figure 3**.

As can be seen in terms of physical symptoms and physical health of college students Theological and Literary physical and engineering sciences and social sciences, and arts and psychology in order to have been better. Results from four mental health scales and symptoms of anxiety and sleep disorders are divided into the following four graphs as shown in **Figure 4**.

Based on these findings in terms of anxiety and sleep disorders in college students Physical and engineering and social sciences, art, literature and psychology were better the situation. The results of the four measures of mental health symptoms and social dysfunction are shown in **Figure 5**.

Diagram 6 to four measures of mental health symptoms in schools heaven compared to that. According to diagram 6 is characterized by symptoms of depression in the Schools Physical and engineering sciences and social sciences and psychology, theology, literature and art are in a more favorable situation as shown in **Figure 6**.

Six charts revealed that symptoms of depressive in The School of Physical Education, Engineering, Theology, Literature, Science, Social Sciences, Psychology and art are in a more favorable situation.

6. Conclusion

Data collection and statistical analysis of the results suggest that student athletes compared to non-athletic

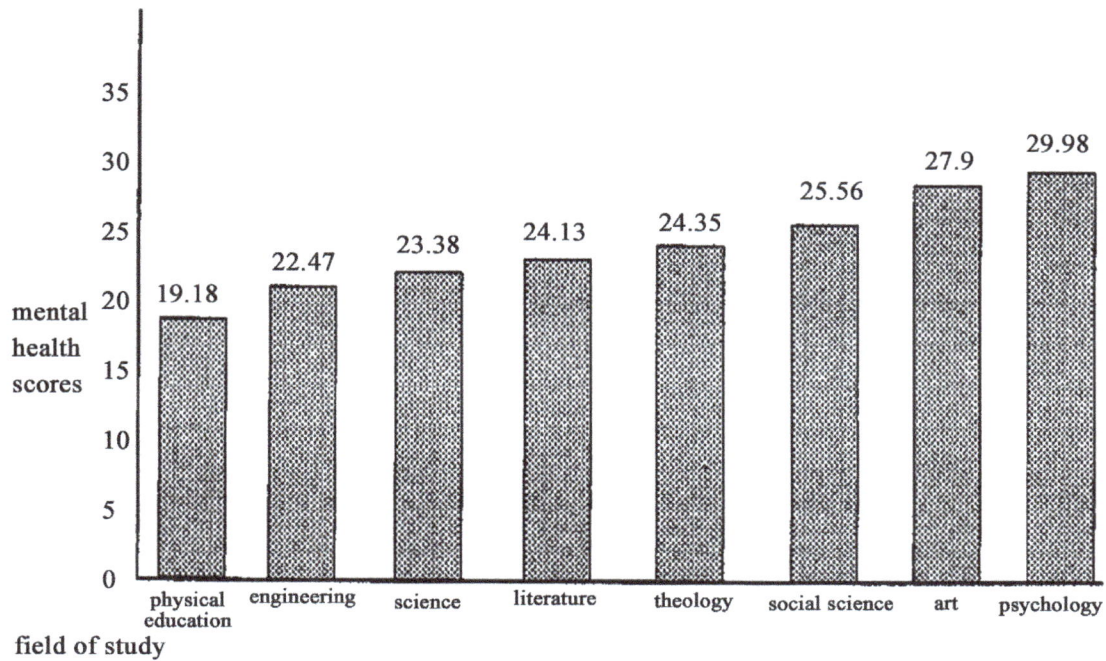

Figure 2. Comparison of the mental health divided into faculty.

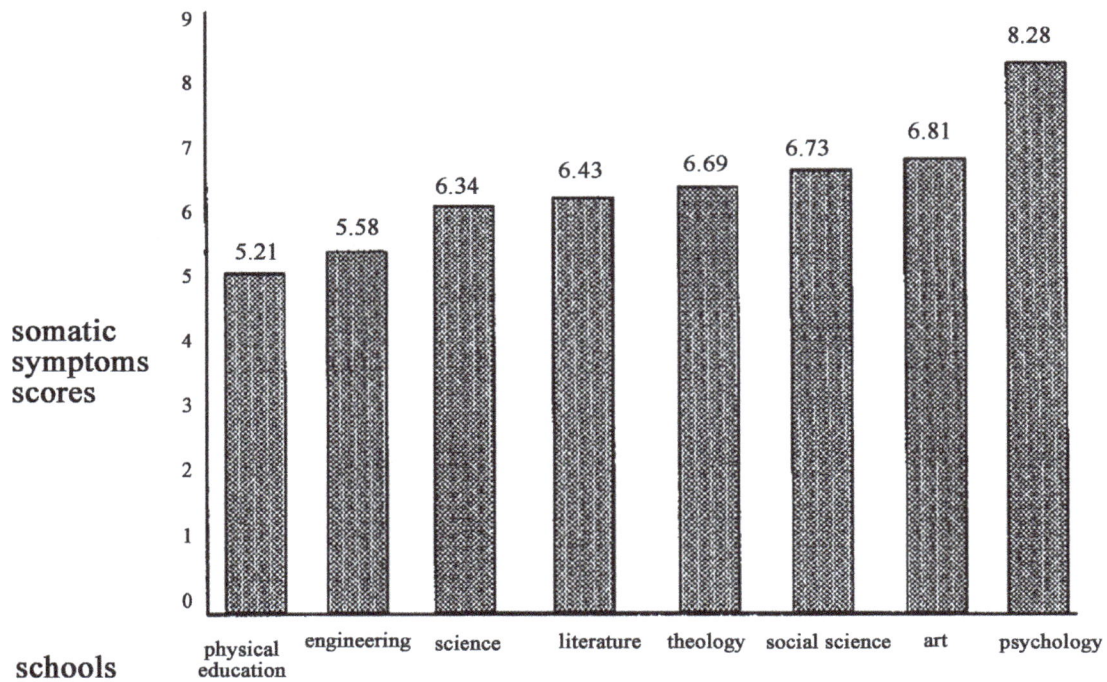

Figure 3. Comparison of physical symptoms Divided into Schools.

students have better mental health significant differences and it was also seen in all aspects of mental health such as physical symptoms and signs and symptoms of anxiety and insomnia, social dysfunction and depressive symptoms. Athletes were significantly different from the non-top {$p < 0/05$}. The results are consistent with similar studies. In this study, it was found that exercise can improve mood and psychological well-being and increased confidence, and physical and mental health is increasing as well. As a result, mental health, and measures

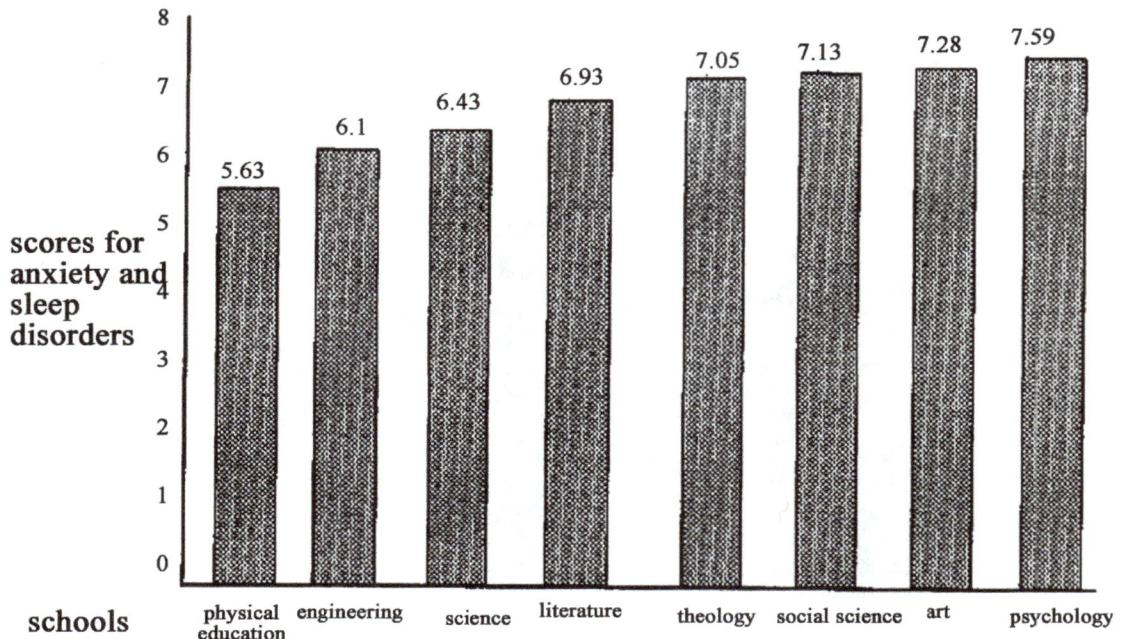

Figure 4. Comparing symptoms of anxiety and sleep disorders Divided into Schools.

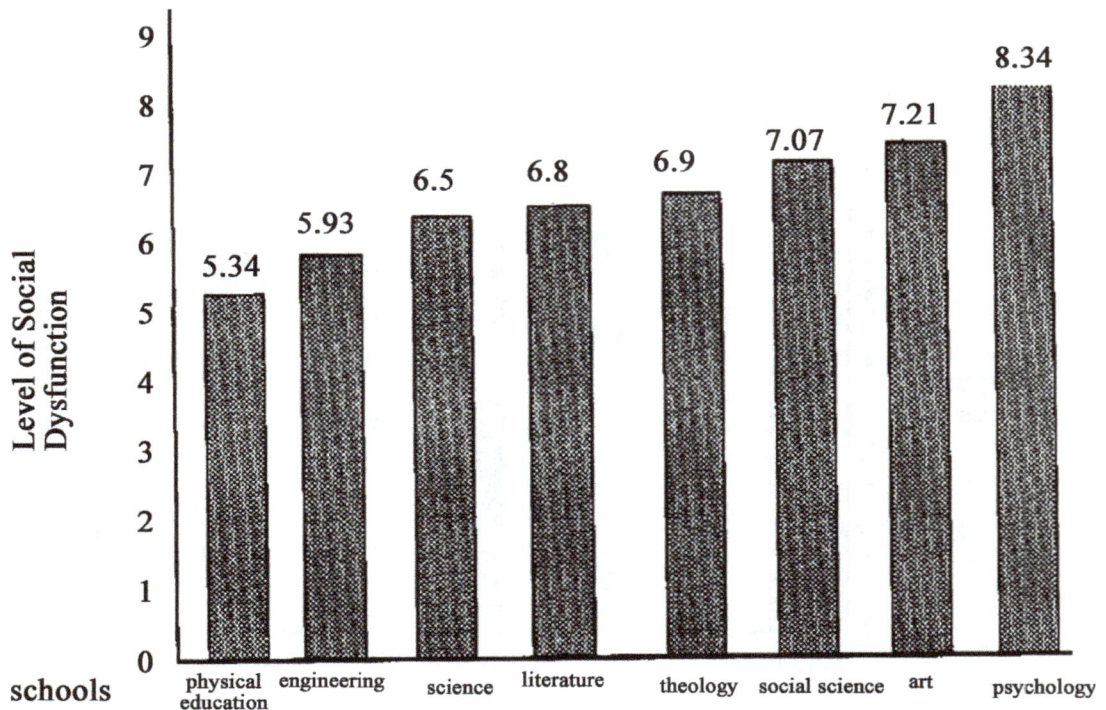

Figure 5. Comparing symptoms of social dysfunction Divided into Schools.

in four different schools are also out. As in the mental faculties Faculty of Physical Education and School Psychology in the best position is at the lowest level. The symptoms of insomnia, anxiety and dysfunction were more frequent in the School of Psychology. Depression scores were registered in the Faculty of Physical Education to be allocated to the lowest rates of depression and depressive symptoms in the highest state of the art

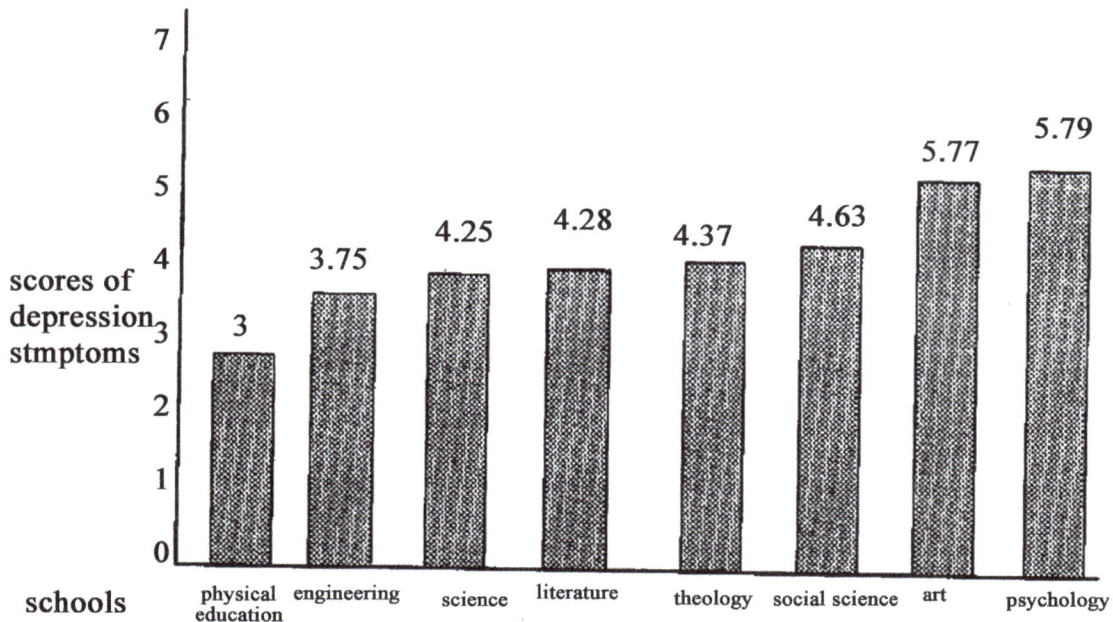

Figure 6. Comparison of symptoms of depression divided into Schools.

school is located. The results are characterized that student athletes in terms of mental health conditions are more favorable. As well as the students physical and mental health of college students are superior to others and the role of physical activity in the student's mental health shows. Hope that all students with physical outdoor activities, and prepare yourself for a healthy life.

References

Brunner, L. S., & Suddarth, D. S. (2004). *Text Book of Medical Surgical Nursing.*12th Edition Company Philadelphia.

Humphreys, R. (2003). The Effect of Professional Sports on Earnings and Employment in the Services and Retail Sectors in US Cities. *Regionsl Scienceand Urban Eco-Nomics, 33,* 175-198. http://dx.doi.org/10.1016/S0166-0462(02)00010-8

Knechtle, B. (2004). Influence of Physical Activity on Mental Well-Being and Psychiatric Disorders. *Schweiz Rundsch Med Prax, 93,* 1403-1411.

Matsudo, S. et al. (2006). Evaluation of a Physical Activity Promotion Program: The Example of Agita São Paulo. *Evaluation and Program Planning, 29,* 301-311. http://dx.doi.org/10.1016/j.evalprogplan.2005.12.006

Pereira, A. C. et al. (2007). An *in Vivo* Correlate of Exercise-Induced Neurogenesis in the Adult Dentate Gyrus. *Proceedings of the National Academy of Sciences of the United States of America, 104,* 5638-5643.

Samad, A. et al. (2004). A Meta-Analysis of the Association of Physical Activity with Reduced Risk of Colorectal Cancer. *Colorectal Disease, 7,* 204-213.

McGannon, K., & Poon, P. (2005). The Effect of Exercise on Global Selfesteem: A Quantitative Review. *Journal of Sport and Exercise, 27,* 311-334.

World Health Organization (2007). Mental Health: A State of Well-Being. *Fact File.*

17

Anxiety, Depression and Coronary Artery Disease among Patients Undergoing Angiography in Ghaem Hospital, Mashhad, Iran

Mohammad Tajfard[1,2], Majid Ghayour-Mobarhan[3], Hamid Reza Rahimi[4],
Mohsen Mouhebati[5], Habibollah Esmaeily[6], Gordon A. A. Ferns[7], Latiffah A. Latiff[2*],
Farzaneh Tajfiroozeh[4], Nagmeh Mokhber[8], Ramin Nazeminezhad[4],
Homa Falsoleyman[5], Ali Taghipour[6], Ahmad Fazli Abdul Aziz[9],
Rosliza A. Manaf[2], Zahra Saghiri[10], Parichehr Hanachi[11]

[1]Health Sciences Research Center, Department of Health and management, School of Health, Mashhad University of Medical Sciences, Mashhad, Iran
[2]Department of Community Health, Faculty of Medicine and Health Sciences, Universiti Putra Malaysia, Serdang, Selangor, Malaysia
[3]Cardiovascular Research Center, School of Medicine, Mashhad University of Medical Sciences, Mashhad, Iran
[4]Student Research Committee, Department of Modern Sciences & Technologies, School of Medicine, Mashhad University of Medical Sciences, Mashhad, Iran
[5]Department of Cardiology, School of Medicine, Mashhad University of Medical Sciences, Mashhad, Iran
[6]Health Sciences Research Center, Department of Biostatistics, School of Health, Mashhad University of Medical Sciences, Mashhad, Iran
[7]Brighton & Sussex Medical School, Falmer, Brighton, UK
[8]Departemet of Psychiatry, School of Medicine, Mashhad University of Medical Sciences, Mashhad, Iran
[9]Department of Medicine, Faculty of Medicine and Health Sciences, University Putra Malaysia, Serdang, Selangor, Malaysia
[10]Department of Biology-Biochemistry, Faculty of Science, Payame Noor University of Mashhad, Mashhad, Iran
[11]Faculty of Science, Biology Department, Biochemistry Unit, Alzahra University, Tehran, Iran
Email: *latiffah.latiff@gmail.com

Abstract

The prevalence of coronary artery disease (CAD) is increasing in Iran. Patients with depression

---

*Corresponding author.

who have a myocardial infarction are more likely to die and patients who have depressive symptoms during hospitalization may have increased cardiovascular events. This study aimed to determine the relationship between anxiety, depression and coronary artery disease among patients undergoing angiography in Ghaem Hospital, Mashhad. This was a case-control study conducted between September 2011 and August 2012 among patients undergoing coronary angiography in Ghaem Hospital, Mashhad, Iran. There were 486 cases that were found to have one or more coronary stenoses, with a stenosis of equal or more than 50% of the diameter of at least one major coronary artery. The other patient group consisted of the patients in whom the coronary artery stenosis was less than 50% in diameter which was classified as angiography negative, and a control group that consisted of 440 healthy adults aged 18 years old and above who were selected among people who attended for routine medical checkup and medical examination of employment. The dependent variables were Beck Anxiety and Depression Inventory scores and the independent factors were coronary artery disease, and socioeconomic profiles. Validated and reliability-tested questionnaires were used for data collection. The mean age of patients was 55.75 ± 10.64 years and in the healthy group was 55.83 ± 8.55 years; there was no significant difference in age between subject groups ($p = 0.897$) nor a significant difference in the gender frequency distribution of subjects ($p = 0.610$). There was a significant difference in anxiety score between the Angio positive and Angio negative patients and healthy control subjects ($p < 0.001$). There was a statistical significant difference between groups for the anxiety score ($p < 0.001$). However, the subjects did not differ significantly for BDI depression score ($p = 0.534$). A significant positive relationship was found between anxiety score and depression score when data were analyzed by Pearson's test ($p < 0.001$, Pearson's correlation = 0.582). Depression and anxiety are associated among patients with CAD undergoing coronary angiography sessions.

Keywords

Coronary Artery Disease, Anxiety, Depression, Angiography

1. Introduction

Coronary artery disease (CAD) is a major problem globally and it is more hazardous for men than for women. The statistic mortality shows that 34% men and 28% women die because of this problem. CAD has a number of risk determinants, such as lifestyle, psychological factors, environment [1] [2], age, emotional status, and smoking [3]. CAD is the end-point of a chronic and progressive condition that leads to heart failure and death [4] [5].

Depression and anxiety are also common disorders within all populations [3], but few studies have paid attention to the influences of depression and anxiety on physical health [6]. Anxiety sensitivity (AS) is different for each person since the symptoms concerning fear are associated with anxiety arousal, and anxiety has negative somatic signs and to a larger extent affects those who are psychologically vulnerable, such as those with depression and depressive symptoms [7]. Studies show that women have a higher prevalence of these symptoms than men [3].

We know that there is an association between depression and physical health and it is thought to be an important risk factor for heart diseases [8], and mood state has been identified as a determinant of quality of life in those who have coronary disease [9]. One out of every five patients with coronary patients has depression symptoms [6] [10] [11]. CAD reduces the life quality of the patient, for example, performance of life activities, ability to use medication and diet therapies [10]. The degree of depression and anxiety is associated with a greater decline in physical functioning of patient with heart failure [6]. Depression and anxiety appear to be highly overlapping with each other and they cause an increased risk more than 80% of CVD following when adjusted for CAD risk factors [12], but we should know that depression and coronary heart diseases are reversible, and coronary heart diseases may lead to depression [13].

Recently studies have shown that patients with depression who have myocardial infarction are more likely to die and the patients who have depressive symptom during hospitalization probably have increased cardiovascular events [8] [14]. Mood state may lead to hospitalization even after correction for demographic and medical factors [6]. Many studies have reported that mood disorders have an important impact on the outcome of cardiac transplantation; depressed patients with heart transplant have a tendency to be less active than those without [15] [16]. Social support is an important factor of psychology and it is useful for influence on heart, for example, patients with heart failure who are unmarried or seldom visit their family or friends have a significantly higher risk of serious impairment in activities [6]. To our knowledge, there are a few data to look at the association between mood status and CAD; therefore, we hope to investigate the association between anxiety and depression in CAD potions based on angiography.

2. Methods & Materials

2.1. Participants and Procedure

Coronary angiograms were undertaken using routine procedures and were performed by a specialist cardiologist. These patients who undergoing coronary angiography, especially for stable angina, and at least as more as one object test of myocardial ischemia such as Dobutamin stress or exercise stress test [17]. 486 patients (247 males and 239 females) were recruited for this study. Patients were selected from adult (>18 years of age). All subjects were without a past clinical history of angiography and heart surgery. The subjects consisted of three groups, patients group and healthy group (control group). The patients were classified into two groups. The first group consisted of the patients whose result of angiography shows one or more stenosis with the occlusion of >50% of the diameter of at least one major coronary artery and so they would be considered as a significant angiography positive (case group). And the second group consists of the patients in whom the coronary artery stenosis was <50% in diameter which is classified as not having significant (angiography negative) [18]-[20]. 440 healthy (231 males and 209 females) from adult (beyond the age of 18) who were selected among people who come for routine medical checkup and employment Medical examination at employment.

All subject full the questionnaires about physical and mental health functioning, smoking, depression, and anxiety test. This study focused on overlapping CAD, depression, and anxiety.

2.2. Anthropometric and Other Measurements

Anthropometric measurements for each subject including height, weight, by using standard protocols were done. The calculation of body mass index (BMI) was performed as weight (Kg) divided by height squared (m^2) [21].

2.3. Assessment of Depression and Anxiety

The Beck Anxiety Inventory (BAI) is a 21-questionstion multiple-choice self-report inventory that is used for measuring the severity of an individual's anxiety [22]. It assesses two factors: somatic, that applied 12 items explaining physiological symptoms, such as, "numbness or tingling", "feeling dizzy or lightheaded" and subjective anxiety and panic, that applied the remaining 9 items of the BAI measures, such as "fear of the worst happening" and "unable to relax" [22]. According to the Anxiety beck questioner score, if a person get 7 or less from this test has minimal anxiety, mild anxiety score is 8 - 15 and moderate anxiety is 16 - 25 and more than 25 is severe anxiety [23] [24]. The Beck Depression Inventory (BDI) is 21-item; self-report rating inventory the measurement of characteristic attitudes and symptoms of depression was done by the Beck. Beck developed a triad of negative cognitions about the world, the future and the self which play a major role in depression. If a person get 15 or less from this test has no depression, mild depression is 16 - 30, moderate depression, score is 31 - 46 and severe depression, is more than 47 [24]. These questioners were given to subjects before any procedures.

2.4. Statistical Analysis

Statistical analysis were used the Statistical Package for Social Sciences version 16. Descriptive statistics (frequency, mean, standard deviation) determined for all variables. Differences in coronary artery stenos is (Angio– or Angio+) were analyzed by the chi-square test for categorical variables. We used categorical depression and anxiety base on score of them. Multivariate analyses were used to examine effects of demographic variable (such as weight, Height, BMI) on coronary artery disease.

3. Results

Nine hundred and twenty six subjects were evaluated for depression and anxiety. Four hundred and eighty six persons had a history of cardiac signs or symptoms and 440 persons were healthy subjects. The mean age of all subjects were 55.79 ± 9.65 years old and there was no significant difference between patients and healthy subjects (p = 0.897) also no statistical significant difference were found in gender of subjects between groups (p = 0.610) (**Table 1**).

When subjects were divided into patient and healthy subjects there was a statistical significant difference between groups in anxiety score (p < 0.001). But the subjects had no significant difference in depression score assessed by the BDI (p = 0.534) (**Table 1**).

A significant statistical effect of gender on depression scores was found for healthy and patient groups (p < 0.001) (**Table 2**).

As shown in **Table 3**, there was a significant difference between angiography positive, negative and healthy subjects in anxiety score and also in the number of persons who had minimal anxiety (p < 0.001). Other category of anxiety score (mild, moderate and severe) had no difference among three groups (p > 0.05) (**Table 3**).

According to that the angiography results subjects can be divided according to the number of involved coronary vessels. Depression and anxiety scores results in **Table 4** based on the number of vessels involved are shown. Again, there were significant differences in anxiety among groups. After post HOC test were performed significant difference was found between healthy and angiography negative group (p < 0.001).

In this study a significant direct linear correlation was found between anxiety score and depression score when data were analyzed by Pearson test (p < 0.001, Pearson correlation = 0.582) (**Figure 1**). This correlation either found in healthy and patients group.

4. Discussion

Depression is one of the main risk factors, which leads to morbidity and mortality resulted from coronary artery disease (CAD). Depressed persons with initially good medical health have an elevated incidence of CHD. In addition, the risk of mortality is increased in people who are depressed after myocardial infarction (MI). Another important point is that depression is also associated with elevated expression of inflammatory biomarkers [25].

According to a recent meta-analysis, perceived stress is associated with the risk of coronary artery disease [26]. Individuals with anxiety disorders or depressed mood are prone to unhealthier lifestyle [27]. This lifestyle might lead to increased cardiovascular risk factors, associated with for example inactivity, smoking, unhealthy nutrition [27].

Table 1. Age, sex, depression score, and anxiety score when subjects were divided to patients and healthy group.

		Patients n = 486	Healthy n = 440	p Value
	Age (year)	55.75 ± 10.64	55.83 ± 8.55	0.897
Sex	Male	247 (50.8)	231 (52.5)	0.610
	Female	239 (49.2)	209 (47.5)	
	Anxiety score	10.62 ± 9.82	8.38 ± 8.62	<0.001
	Depression score	10.37 ± 8.20	10.70 ± 8.38	0.534

Data shown as: Mean ± SD or N (%).

Table 2. Distribution of gender in depression in patients and healthy controls.

Group Sex Depression	Patients n = 486		Healthy n = 440		p Value
	Male	Female	Male	Female	
No depression	215 (87.0)	160 (70)	188 (81.5)	137 (65.5)	p₁ < 0.001
Depressed subject	32 (13.0)	79 (30)	43 (18.5)	72 (34.5)	p₂ < 0.001 p₃ < 0.001

p₁: Compared two groups of healthy, patients for depression and gender overall. p₂: Compared in patients group for gender depression. p₃: Compared in healthy group for gender and depression. Data shown as: N (%).

Table 3. Depression score and anxiety score also their category when subjects were divided to angiography positive, negative and healthy group.

		Patient		Healthy (N = 440)	p Value
		Angio− (N = 201)	Angio+ (N = 285)		
	Depression score	11.27 ± 8.85	9.73 ± 7.66	10.70 ± 8.38	0.108
Depression category	No depression	145 (72.0)	230 (80.7)	325 (74.0)	0.049
	Mild depression	52 (26.0)	50 (17.5)	106 (24.0)	0.051
	Moderate depression	4 (2.0)	5 (2.0)	9 (2.0)	0.961
	Anxiety score	11.53 ± 10.03	9.98 ± 9.63	8.38 ± 8.62	<0.001
Anxiety category	Minimal anxiety	86 (42.8)	143 (50.2)	261 (59.3)	<0.001
	Mild anxiety	62 (30.8)	78 (27.4)	108 (24.5)	0.239
	Moderate anxiety	34 (16.9)	39 (13.7)	46 (10.5)	0.067
	Severe anxiety	19 (9.5)	25 (8.8)	25 (5.7)	0.143

Data shown as: Mean ± SD or N (%).

Table 4. Depression score and anxiety score when subjects were divided to angiography positive (single vessel disease, two vessel disease, three vessel disease), negative and healthy group.

	Patient				Healthy (n = 440)	p Value
	Angio− (n = 201)	SVD (n = 88)	2VD (n = 58)	3VD (n = 139)		
Depression score	11.27 ± 8.85	10.10 ± 7.58	10.71 ± 7.88	9.09 ± 7.60	10.70 ± 8.38	0.181
Anxiety score	11.53 ± 10.03	10.69 ± 9.76	11.03 ± 10.55	9.09 ± 9.12	8.38 ± 8.62	<0.001

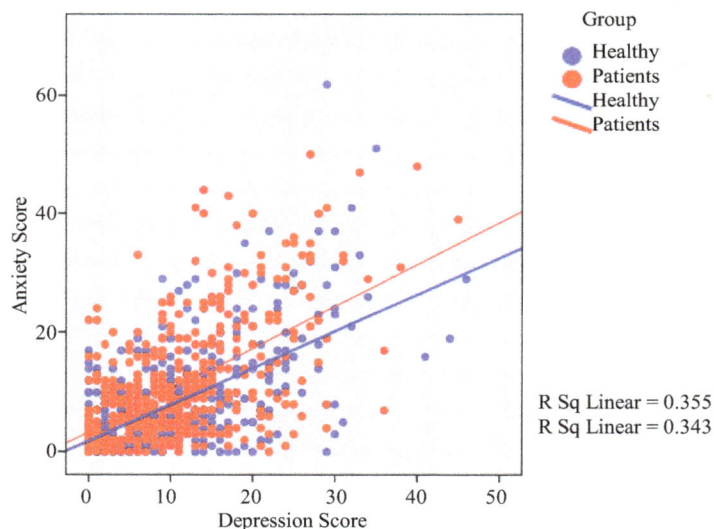

Figure 1. Correlation between anxiety and depression score in healthy and patient group.

In this study 926 healthy and suspected to cardiovascular disease subjects were tested for depression and anxiety by Beck questionnaire. The results of these tests showed that the anxiety is associated with CAD and the angiography positive or negative persons (subjects who had cardiovascular sign and symptoms) had high incidence of anxiety so that the anxiety score and subjects that have minimal anxiety are significant difference between groups ($p < 0.05$). Same findings were reported in some other studies [25] [28] [29].

In Lindeberg's study "exhaustion predicted CHD in both men and women, but its independence from depression and anxiety was demonstrated only in men" [3] an according to **Table 2**, significant difference found between healthy and patients subjects in gender and depression.

Although there is no significant difference between depression score in healthy and patients group but there is statistical significant difference were observed between depression and no depression categories (no < 15 and yes >15) among groups (p < 0.05) (**Table 3**) and also there were a good linear correlation found between anxiety and depression score (**Figure 1**) this correlation are found in both healthy and patient group.

Patients who suffered from severe depression probably have no adequate emotional activity for participate to any researches so it is one of our limitations. Process of in **Table 2** shows that emotional desire in research participation is loss.

5. Conclusion

In conclusion, depression and anxiety Beck scores have great correlation in healthy and CAD patients. We found a good association between anxiety and angiography positive, angiography negative and healthy subjects. So psychiatry visits by specialties in cardiovascular patients are recommended for case fining in depression mood and anxiety disorder.

Acknowledgements

The Mashhad University of Medical Science Research Council supported this research. This paper is the subject thesis of Mr. Mohammad Tajfard, which is the PhD Candidate of the community health in University Putra Malaysia. Authors would like to thank Center for International Scientific Studies and Collaboration for their support.

Ethical Issue

The study was conducted in accordance with the principles of Declaration of Helsinki 1996 version and Good Clinical Practice standards. The study protocol, informed-consent form, and the other study related documents were reviewed and approved by Human Research Ethics Committee of Mashhad University of Medical Sciences (Ethics registration number: MUMS/900671) also Medical Research Ethics Committee of Faculty of Medicine and Health Sciences, Universiti Putra Malaysia (Ethics Committee 15 September 2011).

Conflict of Interest Statement

The authors indicate no potential conflicts of interest.

References

[1] Antonogeorgos, G., Panagiotakos, D.B., Pitsavos, C., Papageorgiou, C., Chrysohoou, C., Papadimitriou, G.N., *et al.* (2012) Understanding the Role of Depression and Anxiety on Cardiovascular Disease Risk, Using Structural Equation Modeling; the Mediating Effect of the Mediterranean Diet and Physical Activity: The ATTICA Study. *Annals of Epidemiology*, **22**, 630-637. http://dx.doi.org/10.1016/j.annepidem.2012.06.103

[2] Murray, C. and Lopez, A. (1996) Summary: The Global Burden of Disease: A Comprehensive Assessment of Mortality and Disability from Diseases, Injuries, and Risk Factors in 1990 and Projected to 2020. Harvard University Press, Cambridge.

[3] Lindeberg, S.I., Rosvall, M. and Ostergren, P.O. (2012) Exhaustion Predicts Coronary Heart Disease Independently of Symptoms of Depression and Anxiety in Men But Not in Women. *Journal of Psychosomatic Research*, **72**, 17-21. http://dx.doi.org/10.1016/j.jpsychores.2011.09.001

[4] Damen, N.L., Pelle, A.J., Szabo, B.M. and Pedersen, S.S. (2012) Symptoms of Anxiety and Cardiac Hospitalizations at 12 Months in Patients with Heart Failure. *Journal of General Internal Medicine*, **27**, 345-350. http://dx.doi.org/10.1007/s11606-011-1843-1

[5] Lloyd-Jones, D., Adams, R., Carnethon, M., De Simone, G., Ferguson, T.B., Flegal, K., *et al.* (2009) Heart Disease and Stroke Statistics—2009 Update: A Report from the American Heart Association Statistics Committee and Stroke Statistics Subcommittee. *Circulation*, **119**, 480-486. http://dx.doi.org/10.1161/CIRCULATIONAHA.108.191259

[6] Shen, B.J., Eisenberg, S.A., Maeda, U., Farrell, K.A., Schwarz, E.R., Penedo, F.J., *et al.* (2011) Depression and Anxiety Predict Decline in Physical Health Functioning in Patients with Heart Failure. *Annals of Behavioral Medicine*, **41**, 373-382. http://dx.doi.org/10.1007/s12160-010-9251-z

[7]   Tull, M.T. and Gratz, K.L. (2008) Further Examination of the Relationship between Anxiety Sensitivity and Depression: The Mediating Role of Experiential Avoidance and Difficulties Engaging in Goal-Directed Behavior When Distressed. *Journal of Anxiety Disorders*, **22**, 199-210. http://dx.doi.org/10.1016/j.janxdis.2007.03.005

[8]   Blumenfield, M., Suojanen, J.K. and Weiss, C. (2012) Public Awareness about the Connection between Depression and Physical Health: Specifically Heart Disease. *Psychiatric Quarterly*, **83**, 259-269. http://dx.doi.org/10.1007/s11126-011-9199-6

[9]   Pedersen, S.S., Herrmann-Lingen, C., de Jonge, P. and Scherer, M. (2010) Type D Personality Is a Predictor of Poor Emotional Quality of Life in Primary Care Heart Failure Patients Independent of Depressive Symptoms and New York Heart Association Functional Class. *Journal of Behavioral Medicine*, **33**, 72-80. http://dx.doi.org/10.1007/s10865-009-9236-1

[10]   Steinberg, G., Lossnitzer, N., Schellberg, D., Mueller-Tasch, T., Krueger, C., Haass, M., *et al.* (2011) Peak Oxygen Uptake and Left Ventricular Ejection Fraction, But Not Depressive Symptoms, Are Associated with Cognitive Impairment in Patients with Chronic Heart Failure. *International Journal of General Medicine*, **4**, 879-887.

[11]   Rutledge, T., Reis, V.A., Linke, S.E., Greenberg, B.H. and Mills, P.J. (2006) Depression in Heart Failure a Meta-Analytic Review of Prevalence, Intervention Effects, and Associations with Clinical Outcomes. *Journal of the American College of Cardiology*, **48**, 1527-1537. http://dx.doi.org/10.1016/j.jacc.2006.06.055

[12]   Gallagher, D., O'Regan, C., Savva, G.M., Cronin, H., Lawlor, B.A. and Kenny, R.A. (2012) Depression, Anxiety and Cardiovascular Disease: Which Symptoms Are Associated with Increased Risk in Community Dwelling Older Adults? *Journal of Affective Disorders*, **142**, 132-138. http://dx.doi.org/10.1016/j.jad.2012.04.012

[13]   Gilani, K.A., Fallahi, B., Jamak, M.E. and Mahani, M.S. (2006) Effects of Depression on Myocardial Perfusion Scintigraphy [Persian]. *Iranian Journal of Nuclear Medicine*, **4**, 1-7.

[14]   Burg, M.M. and Abrams, D. (2001) Depression in Chronic Medical Illness: The Case of Coronary Heart Disease. *Journal of Clinical Psychology*, **57**, 1323-1337. http://dx.doi.org/10.1002/jclp.1100

[15]   Madan, A., White-Williams, C., Borckardt, J.J., Burker, E.J., Milsom, V.A., Pelic, C.M., *et al.* (2012) Beyond Rose Colored Glasses: The Adaptive Role of Depressive and Anxious Symptoms among Individuals with Heart Failure Who Were Evaluated for Transplantation. *Clinical Transplantation*, **26**, E223-E231. http://dx.doi.org/10.1111/j.1399-0012.2012.01613.x

[16]   Spaderna, H., Zahn, D., Schleithoff, S.S., Stadlbauer, T., Rupprecht, L., Smits, J.M., *et al.* (2010) Depression and Disease Severity as Correlates of Everyday Physical Activity in Heart Transplant Candidates. *Transplant International*, **23**, 813-822. http://dx.doi.org/10.1111/j.1432-2277.2010.01056.x

[17]   Alamdari, D.H., Ghayour-Mobarhan, M., Tavallaie, S., Parizadeh, M.R., Moohebati, M., Ghafoori, F., *et al.* (2008) Prooxidant-Antioxidant Balance as a New Risk Factor in Patients with Angiographically Defined Coronary Artery Disease. *Clinical Biochemistry*, **41**, 375-380. http://dx.doi.org/10.1016/j.clinbiochem.2007.12.008

[18]   Kazemi-Bajestani, S.M., Ghayour-Mobarhan, M., Ebrahimi, M., Moohebati, M., Esmaeili, H.A. and Ferns, G.A. (2007) C-Reactive Protein Associated with Coronary Artery Disease in Iranian Patients with Angiographically Defined Coronary Artery Disease. *Clinical Laboratory*, **53**, 49-56.

[19]   Geluk, C.A., Post, W.J., Hillege, H.L., Tio, R.A., Tijssen, J.G., van Dijk, R.B., *et al.* (2008) C-Reactive Protein and Angiographic Characteristics of Stable and Unstable Coronary Artery Disease: Data from the Prospective PREVEND Cohort. *Atherosclerosis*, **196**, 372-382. http://dx.doi.org/10.1016/j.atherosclerosis.2006.11.013

[20]   Nezhad, M., Ghanbari, P., Shahryari, B. and Aghasadeghi, K. (2009) C-Reactive Protein in Angiographically Documented Stable Coronary Disease. *Iranian Cardiovascular Research Journal*, **3**, 97-101.

[21]   Kazemi-Bajestani, S.M., Ghayour-Mobarhan, M., Ebrahimi, M., Moohebati, M., Esmaeili, H.A., Parizadeh, M.R., *et al.* (2007) Serum Copper and Zinc Concentrations Are Lower in Iranian Patients with Angiographically Defined Coronary Artery Disease Than in Subjects with a Normal Angiogram. *Journal of Trace Elements in Medicine and Biology*, **21**, 22-28. http://dx.doi.org/10.1016/j.jtemb.2006.11.005

[22]   Leyfer, O.T., Ruberg, J.L. and Woodruff-Borden, J. (2206) Examination of the Utility of the Beck Anxiety Inventory and Its Factors as a Screener for Anxiety Disorders. *Journal of Anxiety Disorders*, **20**, 444-458. http://dx.doi.org/10.1016/j.janxdis.2005.05.004

[23]   Beck, A.T., Steer, R.A. and Carbin, M.G. (1998) Psychometric Properties of the Beck Depression Inventory: Twenty-Five Years of Evaluation. *Clinical Psychology Review*, **8**, 77-100. http://dx.doi.org/10.1016/0272-7358(88)90050-5

[24]   Beck, A.T., Ward, C.H., Mendelson, M., Mock, J. and Erbaugh, J. (1961) An Inventory for Measuring Depression. *Archives of General Psychiatry*, **4**, 561-571. http://dx.doi.org/10.1001/archpsyc.1961.01710120031004

[25]   Miller, G.E., Freedland, K.E., Carney, R.M., Stetler, C.A. and Banks, W.A. (2003) Pathways Linking Depression, Adiposity, and Inflammatory Markers in Healthy Young Adults. *Brain, Behavior, and Immunity*, **17**, 276-285. http://dx.doi.org/10.1016/S0889-1591(03)00057-6

[26] Richardson, S., Shaffer, J.A., Falzon, L., Krupka, D., Davidson, K.W. and Edmondson, D. (2012) Meta-Analysis of Perceived Stress and Its Association with Incident Coronary Heart Disease. *American Journal of Cardiology*, **110**, 1711-1716. http://dx.doi.org/10.1016/j.amjcard.2012.08.004

[27] Rozanski, A., Blumenthal, J.A. and Kaplan, J. (1999) Impact of Psychological Factors on the Pathogenesis of Cardiovascular Disease and Implications for Therapy. *Circulation*, **99**, 2192-2217. http://dx.doi.org/10.1161/01.CIR.99.16.2192

[28] Kawachi, I., Sparrow, D., Vokonas, P.S. and Weiss, S.T. (1994) Symptoms of Anxiety and Risk of Coronary Heart Disease. The Normative Aging Study. *Circulation*, **90**, 2225-2229. http://dx.doi.org/10.1161/01.CIR.90.5.2225

[29] Kawachi, I., Colditz, G.A., Ascherio, A., Rimm, E.B., Giovannucci, E., Stampfer, M.J., *et al.* (1994) Prospective Study of Phobic Anxiety and Risk of Coronary Heart Disease in Men. *Circulation*, **89**, 1992-1997. http://dx.doi.org/10.1161/01.CIR.89.5.1992

18

Effect of *Citrus aurantium* L. Essential Oil and Its Interaction with Fluoxetine on Anxiety in Male Mice

Sorin Saketi[1], Maryam Bananej[1], Mahsa Hadipour Jahromy[2*]

[1]Biology Department, Faculty of Biological Sciences, Islamic Azad University, North Tehran Branch, Tehran, Iran
[2]Medical Sciences Research Centre, Tehran Medical Sciences Branch, Islamic Azad University, Tehran, Iran
Email: *jahromymh@yahoo.com

Abstract

Anxiety is a very common mental disorder among neurological diseases. Some herbs have soothing effects and play an important role in reducing anxiety. The purpose of this study is to investigate the effect of *Citrus aurantium* L. essential oil on anxiety and its interference with serotonergic pathway. Sixty male mice were assigned into control, sham (saline and olive oil), and experimental groups. Intraperitoneal injection of *Citrus aurantium* L. essential oil was applied at doses of 0.5, 2.5, and 5 percent for 5 days. In another set of experiments, after intraperitoneal injection of *Citrus aurantium* L. essential oil at doses of 0.5, 2.5, and 5 percent for 5 days, on the 5th day, 30 minutes before applying essential oil, fluoxetine (2 mg/kg) was injected. Then, the anxiety-related behavior was assessed using elevated plus maze test. The results revealed that injection of essential oil of *Citrus aurantium* L. alone or along with fluoxetine led to increasing the number of entries into the open arms and the time spent in open arms that was significantly different compared with control and sham groups ($P < 0.001$). Besides, further effects revealed when fluoxetine added to essential oils, however no more effects obtained when compared to fluoxetine alone. It is concluded that *Citrus aurantium* L. essential oil can reduce the anxiety in male mice and due to fluoxetin potentiation and maximum response observed, the herb may express its anxiolytic effects in part, via serotonergic system.

Keywords

Anxiety, Essential Oil, *Citrus aurantium* L., Fluoxetine

---

*Corresponding author.

1. Introduction

Anxiety is a very common mental disorder. Stressful life events are one of the causes of anxiety [1]. There are some effective medicinal and behavioral treatments for anxiety. Antianxiety effects of various medicines applying in different treatment methods have been investigated. It is believed that selective serotonin reuptake inhibitors (SSRIs) such as fluoxetine, citalopram, paroxetine, are appropriate substitutes for traditional treatments of anxiety [2].

Serotonin, a neurotransmitter exists in the brain neurons, also known as 5-hydroxytryptamine (5-HT) possesses several roles in maintaining normal physiological functions [3]. Serotonergic system is involved in expressing fear and anxiety. Fluoxetine is one of the antagonists of 5-HT3 receptors that is effective in treatment of acute depression (including children's depression), phobia disorder (among children and adults), and obsessive-compulsive disorder [4].

Many traditional herbs such as the family of rutaceae, is known to have beneficial effects on anxiety for many years [5]. The effects of brewed and boiled flowers and leaves of the family of rutaceae have been studied to treat nervous system disorders [6]. They are very helpful in reduction of anxiety and insomnia symptoms, and recently *Citrus aurantium* L. is suggested as a medication for depression [6]. The results of analytical chemistry have shown that *Citrus aurantium* L. contains phenolic compounds and flavonoids that possess antioxidant, anticonvulsant, and anticancer properties [5].

Therefore, in this study anxiolytic effect of *Citrus aurantium* L. along with fluoxetine as a 5-HT receptor modulator was investigated on adult male mice in elevated plus maze test.

2. Methods and Materials

2.1. Animals

Male albino mice weighed 22 to 28 g supplied from Pasteur Institute were used in this study. The mice were kept in animal room of the Medical Faculty of Baghiatallah University. Sixty mice were assigned into 10 groups of six. Animals housed under the following laboratory conditions: temperature 22°C ± 1°C, humidity 40% - 60%, 12 h Light/Dark cycle, lights on at 07:00 h. Mice were maintained in polyethylene cages with enough food and water available *ad libitum*. All measurements were performed between 9:00 and 15:00 h in the animal testing room. Mice were treated in accordance with the National Institutes of Health (NIH) Guide for Care and Use of Laboratory Animals.

2.2. Essential Oil Preparation

Collected *Citrus aurantium* L. flowers were bought from local market of Shiraz and dried in darkness and pulverized. 300 g of the dried powder were extracted with maceration. Essential oil was collected using n-hexane and sodium sulfate, then, exposure to open air till n-hexane vaporized. The oils were kept in a cool place till used (35% W/V). The essential oil dissolved in olive oil to make different concentrations of 0.5, 2.5, and 5 percent.

2.3. Drugs and Treatments

Fluoxetine was supplied from Damavand-Darou Company and injected intraperitoneally, using sodium chloride 9% (normal saline).

Intraperitoneal injection of *Citrus aurantium* L. essential oil was applied for the experimental group at doses of 0.5, 2.5, and 5 percent at a certain hour for 5 days. According to different studies and based on our previous experimental experiences, it is decided to use low dose of fluoxetine (2 mg/kg) that shows anxiolytic effects, and thirty minutes interval for injections. Therefore, in another set of experiments, after intraperitoneal injection of *Citrus aurantium* L. essential oil at doses of 0.5, 2.5, and 5 percent for 5 days, on the 5th day, 30 minutes before applying the last injection of essential oil, fluoxetine (2 mg/kg) was injected to evaluate its modulator action. Thirty minutes after the injection of essential oil of *Citrus aurantium* L., the anxiety-related behavior of mice was assessed using elevated plus maze (EPM) test.

2.4. EPM Test

The studies were carried out on mice according to the method of Lister [7]. The plus-maze apparatus was made of Plexiglas and consisted of two open (30×5 cm) and two closed ($30 \times 5 \times 15$ cm) arms. The arms extended from a central platform of 5×5 cm. The apparatus was mounted on a Plexiglas base raising it 38.5 cm above the floor. The test consisted in placing a mouse in the center of the apparatus (facing a closed arm) and allowing it to freely explore. All experiments recorded using personal camcorder. The number of entries into the open arms and the time spent in these arms were scored for a 5-min test period. An entry was defined as placing all four paws within the boundaries of the arm. The following measures were obtained from the test: the total number of arm entries; the percentage of arm entries into the open arms; the time spent in the open arms expressed as a percentage of the time spent in both the open and closed arms. Anxiolytic activity was indicated by increases in time spent in open arms or in number of open arm entries. Total number of entries into either type of arm was used as a measure of overall motor activity.

2.5. Statistical Analysis

All values were expressed as mean ± SEM from six animals. The results were subjected to statistical analysis using Unpaired-t test to calculate the significance difference if any among the groups. $P < 0.05$ was considered significant (Origin IV software).

3. Results

Figure 1 illustrates that in terms of the applied doses, the intraperitoneal injection of the essential oil of *Citrus aurantium* L. at doses of 0.5, 2.5, and 5 percent, increases the time spent in open arms. Also, significant differences were observed between the groups that received doses of 2.5 and 5 percent and control group in the time spent in open arms ($P < 0.001$); this difference was less in the group that received lower dose ($P < 0.05$).

Figure 2 illustrates that intraperitoneal injection of fluoxetine (2 mg/kg) results in increased spent time in open arms. Significant differences were observed between experimental group and control group ($P < 0.001$). Injection of essential oil of *Citrus aurantium* L. along with fluoxetine (at doses of 0.5, 2.5, and 5 percent) resulted in significant increased spent time in open arms ($P < 0.001$).

Figure 3 illustrates that intraperitoneal injection of essential oil of *Citrus aurantium* L. (at dose of 5 percent) results in significant differences $^*P < 0.05$ between experimental group and control group in the number of entries to the open arms.

Figure 4 illustrates that intraperitoneal injection of fluoxetine (2 mg/kg) results in increased number of entries to the open arms. Significant differences were observed between the experimental groups and control group in the number of entries to the open arms ($P < 0.001$). Also, the injection of *Citrus aurantium* L. (at doses of 0.5,

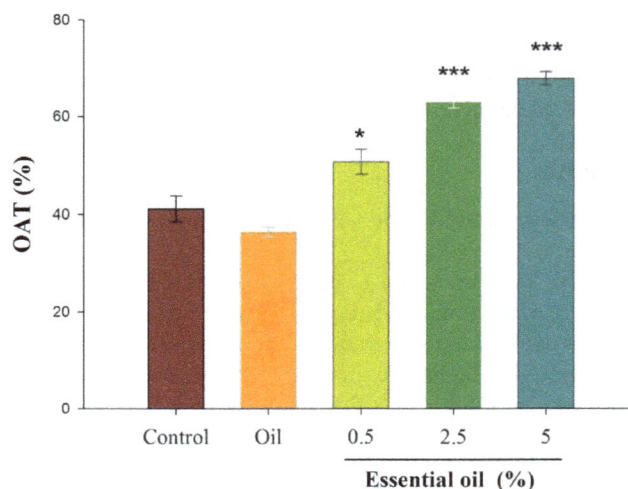

Figure 1. Comparison between experimental groups (received essential oil of *Citrus aurantium* L. at doses of 0.5, 2.5, and 5 percent), control and sham groups (received olive oil) in antianxiety effect of *Citrus aurantium* L. essential oil. Mean ± S.E.M. $n = 6$. $^*P < 0.05$ and $^{***}P < 0.001$. OAT is the spent time in open arms.

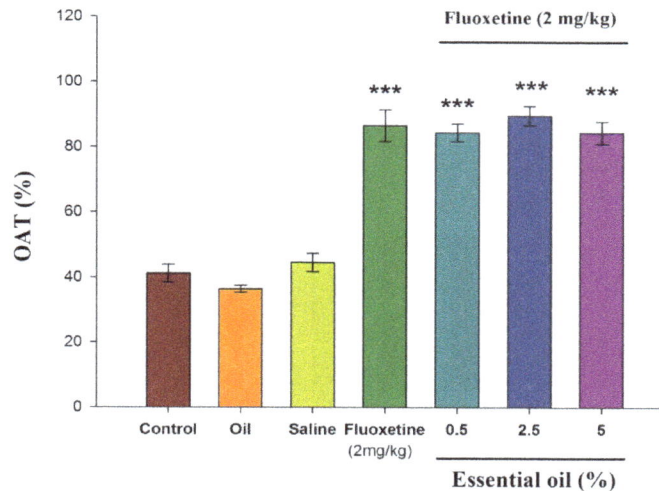

Figure 2. Comparison between experimental groups (received essential oil of *Citrus aurantium* L. at doses of 0.5, 2.5, and 5 percent along with fluoxetine), control group and sham group (received olive oil) in antianxiety effect of *Citrus aurantium* L. essential oil. Mean ± S.E.M. $n = 6$. $^{***}P < 0.001$. OAT is the spent time in open arms.

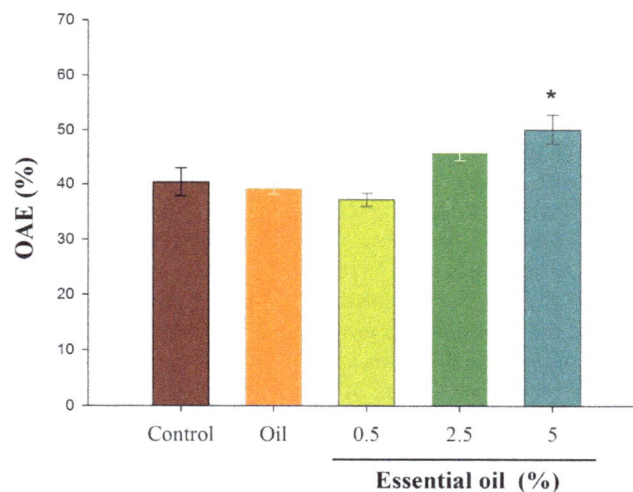

Figure 3. Comparison between experimental groups (received essential oil of *Citrus aurantium* L. at doses of 0.5, 2.5, and 5 percent), control group and sham group (received olive oil) in antianxiety effect of *Citrus aurantium* L. essential oil. Mean ± S.E.M. $n = 6$. $^{*}P < 0.05$. OAE is the number of entries to the open arms.

2.5, and 5) along with fluoxetine resulted in significant increased number of entries to the open arms in the experimental group compared with the control group ($P < 0.001$).

4. Discussion

The results revealed that applying *Citrus aurantium* L. alone or along with fluoxetine affect the anxiety behavior in mice.

The role of serotonin in changing anxiety behavior has been shown in previous studies. The reduction of serotonin in the synaptic cleft results in increased anxiety disorders and depression. The shortage of serotonin is not the only reason of development of anxiety disorders [8]. Preclinical studies have proposed that through agonist and antagonist drugs, specific 5-HT receptors may increase anxiloytic responses. Several studies have shown that antagonists of 5-HT3 receptor have a role in mood and anxiety disorders [9].

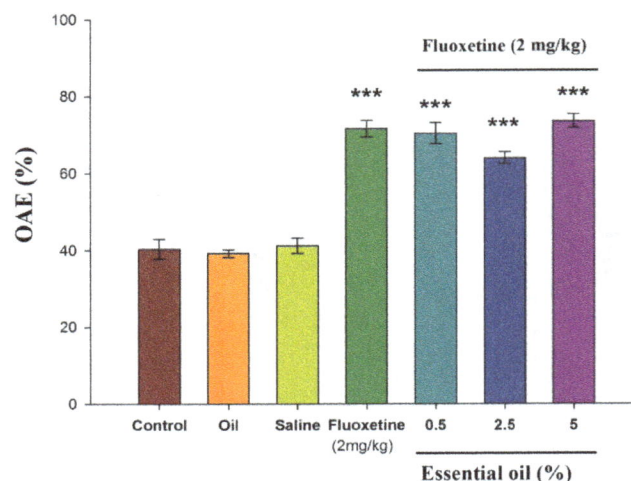

Figure 4. comparison between experimental groups (received essential oil of *Citrus aurantium* L. at doses of 0.5, 2.5, and 5 percent along with fluoxetine), control group and sham group (received olive oil) in antianxiety effect of *Citrus aurantium* L. essential oil. Mean ± S.E.M. n = 6. [***]$P < 0.001$. OAE is the number of entries to the open arms.

5-HT3 receptors distributed in amygdala have a key role in the physiopathology of anxiety [10]. The local injection of 5-HT3 receptor antagonists in the amygdala of mice resulted in decreased responses while 5-HT3 receptor agonists showed the opposite effect [11].

According to different studies and based on our previous experimental experiences, it is decided to use low dose of fluoxetine (2 mg/kg) that shows anxiolytic effects, and thirty minutes interval for injections considered for complete absorption of injected materials. In this study, apparently, fluoxetine (2 mg/kg) acted as 5-HT3 receptor agonist. According to the results, intraperitoneal injection of fluoxetine into the mice results in the increased number of entries to the open arms ($P < 0.001$) and the spent time in open arms. Also, this study investigated the antianxity effect of *Citrus aurantium* L. and its interference in serotonergic pathway. As shown in the **Figures 1-4**, different doses of essential oil *Citrus aurantium* L. result in increased spent time in open arms dose-dependently. In terms of the number of entries to the open arms, only at a dose of 5 percent there was a significant difference between the experimental group and control group ($P < 0.05$).

It is reported that fluoxetine prevents the connection of 5HT-3 receptor antagonists [12]. However some other studies showed that fluoxetine blocks the release of 5-HT from dorsal raphe nucleus [13].

Citrus aurantium L. contains various compounds that have positive effects on organs' activity, especially in the nervous system. The antianxiety effects of *Citrus aurantium* L. have been investigated in some studies. Carvalho *et al*. (2002) have reported that *Citrus aurantium* L. potentiates the sleep caused by barbiturates and reduces anxiety [14]. Mahmoudi *et al*. (1384) investigated that flavonoids in *Citrus aurantium* L. have antianxiety and tranquilizing effects [15]. Also, Lehner (2000) reported that the spray of *Citrus aurantium* L. essential oil in a dental office leads to decreased anxiety of patients [7]. Shabanian *et al*. (1387) showed that *Citrus aurantium* L. can be applied as a premedication to reduce the anxiety of patients before surgery [16]. *Citrus aurantriun* contains various compounds such as linanol, linalyl acetate, myrcene, limonene, and flavonoids [17]. Antianxiety effects of some of these compounds individually, also have been reported. Limonene reduces the activity of the central nervous system and decreases anxiety [18]. Another study has reported that limonene and myrcene exhibit inhibitory actions in the central nervous system and has antianxiety and antiepileptic effects through suppressing the central nervous system [19]. Other anxiolytic compound of *Citrus aurantium* L. is coumarin. Pereira (2009) reported that coumarin can have a specific inhibitory effect on the central nervous system and prevent epileptic attacks and seizures [20]. Linanol inhibits the release of acetylcholine and has antiepileptic effects [19]. Generally, flavonoids affect benzodiazepine receptors and result in suppression of nervous system [15].

5. Conclusion

It is concluded that certain compounds of *Citrus aurantium* L. reinforce serotonergic pathways and increase the effect of serotonin in synaptic clefts, which leads to maintain tranquility and reduce the anxiety of laboratory animals.

Acknowledgements

We would like to thank Dr. Hedayat Sahrai for his valuable help and guide.

References

[1] Brown, G.W. and Harris, T.O. (1989) Depression. In Brown, G.W. and Harris, T.O., Eds., *Life Events and Illness*, The Guilford, New York, 49-93.

[2] Kulkarni, S.K., Singh, K. and Bishnoi, M. (2008) Comparative Behavioural Profile of Newer Antianxiety Drugs on Different Mazes. *Indian Journal of Experimental Biology*, **46**, 633-638.

[3] Aghajanian, G.K. and Sanders-Bush, E. (2002) Serotonin. *Neuropsychopharmacology*, **35**, 15-35.

[4] Hagerman, R.J. (1999) Neurodevelopmental Disorders: Diagnosis and Treatment. Oxford University Press, Oxford.

[5] Karimi, E., Oskoueian, E., Hendra, R., Oskoueian, A. and Jaafar, H. (2012) Phenolic Compounds Characterization and Biological Activities of *Citrus aurantium* Bloom. *Molecules*, **17**, 1203-1218. http://dx.doi.org/10.3390/molecules17021203

[6] Costa, C.A., Cury, T.C., Cassettari, B.O., Takahira, R.K., Flório, J.C. and Costa, M. (2013) *Citrus aurantium* L. Essential Oil Exhibits Anxiolyticlike Activity Mediated by 5-HT1A-Receptors and Reduces Cholesterol after Repeated Oral Treatment. *BMC Complementary and Alternative Medicine*, **13**, 42. http://dx.doi.org/10.1155/2013/841580

[7] Lehrner, J., Eckersberger, C., Walla, P., Pötsch, G. and Deecke, L. (2000) Ambient Odor of Orange in a Dental Office Reduces Anxiety and Improves Mood in Female Patients. *Physiology Behavior*, **71**, 83-86. http://dx.doi.org/10.1016/S0031-9384(00)00308-5

[8] Turner, E.H., Loftis, J.M. and Blackwell, A.D. (2006) Serotonin a la carte: Supplementation with the Serotonin Precursor 5-Hydroxytryptophan. *Pharmacology & Therapeutics*, **109**, 325-338. http://dx.doi.org/10.1016/j.pharmthera.2005.06.004

[9] Artigas, F., Adell, A. and Celada, P. (2006) Pindolol Augmentation of Antidepressant Response. *Current Drug Targets*, **7**, 139-147. http://dx.doi.org/10.2174/138945006775515446

[10] Ninan, P.T. (1999) The Functional Anatomy, Neurochemistry, and Pharmacology of Anxiety. *Journal of Clinical Psychiatry*, **60**, 12-17.

[11] Higgins, G.A., Jones, B.J., Oakley, N.R. and Tyers, M.B. (1991) Evidence That the Amygdala Is Involved in the Disinhibitory Effects of 5-HT3 Receptor Antagonists. *Psychopharmacology* (*Berlin*), **104**, 545-551. http://dx.doi.org/10.1007/BF02245664

[12] Lucchelli, A., Santagostino-Barbone, M.G., Barbieri, A., Candura, S.M. and Tonini, M. (1995) The Interaction of Antidepressant Drugs with Central and Peripheral (Enteric) 5-HT3 and 5-HT4 Receptors. *British Journal of Pharmacology*, **114**, 1017-1025. http://dx.doi.org/10.1111/j.1476-5381.1995.tb13307.x

[13] Bagdy, E., Solyom, S. and Harsing Jr., L.G. (1998) Feedback Stimulation of Somatodendritic Serotonin Release: A 5-HT3 Receptor-Mediated Effect in the Raphe Nuclei of the Rat. *Brain Research Bulletin*, **45**, 203-208. http://dx.doi.org/10.1016/S0361-9230(97)00340-7

[14] Carvalho-Freitas, M.I. and Costa, M. (2002) Anxiolytic and Sedative Effects of Extracts and Essential Oil from *Citrus aurantium* L. *Biological Pharmaceutical Bulletin*, **25**, 1629-1633.

[15] Mahmoudi, M., Shamsi, M., Froumadi, A. Raftari, Sh. and Asadi Shekari, M. (2005) The Effects of Essential Oil of *Citrus aurantium* on the Prevention of Pseudo Depression Caused by the Injection of Lipopolysaccharide in Rats. *Kerman Medical Sciences Journal*, **12**, 244-251.

[16] Shabanian, Gh., Pouria Monfared E. and Akhlaghi M. (2008) A Comparison between the Effects of *Citrus aurantium* and Diazepam on Reducing Anxiety before Surgery. *Shahrekord Medical Sciences University Magazine*, **4**, 13-18.

[17] Lopes Campêlo, L.M., Gonçalves e Sá, C., de Almeida, A.A.C., *et al.* (2011) Sedative, Anxiolytic and Antidepressant Activities of *Citrus limon* (Burn) Essential Oil in Mice. *Pharmazie*, **66**, 623-627.

[18] Re, L., Barocci, S., Sonnino, S., *et al.* (2000) Linalool Modifies the Nicotinic Receptor-Ion Channel Kinetics at the Mouse Neuromuscular Junction. *Pharmacological Research*, **42**, 177-181. http://dx.doi.org/10.1006/phrs.2000.0671

[19] Deckers, C.L.P., Genton, P., Sills, G.J. and Schmidt, D. (2003) Current Limitations of Antiepileptic Drug Therapy: A Conference Review. *Epilepsy Research*, **53**, 1-17. http://dx.doi.org/10.1016/S0920-1211(02)00257-7

[20] Pereira, E.C., Lucetti, D.L. and Barbosa Filho, J.M. (2009) Coumarin Effects on Amino Acid Levels in Mice Prefrontal Cortex and Hippocampus. *Neuroscience Letters*, **454**, 139-142. http://dx.doi.org/10.1016/j.neulet.2009.03.009

19

Description of the General Procedure of a Stress Inoculation Program to Cope with the Test Anxiety

Isabel Serrano Pintado[1], María del Camino Escolar Llamazares[2]

[1]Department Personalidad, Evaluación y Tratamiento Psicológico, Facultad de Psicología, Universidad de Salamanca, Salamanca, España
[2]Department Personalidad, Evaluación y Tratamiento Psicológico, Facultad de Humanidades y Educación, Universidad de Burgos, Burgos, España
Email: serrano@usal.es, cescolar@ubu.es

Abstract

We set out the stages in the general procedure of a stress inoculation program for the treatment of test anxiety in university students, with the aim of adapting it to the characteristics of each participant. Research has previously been conducted to that end (Serrano, Delgado, & Escolar, 2010; Serrano, Escolar, & Delgado, 2002; Serrano, Escolar, & Delgado, 2011) on dismantling strategies in a real clinical field. We conclude that there are individual response patterns to test anxiety, so it is therefore necessary to adapt the intervention to the principle variable that is affected in each individual (Escolar & Serrano, 2012). We do not consider that training in study skills is appropriate, when treating problems of irrational anxiety.

Keywords

Stress Inoculation, Irrational Test Anxiety, Worry-Emotionality, Individual Response Patterns

1. Introduction

The evaluation anxiety represents a prolific line of research that has generated many areas of psychological intervention (Iruarrizaga & Salvador, 1999; Miralles & Hernández, 2012; Miralles & Sanz, 2011; Ramirez & Beilock, 2011).

The significant and debilitating effects of tests in modern society on individuals' emotional well-being and cognitive performance (Amutio & Smith, 2008; Bonaccio, Reeve, & Winford, 2012; Conley & Lehman, 2012;

Gutiérrez-Calvo, 1996; Miralles & Hernández, 2012; Miralles & Sanz, 2011; Nemati & Habibi, 2012; Piemontesi & Heredia, 2009; Polo, Hernández, & Pozo, 1996; Rosário et al., 2008; Spielberger & Vagg, 1987; Szafranski, Barrera, & Norton, 2012) have led to the extensive development of "test anxiety" programs, as described by Escolar and Serrano (2012). These treatments have provided adaptive strategies for students with test anxiety to face the exam situation rather than to avoid it, and so prevent a significant decrease in academic achievement (Serrano & Delgado, 1990; Serrano & Delgado, 1991; Serrano, Delgado, & Escolar, 2010; Serrano & Escolar, 2011; Serrano, Escolar, & Delgado, 2002; Serrano, Escolar, & Delgado, 2011).

Moreover, many studies have been completed on the treatment of test anxiety with the objective of demonstrating that one particular treatment is effective at reducing this type of anxiety and/or at improving the cognitive performance of students (Escolar & Serrano, 2012).

In this direction, Zeidner (2007), considered necessary to set up a program of intervention directed at the control of this type of anxiety and to develop effective therapeutic methods for their treatment, specifically based on studies of efficiency.

Thus, authors such as Furlan, Sánchez, Heredia, Piemontesi and Illbele (2009), Martínez-Monteagudo, Inglés, Cano-Vindel and García-Fernández (2012), Miralles and Hernández (2012), Miralles and Sanz (2011), Onwuegbuzie and Daley (1996), and Zeidner (1998) have all proposed the need to adapt the coping strategy to the type of response that is principally affected in each individual (cognitive and/or emotional), as the same therapeutic procedures may not be successful for all students who suffer from test anxiety (Escolar & Serrano, 2012). Zeidner (1998) considered that therapeutic interventions and techniques would be effective if they could be adjusted to the needs of different types of students with test anxiety, as each one may be characterized by different problems and concerns. Clearly, a one-size-fits-all program of treatment can never be expected to be equally effective.

Given this situation, the objective of our research (Serrano et al., 2002, 2010, 2011) has been to study the differential efficacy of coping strategies in the reduction of test anxiety, as a function of the variable predominantly affected in the student: the cognitive variable or the emotional variable.

For this end, we adapt the characteristics of each participant to a stress inoculation program (IEA) for the treatment of test anxiety, with dismantling strategies in a real clinical field. These participants were students enrolled in the Salamanca University (Spain). The IEA was designed to develop coping skills. According to Meichenbaum (1985), he combines elements of didactic teaching, socratic discussion, cognitive restructuring, problem solving and relaxation training, behavioral rehearsal imagined, self-recording, self-instruction and reinforcement. It consists of three stages: the first, conceptualization, the second, skill acquisition and practice and the third stage consolidation.

The test anxiety in our work is understood within the conceptual framework of Spielberger (1972a, 1972b), which has also been recently used by authors such as Can, Dereboy and Eskin (2012), Cunha and Paiva (2012), Nemati and Habibi (2012), Piemontesi, Heredia, Furlan, Sanchéz-Rosas and Martínez (2012) and Putwain and Sysmes (2012) among others. We therefore understand that the construct of test anxiety is defined as a specific type of anxiety that reflects the predisposition to manifest anxiety responses in educational situations in which the individuals are or feel evaluated. Moreover, we accept the distinction between irrational anxiety and rational anxiety proposed by Wolpe (1958). That is, we differentiate between students without study skills and without self-control skills over their study behavior, and students who have these skills in their behavioral repertoire and put them into practice. In the first case, we are talking about *rational anxiety* and in the second case about *irrational anxiety*. Thus, we considered that the students who suffer test anxiety come under the concept of irrational anxiety. They are in other words, students who know how to study and do so in an acceptable manner but, who feel uneasy in real or imagined situations to do with tests that are present, anticipated or remembered. It is therefore a question of students who, in an exam situation, despite preparing themselves in an acceptable way for the test, experience debilitating fear, as a consequence of which their academic performance is below their optimum level, and students who even display avoidance behaviors (Serrano & Delgado, 1990; Serrano et al., 2010, 2011). These are clearly students who come under the first type referred to by Naveh-Benjamin (1991) and Naveh-Benjamin, McKeachie & Lin (1987), in other words, those students with good study skills whose poor performance is related to problems of information recall.

In this paper we present: a) a description of the general procedure of a stress inoculation program to cope with the test anxiety used in the authors' previous research, and b) a summary of main findings that make clear how this test anxiety intervention can be tailored to an individual client's need.

2. Stages in the General Procedure

The general procedure and its different stages detailed in Escolar (2007) are listed below:

2.1. Selection of Participants Distinguishing between Deterioration in Performance and Poor Study Skills

A public invitation, over eight academic years, has been addressed to all students at the University of Salamanca who requested assistance with test anxiety problems. They were informed in this public invitation (initial session) that it involved the offer of group treatment, of an approximate duration of 12 - 14 sessions arranged over various months, during which time they would learn strategies and skills to confront test anxiety and to resolve the problems it caused.

They were then administered a general questionnaire on anxiety, specifically, the trait version of the State/ Trait Anxiety Inventory (STAI) (STAI E/R; Spielberger, Gorsuch, & Lushene, 1970). This inventory has good validity and reliability, Spielberger (1983) reported validity measures from 75 - 85 and measures of test-retest reliability from 73 - 86 (Sapp, 1999).

In addition, they were administered:

-The Test Anxiety Inventory (TAI; Spielberger, 1980), which measures the trait test anxiety responses in its physiological and cognitive manifestations. It has a reliability index, according to the Cronbach's Alpha coefficient, of 0.92.

-The Test Anxiety Scale (TAS; Sarason, 1978), which measures the trait test anxiety response in its physiological and cognitive contexts. The test-retest reliability index is 0.87 (Wagaman, Cornier, & Cornier, 1975).

-The Cuestionario de Ansiedad ante los Exámenes [Questionnaire on the assessment of anxiety behaviours in exams] (CAEX) by Valero, 1997 (cited in Valero, 1999), which covers a variety of motor, verbal, cognitive, and physiological responses that usually appear in test anxiety, together with the typology of the most frequent tests. According to the author, the internal consistency of Cronbach's Alpha is 0.92.

-The Inventario de Hábitos de Estudio [Study Habits Inventory] (IHE; Pozar, 1979) evaluates the work and study habits of students on four scales. Scale I: Study Environmental Conditions; Scale II: Planning Study; Scale III: Use of Materials; Scale IV: Assimilation of Contents, and Sincerity Scale (additional scale). The IHE according to the two-halves model has a reliability index of over 0.91.

This permits us to evaluate anxiety over untreated themes, the trait test anxiety response and study habits in pre-treatment situations.

At the end of this initial session, it was explained that the program targets those students whose academic performance is weakened due to anxiety and not those with poor study behavior (in coherence with our definition of test anxiety).

2.2. Evaluation Pre-Treatment of Situational Test Anxiety

We contacted the students during the first term, to inform them that. Thus, immediately after finishing one of the exams judged by them as "the most difficult", we evaluated their state test anxiety, with:

-The Inventory of Test Anxiety (ITA; Osterhouse, 1969), which measures the state test anxiety response, in its physiological and cognitive manifestation. Osterhouse specifically developed it to measure the effects of treatment directed at the reduction of test anxiety. The reliability obtained by the two-halves method was 0.92 (McMillan & Osterhouse, 1972; Osterhouse, 1972).

-The Cognitive Interference Questionnaire (CIQ; Sarason, 1984), which measures the response of the test anxiety state, in its cognitive manifestation. Specifically, it measures the frequency of adverse and irrelevant thoughts for the task at hand.

-An inventory of general anxiety in its state version, in concrete The State-Trait Anxiety Inventory (STAI E/R; Spielberger et al., 1970).

2.3. Selection of the Sample

The two aforementioned evaluation stages permit us to establish the degree of state-trait anxiety levels on topics unrelated to exams, the levels of state-trait test anxiety, and the study habits of each student. The students who were selected had the highest scores in: a) the questionnaire on general anxiety: The State/Trait Anxiety Inventory (STAI) (STAI E/R; Spielberger et al., 1970) (above the average of 5.50 on the decatype scale); b) the questionnaires on trait test anxiety: The Test Anxiety Inventory (TAI; Spielberger, 1980) (those participants with medium and high scores); and the Test Anxiety Scale (TAS; Sarason, 1978) (those participants with medium and high scores); and c) in particular, the questionnaires on state test anxiety: The Inventory of Test Anxiety (ITA; Osterhouse, 1969) (those participants with medium and high scores) and the Cognitive Interference Questionnaire (CIQ; Sarason, 1984) (those participants with medium and high scores). Moreover, none of the students presented poor study habits evaluated with the Inventario de Hábitos de Estudio (IHE; Pozar, 1979) (participants with scores of normal, good, and excellent on the scale). The results of the Cuestionario de Ansiedad ante Exámenes (CAEX) proposed by Valero, 1997 (cited in Valero, 1999) assisted us in our decision taking (participants with scores over the average score in all the scales). All of this in accordance with our definition of test anxiety construct.

We assessed the scores of the selected participants, under the components of emotionality and worries in the aforementioned questionnaires. Thus, some individuals presented high and average scores for emotionality and high, average and low scores for worry, and others presented high and average scores for worry and high, average and low scores for emotionality. Logically, there were no individuals with low scores for both components. In this context, in accordance with Liebert and Morris (1967), we understand emotionality to be the affective-physiological experience generated by autonomous activation (Serrano et al., 2010).

2.4. Assignation of Participants to Experimental Groups

We assigned the 104 participants who had been selected to the three experimental groups by means of simple random sampling. One group, referred to as "Treatment group 1", would receive cognitive training; a second group, referred to as "Treatment group 2", would receive training in relaxation strategies; and the third group, referred to as "Treatment group 3", would receive training in relaxation strategies and cognitive training.

The dismantling strategy that was carried out may be observed in this section. We systematically dismantled specific components of the stress-inoculation program in three types of intervention, with the final objective of adapting it to the characteristics of each patient.

2.5. Application of the Program

The program has three stages: educational, practical, and in application.

a) Educational stage. The concept of test anxiety was separately explained to the three treatment groups. Information was also collected on the way in which the problem appeared to each participant, at the three response levels (cognitive, somatic and behavioral). Subsequently, participants were informed about the desired outcome of the treatment, and the procedures in use to arrive at the proposed objectives were explained and justified.

"Treatment group 1" received an explanation of cognitive restructuring and thought stopping (cognitive treatment) as the sole strategies with which to control negative self-verbalizations and in this way, to control the physiological activation linked with them, and in consequence the behavioral response. "Treatment group 2" received relaxation as the sole strategy with which to control the physiological activation of the anxiety response and by doing so, to confront the other two manifestations of anxiety: the cognitive and the behavioral. "Treatment group 3" received two coping strategies: relaxation, with which to control physiological activation and cognitive training with which they could confront negative self-verbalizations, changing them into positive self-verbalizations.

b) Practical stage. During this stage, the participants learnt about and practiced the skills that have been described over fourteen sessions.

b.1. Training in relaxation

Both the participants in "Treatment group 2" and those in "Treatment group 3" received relaxation training over six sessions. This relaxation training was done following the progressive relaxation scheme of Jacobson (1938), but using a very much briefer version than that of Bernstein and Borkovec (1983), developed by the authors.

b.2. Training in domain of Subjective Units of Anxiety (SUAs)

The participants of the three treatment groups were also instructed in the use of the SUA scale. The objective was to evaluate the subjective experience of the level of anxiety before and after carrying out the confrontations in the hierarchical situations and to communicate them. The relaxation level achieved after the practice was also assessed in the case of the participants in "Treatment group 2" and in "Treatment group 3". A scale of 0, for completely relaxed, to 100, extremely tense, was used.

b.3. Training in the control of self-verbalizations

This training was carried out with the participants in "Treatment groups 1-3" over approximately eight sessions. The negative effect of certain sorts of self-verbalizations pronounced before the test situation, and how they could make use of alternative self-verbalizations was explained to them to confront those negative effects. Subsequently, they were invited to identify the negative self-verbalizations that they pronounced when preparing for an exam: before, during and after them.

All of the self-verbalizations were submitted one by one to logical questions in a process of Socratic dialogue, between the members of the group, in order to analyze their validity and utility. Group formulating another alternative self-verbalization/s of a positive and rational, task-oriented nature.

The last step was to train the groups in thought-stopping and in the substitution of self-verbalizations with external subvocal cues and hidden cues

b.4. Construction of hierarchies

A shared hierarchy was established for all participants in each of the treatment groups, of approximately 10 anxiogenic situations hierarchically organized by SUAs (Subjective Units of Anxiety), usually in accordance with the temporal proximity of a test and its subsequent consequences.

c) *Application stage*. In this stage, coping skills were used, which had been learnt to face the anxiogenic situations of the respective hierarchies in the imagination. One session was dedicated to training the participants from the three treatment groups in the use of the imagination.

The practical guide for the participants of "Treatment group 1" consisted of the presentation of each hierarchical and coping situation through cognitive restructuring and thought stopping.

The guided practice with the participants of "Treatment group 2" consisted in the presentation of each of the hierarchical and coping situations through the relaxation of the anxiety experienced in each of the tests, until the stress had abated.

The guided practice with the participants of "Treatment group 3" consisted in the presentation of each hierarchical and coping situation, through relaxation and thought-stopping, relating to the anxiety experienced in each of the tests, until they had reduced the stress.

When the participants of all the groups were accustomed to mastering the anxiety provoked by those situations in their imagination, they were confronted with real anxiogenic situations relating to tests. In the last session, they were asked for a list showing the dates of the final tests corresponding to the second term, ordered by their degree of difficulty.

2.6. Post-Treatment Evaluation

Immediately after starting the final exams in their second term, we once again measured the degree of anxiety that the students experienced through the following questionnaires: The State/Trait Anxiety Inventory (with the trait version) (STAI E/R; Spielberger et al., 1970), the Test Anxiety Inventory (TAI; Spielberger, 1980), the Test Anxiety Scale (TAS; Sarason, 1978) and the Cuestionario de Ansiedad ante Exámenes (CAEX) by Valero, 1997 (cited in Valero, 1999). We also recorded the study habits by means of the Inventario de Hábitos de Estudio (IHE; Pozar, 1979)[1].

In the same way as we did for the pre-treatment evaluation, we contacted each of the participants immediately after they had completed what they considered one of their most difficult exam, so as to record the degree of anxiety that they experienced. They therefore responded to the state test anxiety questionnaires: The Inventory of Test Anxiety (ITA; Osterhouse, 1969), the Cognitive Interference Questionnaire (CIQ; Sarason, 1984), and the State/Trait Anxiety Inventory (in its state version) (STAI E/R; Spielberger et al., 1970). There was an interval of between six-to-nine days, from the evaluation of the anxiety trait and the evaluation of the component state, for all participants.

Finally, information was collected orally from participants on their mastery of the situations *in vivo*.

Having completed the research, the results of which may be found in Serrano et al. (2010, 2011), we verified the adjustment of different strategies to the different characteristics of the patients. In particular, we noted that

---

[1]The reason for the post-intervention measurement of study habits was to test whether anxiety control might have some sort of influence on improving study habits.

the individuals classified as "more emotional" in the pre-treatment observations, benefitted mainly from the combined treatment (Treatment group 3: physiological and cognitive treatment). While the subjects classified as "more worried" (suffer more anxiety at a cognitive level) benefitted equally from the three types of intervention. We therefore considered it sufficient to apply one of the treatments in isolation.

3. Discussion

We see, in what follows, a reflection of the results of this program, first of all, for more worried individuals, in second place, for more emotional individuals and thirdly, on the advisability or otherwise of using training in study skills in these programs.

With regard to the subjects classified as more worried, we consider that our results are in accordance with those obtained by Morris, Davis and Hutchings (1981), who established that worry-state test anxiety responded well to the majority of treatments (significant reductions were obtained).

So, as the more worried subjects will benefit equally from the three types of intervention, we consider it sufficient to select one of the two individual treatments (Serrano et al., 2002, 2010). In particular, we considered the advantages of the physiological intervention instead of the cognitive one, for various motives: a) because with this intervention, greater improvements were obtained in our studies (Serrano et al., 2002, 2010, 2011) than with the cognitive treatment, and because the physiological treatment is not negative for any of the participants, as happens with the cognitive treatment in participants with high levels of both emotionality and worry; and, b) because of the results obtained by Serrano and Delgado (1991), in which it may be noted that students with high levels of worry can suffer possible interferences of an attentional nature with the cognitive treatment. We may also recall that, in this regard, various researchers have demonstrated that people exposed to stressful situations have difficulty executing complex mental operations that they confront with stress (Gaudry & Spielberger, 1971). And, on the contrary, the relaxation treatment (Hernández, Pozo, & Polo, 1994; Spielberger & Vagg, 1995) applied during the evaluation counteracted the activated state of the individual and reduced subjectively experienced anxiety, as well as stress. In other words, possibly in these more worried participants the physiological treatment in addition to decreasing the physiological response of anxiety acted positively on cognitive manifestation.

As well, some studies (Fletcher & Spielberger, 1995; Gonzalez, 1995; Parker, Vagg, & Papsdorf, 1995) suggest that cognitively focused treatments have consistently been more successful than emotionally focused treatments in the reduction of test anxiety and its components of emotionality and worry. However, it is highly relevant to point out that none of the studies took prior account of the intra-individual variability among these students, which is included in our study.

With regard to the subjects classified as more emotional, where we see the need to apply the combined treatment (Serrano et al., 2010, 2011), it may be observed that some authors such as Morris et al. (1981) found no connection between the type of treatment in use and its effectiveness in the emotionality state. However, other authors such as Kaplan, McCordick and Twitchell (1979) found differential effects in the treatments, the cognitive being superior (Morris et al., 1981). On the other hand, Naveh-Benjamin (1991) observed that the treatments directed at reducing emotional reactions during test situations, such as systematic desensitization, reduced the emotionality state of test anxiety, but had less effect on academic performance.

In these studies we can see that data on the emotionality of the test anxiety concept are confusing. We therefore think that we have taken a step forward with this research, in so far as we have shown in our work (Escolar & Serrano, 2012; Serrano et al., 2002, 2010, 2011; Serrano & Escolar, 2011) that a complete intervention is needed, both of a physiological and of a cognitive type, for subjects with high emotionality.

Some authors have pointed to the complexity of the affective facet of this construct, for example, Liebert and Morris (1967) and Cassady and Johnson (2002). The latter two considered that emotionality is the subjective knowledge that individuals have on their higher autonomic activation. Others, such as Zeidner (1998), have pointed out that it also involves objective somatic symptoms of physiological activation, such as more subjective expressions of emotional activation and of stress and that it is useful for researchers to differentiate between the real physiological reactions and the person's own personal perception of these reactions. These differences have meant that the term "emotionality" is used to refer to the knowledge and to the interpretation that a person has and makes of physiological activation and of the corporal changes that are experienced in evaluative situations, as against "physiological activation" in itself (Deffenbacher, 1980; Holroyd & Appel, 1980; Liebert & Morris,

1967). Therefore, emotionality implies a considerable degree of cognitive processes; for example, attention that is paid and the interpretations made of affective/physiological activation.

With regard to the pertinence or otherwise of training in study skills, in our experience, the patients who ask for help do so because they either fail to attend exams or because they are unable to pass them. And having received the treatment, they told us that had they managed to sit the exams and that they passed them. Our findings confirm the existence of this irrational anxiety and support the affirmations of authors such as Gonzalez (1995) with regard to the inadvisability of training in study skills, due to the saturation effect on the individual (Serrano et al., 2002, 2010, 2011; Serrano & Escolar, 2011). This is the reason why in no case did we train patients in study skills in our research. Those who presented rational anxiety were channeled towards training programs in study skills or in self-control of this type of behaviours.

So, we therefore consider that our findings (Serrano et al., 2002, 2010, 2011) are clearly pertinent and decisive for the stage in which an appropriate training is sought for the patient throughout the therapeutic process.

4. Conclusion

On the basis of our observations of each individual treated in our studies, we may therefore affirm that individual response patterns do exist in relation to test anxiety. It is therefore necessary to adjust the intervention to the variable that is principally affected in each individual. In other words, we assume that both worry and emotionality can have a negative influence on academic performance. This influence will depend on whether one or another component has affected the student and will be the definitive guide to possible therapeutic interventions (Escolar & Serrano, 2012; Serrano et al., 2002, 2010, 2011; Serrano & Escolar, 2011).

Finally, we consider that a careful diagnostic evaluation of the specific weaknesses of students with this type of anxiety is necessary, with a view to further research into test anxiety treatments and their optimization. This requires an evaluation of individual differences in willingness to experience cognitive processes of worry and emotional reactions in test situations and the measurement of attitudes towards study skills and routines. Only then will it be possible to prepare treatment programs in accordance with the specific needs and specific problems of our students.

Acknowledgements

The authors thank the Psychological Care Unit at the Faculty of Psychology at the University of Salamanca for starting test anxiety treatment groups and allow us to carry them out. Consequently, we would like to thank the ninety-four students that have been the sample for this research for the trust they have placed in our work as a way to alleviate their fears and anxieties.

References

Amutio, A., & Smith, J. C. (2008). Stress and Irrational Beliefs in College Students. *Ansiedad y Estrés, 14,* 211-220.

Bernstein, D. A., & Borkovec, T. D. (1983). *Entrenamiento en relajación progresiva* (9th ed.). Bilbao: Desclée de Brouver.

Bonaccio, S., Reeve, C. L., & Winford, E. C. (2012). Text Anxiety on Cognitive Ability Test Can Result in Differential Predictive Validity of Academic Performance. *Personality and Individual Differences, 52,* 497-502. http://dx.doi.org/10.1016/j.paid.2011.11.015

Can, P. B., Dereboy, C., & Eskin, M. (2012). Comparison of the Effectiveness of Cognitive Restructuring and Systematic Desensitization in Reducing High-Stakes Test Anxiety. *Turkish Journal of Psychiatry, 23,* 9-17.

Cassady, J. C., & Johnson, R. E. (2002). Cognitive Test Anxiety and Academic Performance. *Contemporary Educational Psychology, 27,* 270-295. http://dx.doi.org/10.1006/ceps.2001.1094

Conley, K. M., & Lehman, B. J. (2012). Test Anxiety and Cardiovascular Responses to Daily Academic Stressors. *Stress and Health, 28,* 41-50. http://dx.doi.org/10.1002/smi.1399

Cunha, M., & Paiva, M. J. (2012). Text Anxiety in Adolescents: The Role of Self-Criticism and Acceptance and Mindfulness Skills. *The Spanish Journal of Psychology, 15,* 533-543. http://dx.doi.org/10.5209/rev_SJOP.2012.v15.n2.38864

Deffenbacher, J. L. (1980). Worry and Emotionality in Test Anxiety. In I. G. Sarason (Ed.), *Test Anxiety: Theory, Research, and Applications* (pp. 111-128). Hillsdale, NJ: Lawrence Erlbaum Associates.

Escolar, M. C. (2007). *Eficacia diferencial de estrategias de afrontamiento de la ansiedad ante los exámenes universitarios en función de la variable principalmente afectada.* Unpublished Doctoral Thesis, Universidad de Salamanca, Spain.

Escolar, M. C., & Serrano, I. (2012). Eficacia de las herramientas cognitivo-conductuales para disminuir la ansiedad en el ámbito educativo. *Boletín de la SEAS, 37,* 8-21.

Fletcher, T. M., & Spielberger, C. D. (1995). Comparison of Cognitive Therapy and Rational-Emotive Therapy in the Treatment of Test Anxiety. In C. D. Spielberger, & P. R. Vagg (Eds.), *Test Anxiety: Theory, Assessment, and Treatment* (pp. 153-169). Washington DC: Taylor & Francis.

Furlan, L. A., Sanchez Rosas, J., Heredia, D., Piemontesi, S., & Illbele, A. (2009). Estrategias de aprendizaje y ansiedad ante los exámenes en estudiantes universitarios. *Pensamiento Psicológico, 5,* 117-124.

Gaudry, E., & Spielberger, C. D. (1971). *Anxiety and Educational Achievement.* New York: Wiley.

Gonzalez, H. P. (1995). Systematic Desensitization, Study Skills Counseling, and Anxiety-Coping Training in the Treatment of Test Anxiety. In C. D. Spielberger, & P. R. Vagg (Eds.), *Test Anxiety: Theory, Assessment, and Treatment* (pp. 117-132). Washington DC: Taylor & Francis.

Gutiérrez-Calvo, M. (1996). Ansiedad y deterioro cognitivo: Incidencia en el rendimiento académico. *Ansiedad y Estrés, 2,* 173-194.

Hernández, J. M., Pozo, C., & Polo, A. (1994). *Ansiedad ante los exámenes: Un programa para su afrontamiento de forma eficaz.* Valencia: Promolibro.

Holroyd, K. A., & Appel, M. A. (1980). Test Anxiety and Physiological Responding. In I. G. Sarason (Ed.), *Test Anxiety: Theory, Research, and Applications* (pp. 129-151). Hillsdale, NJ: Lawrence Erlbaum Associates.

Iruarrizaga, I., & Salvador, M. E. (1999). Intervención cognitivo conductual en los problemas de ansiedad de evaluación. Tratamiento de un caso. Psicología. http://www.psiquiatria.com/revistas/index.php/psicologiacom/article/view/640/

Jacobson, E. (1938). *Progressive Relaxation.* Chicago, IL: University of Chicago Press.

Kaplan, R. M., McCordick, S. M., & Twitchell, M. (1979). Is It the Cognitive or the Behavioral Component Which Makes Cognitive-Behavior Modification Effective in Test Anxiety? *Journal of Counseling Psychology, 26,* 371-377. http://dx.doi.org/10.1037/0022-0167.26.5.371

Liebert, R. M., & Morris, L. W. (1967). Cognitive and Emotional Components of Test Anxiety: A Distinction and Some Initial Data. *Psychological Reports, 20,* 975-978. http://dx.doi.org/10.2466/pr0.1967.20.3.975

Martínez-Monteagudo, M. C., Inglés, C. J., Cano-Vindel, A., & García-Fernández, J. M. (2012). Estado actual de la investigación sobre la teoría tridimensional de la ansiedad de Lang. *Ansiedad y Estrés, 18,* 201-219.

McMillan, J. R., & Osterhouse, R. A. (1972). Specific and Generalized Anxiety as Determinants of Outcome with Desensitization of Text Anxiety. *Journal of Counseling Psychology, 19,* 518-521. http://dx.doi.org/10.1037/h0033583

Meichenbaum, D. (1985). *Stress Innoculation Training.* Oxford: Pergamon Press Inc.

Miralles, F., & Hernández, I. (2012). La ansiedad ante los exámenes. *Boletín de la SEAS, 36,* 9-16.

Miralles, F., & Sanz, M. C. (2011). *Cómo enfrentarse con éxito a exámenes y oposiciones.* Madrid: Ediciones Pirámide.

Morris, L. W., Davis, M. A., & Hutchings, C. H. (1981). Cognitive and Emotional Components of Anxiety: Literature Review and a Revised Worry-Emotionality Scale. *Journal of Educational Psychology, 73,* 541-555. http://dx.doi.org/10.1037/0022-0663.73.4.541

Naveh-Benjamin, M. (1991). A Comparison of Training Programs Intended for Different Types of Test-Anxious Students: Further Support for an Information-Processing Model. *Journal of Educational Psychology, 83,* 134-139. http://dx.doi.org/10.1037/0022-0663.83.1.134

Naveh-Benjamin, M., McKeachie, W. J., & Lin, Y. G. (1987). Two Types of Test-Anxious Students: Support for an Information Processing Model. *Journal of Educational Psychology, 79,* 131-136. http://dx.doi.org/10.1037/0022-0663.79.2.131

Nemati, A., & Habibi, P. (2012). The Effect of Practicing Pranayama on Test Anxiety and Test Performance. *Indian Journal of Science and Technology, 5,* 2645-2650.

Onwuegbuzie, A. J., & Daley, C. E. (1996). The Relative Contributions of Examination-Taking Coping Strategies and Study Coping Strategies to Test Anxiety: A Concurrent Analysis. *Cognitive Therapy and Research, 20,* 287-303. http://dx.doi.org/10.1007/BF02229239

Osterhouse, R. A. (1969). *A Comparison of Desensitization and Study-Skills Training for the Treatment of Two Kinds of Test-Anxious Students.* Unpublished Doctoral Dissertation, Columbus, OH: Ohio State University.

Osterhouse, R. A. (1972). Desensitization and Study-Skills Training as Treatment for Two Types of Test-Anxious Students. *Journal of Counseling Psychology, 19,* 301-307. http://dx.doi.org/10.1037/h0034177

Parker, J. C. I., Vagg, P. R., & Papsdorf, J. D. (1995). Systematic Desensitization, Cognitive Coping, and Biofeedback in the Reduction of Test Anxiety. In C. D. Spielberger, & P. R. Vagg (Eds.), *Test Anxiety: Theory, Assessment, and Treatment* (pp. 171-182). Washington DC: Taylor & Francis.

Piemontesi, S. E., & Heredia, D. E. (2009). Afrontamiento ante exámenes: Desarrollo de los principales modelos teóricos para su definición y medición. *Anales de Psicología, 25,* 102-111.

Piemontesi, S., Heredia, D., Furlan, L., Sanchéz-Rosas, J., & Martínez, M. (2012). Ansiedad ante los exámenes y estilos de afrontamiento ante el estrés académico en estudiantes universitarios. *Anales de Psicología, 28,* 89-96.

Polo, A., Hernández, J. M., & Pozo, C. (1996). Evaluación del estrés académico en estudiantes universitarios. *Ansiedad y Estrés, 2,* 159-172.

Pozar, F. F. (1979). *Inventario de hábitos de estudio: IHE.* Madrid: TEA.

Putwain, D. W., & Sysmes, W. (2012). Achievement Goals as Mediators of the Relationship between Competence Beliefs and Test Anxiety. *British Journal of Educational Psychology, 82,* 207-224. http://dx.doi.org/10.1111/j.2044-8279.2011.02021.x

Ramirez, G., & Beilock, S. L. (2011). Writing about Testing Worries Boosts Exam Performance in the Classroom. *Science, 331,* 211-213. http://dx.doi.org/10.1126/science.1199427

Rosário, P., Núñez, J. C., Salgado, A., González-Pienda, J. A., Valle, A., & Joly, C. (2008). Ansiedad ante los exámenes: Relaciones con variables personales y familiares. *Psicothema, 20,* 563-570.

Sapp, M. (1999). *Test Anxiety. Applied Research, Assessment, and Treatment Interventions.* Lanham, MD: University Press of America.

Sarason, I. G. (1978). The Test Anxiety Scale: Concept and Research. In C. D. Spielberger, & I. G. Sarason (Eds.), *Stress and Anxiety* (Vol. 5, pp. 193-216). Washington DC: Hemisphere.

Sarason, I. G. (1984). Stress, Anxiety, and Cognitive Interference: Reactions to Test. *Journal of Personality and Social Psychology, 46,* 929-938. http://dx.doi.org/10.1037/0022-3514.46.4.929

Serrano, I., & Delgado, J. (1990). Ansiedad ante los exámenes, ¿estado o rasgo? Tratamiento conductual. *Studia Paedagogica, 22,* 81-93.

Serrano, I., & Delgado, J. (1991). Estrategias de afrontamiento y ansiedad ante los exámenes. *Revista de Psicología General y Aplicada, 44,* 447-456.

Serrano, I., & Escolar, M. C. (2011). Psicopatología de la ansiedad ante los exámenes: Dimensiones y componentes. *Escuela y Psicopatología, 2,* 135-168.

Serrano, I., Delgado, J., & Escolar, M. C. (2010). Eficacia diferencial de estrategias de afrontamiento en la reducción de la ansiedad ante los exámenes en función del tipo de variable principalmente afectada. *Ansiedad y Estrés, 16,* 109-126.

Serrano, I., Escolar, C., & Delgado, J. (2002). Eficacia diferencial de estrategias de afrontamiento en la reducción de la ansiedad ante los exámenes. *Análisis y Modificación de Conducta, 28,* 523-550.

Serrano, I., Escolar, M. C., & Delgado, J. (2011). Eficacia de tres estrategias de afrontamientos en la reducción de la ansiedad ante los exámenes en función del tipo de variable principalmente afectada. In J. M. Román, M. A. Carbonero, & J. D. Valdivieso (Eds.), *Educación, aprendizaje y desarrollo en una sociedad multicultural* (pp. 1115-1133). Madrid: Ediciones de la Asociación Nacional de Psicología y Educación.

Spielberger, C. D. (1972a). Anxiety as an Emotional State. In C. D. Spielberger (Ed.), *Anxiety: Current Trends in Theory and Research* (Vol. 1, pp. 23-49). New York: Academic Press. http://dx.doi.org/10.1016/B978-0-12-657401-2.50009-5

Spielberger, C. D. (1972b). Conceptual and Methodological Issues in Anxiety Research. In C. D. Spielberger (Ed.), *Anxiety: Current Trends in Theory and Research* (Vol. 2, pp. 481-493). New York: Academic Press. http://dx.doi.org/10.1016/B978-0-12-657402-9.50013-2

Spielberger, C. D. (1980). *Test Anxiety Inventory.* Palo Alto, CA: Consulting Psychologists Press.

Spielberger, C. D. (1983). *Manual for the State-Trait Anxiety Inventory (STAI).* Palo Alto, CA: Consulting Psychologists Press.

Spielberger, C. D., & Vagg, P. R. (1987). The Treatment of Test Anxiety: A Transactional Process Model. In R. Schwarzer, H. M. Van Der Ploeg, & C. D. Spielberger (Eds.), *Advances in Test Anxiety Research* (Vol. 5, pp. 179-186). Lisse/Hillsdale, NJ: Swets and Zeitlinger/Erlbaum Associates.

Spielberger, C. D., & Vagg, P. R. (1995). Test Anxiety: A Transactional Process Model. In C. D. Spielberger, & P. R. Vagg (Eds.), *Test Anxiety: Theory, Assessment and Treatment* (pp. 3-14). Washington DC: Taylor & Francis.

Spielberger, C. D., Gorsuch, R. L., & Lushene, R. D. (1970). *Manual for the State-Trait Anxiety Inventory.* Palo Alto, CA: Consulting Psychologists Press.

Szafranski, D. D., Barrera, T. L., & Norton, P. J. (2012). Test Anxiety Inventory: 30 Years Later. *Anxiety, Stress, & Coping: An International Journal, 25,* 667-677. http://dx.doi.org/10.1080/10615806.2012.663490

Valero, L. (1999). Evaluación de ansiedad ante exámenes: Datos de aplicación y fiabilidad de un cuestionario CAEX. *Anales de Psicología, 15,* 223-231.

Wagaman, G. L., Cornier, W. H., & Cornier, L. S. (1975). Cognitive Modification on Test-Anxious Students. *Paper Presented at the Meeting of the American Educational Research Association,* Washington DC.

Wolpe, J. (1958). *Psychotherapy by Reciprocal Inhibition.* Stanford, CA: Stanford University Press.

Zeidner, M. (1998). *Test Anxiety: The State of the Art.* New York: Plenum Press.

Zeidner, M. (2007). Test Anxiety in Educational Contexts: Concepts, Findings, and Future Directions. In P. A. Schutz, & R. Pekrun (Eds.), *Emotion in Education* (pp. 165-184). Boston, MA: Elsevier Academic Press. http://dx.doi.org/10.1016/B978-012372545-5/50011-3

20

Prevalence and Sex Distribution of Temporomandibular Disorder and Their Association with Anxiety and Depression in Indian Medical University Students

Kaberi Majumder[1], Shalender Sharma[2]*, Dayashankara Rao JK[2], Vijay Siwach[2], Varun Arya[2], Sunil Gulia[2]

[1]Department of Orthodontics, SGT Dental College, Gurgaon, India
[2]Department of Oral and Maxillofacial Surgery, SGT Dental College, Gurgaon, India
Email: *sharma.shalender@rediffmail.com

Abstract

Objectives: The term TMD refers to a group of disorders characterized by pain in the temporomandibular joint and associated structures. The aim of this study was designed to evaluate prevalence, severity and sex distribution of sign and symptoms of TMD and to evaluate their relation with anxiety and depression among the students. Material and Methods: A total of 1000 university students were enrolled in the study (550 females; 450 males), with ages ranged between 18 and 28 years. Helkimo anamnestic index (Ai) and clinical dysfunction index (Di) were used to determine symptoms and signs respectively. For the association of TMD with anxiety and depression, HAD (Hospital Anxiety and Depression) scale was used. Results showed that prevalence of one or more symptoms of TMD was 27.7%, while the prevalence of one or more signs of TMD was 64.4% which was mild in severity. Mild anamnestic symptoms (AiI) were found in 19.8% and severe symptoms (AiII) were found in 7.6%, while mild clinical sign (DiI), moderate clinical (DiII) and severe clinical sign (DiIII) were found in 49.7%, 12.2% and 2.4% respectively. Statistically there was no gender difference in these two scales. Regarding the association between TMD with anxiety and depression, 206 of the 311 students (66.2%) with TMD symptoms also had signs of anxiety and depression (P < 0.001). Conclusion: These findings confirmed that students had high prevalence of TMD which was significantly associated with anxiety and depression.

Keywords

TMD, Helkimo Index, HAD Scale, Anxiety

*Corresponding author.

1. Introduction

Temporomandibular joint disorders (TMD) are a group of conditions that cause pain and dysfunction in the jaw joint and the muscles that control jaw movement. Bell suggested the term temporomandibular disorders. The wide variety of terms used has contributed to the great amount of confusion that exists in this already complicated field. Therefore, the American Dental Association has adopted the term temporomandibular disorders. The movement of the mandible needs coordination among them to maximize function and minimize the damage to surrounding structures [1].

It has been well established, by means of epidemiological studies in which signs and symptoms of TMDs are common in adults of all ages [2]. Reports have shown that signs and symptoms of temporomandibular disorder (TMD) increase with age [3]; however, other studies have shown a decrease in symptoms with increasing age [4]. Over a 20-year period, investigations on TMD have revealed predominately mild signs and symptoms already present in childhood. An increase in symptoms occurs until young adulthood, after which they level out [5]. The concept of TMD may be attributable to specific genes that are inheritable.

There is some evidence to suggest that anxiety, stress, and other emotional disturbances may exacerbate TMDs, especially in patients who clinically experience chronic pain. Nevertheless, the cause of the signs and symptoms of TMDs is not clearly understood and various opinions on their etiology have been offered [6].

Evidence indicates that myofascial pain and functional somatic syndromes such as fibromyalgia and chronic fatigue syndrome are comorbidities of the muscular pain that may be due to psychosocial factors. The manifestations of myofascial pain and discomfort coincide with moments of tension and stress, which causes muscular hyperactivity, and this tension can lead to parafunctional habits. Thus, psychosocial factors such as anxiety, stress, and depression might be important in the pathogenesis of TMD [7].

It is evident from the numerous epidemiologic studies on the occurrence of temporomandibular disorders that signs of temporomandibular disorders appear in about 60% - 70% of the general population and yet only about one in four people with signs are actually aware of or report any symptoms [8].

The frequency of severe disorders that are accompanied by headache and facial pain characterized by urgent need of treatment is 1% - 2% in children, about 5% in adolescents and 5% - 12% in adults [9].

In epidemiological studies of TMD, Helkimo found that prevalence was between 12% and 57% for anamnestic symptoms and between 28% and 88% for clinical signs [10]. In Asia, Shiau [11] reported that 43% of Taiwanese university students had a prevalence of one or more signs of TMD. Jagger [12] found that more than 19% had anamnestic symptoms and that over 36% showed clinical sign in university students. The lack of standardized criteria in the evaluation of TMD, however, makes comparison among different studies difficult. This problem was addressed by Helkimo [13] in 1974 and it was the basis for the development of his anamnestic (reported) and clinical dysfunction index which probably still remained the most widely applied system in epidemiological studies of TMD.

The aim of this study was to estimate the prevalence of TMD in SGT university students and to evaluate its association with anxiety and depression.

2. Material and Methods

2.1. Study Design

Sample consisted of 1000 students from five different colleges of SGT University. Only those students were enrolled in the study who signed a consent form agreeing to participate in the study. This study was approved by the SGT University IRB.

Out of 1000 students, 550 were females and 450 were males. Age ranged between 18 to 28 years with mean age of 23.4 years. The study population was students of the following institutions: SGT Dental College, SGT Medical College, SGT College of Pharmacy, SGT College of Physiotherapy and SGT College of Nursing. All students who agreed to participate were eligible for inclusion regardless of age or sex.

For evaluating the prevalence of severity and sex distribution of TMD Helkimo anamnestic dysfunction index was the instrument of choice. For evaluating the association of TMD symptoms with anxiety and depression Hospital Anxiety and Depression (HAD) scale was used.

2.2. Data Collection

Helkimo anamnestic index was one of the first instruments to be confirmed as reliable in identifying TMD sign and symptoms [14]. For the assessment of symptoms this index was classified into three grades;

(Ai0) denotes complete absence of subjective symptoms of dysfunctions of the masticatory system. (AiI) denotes mild symptoms; one or more of the following symptoms were reported in anamnesis: joint sound, feeling of fatigue, feeling of stiffness of the jaws on awaking. (AiII) denotes severe symptoms of dysfunction; one or more of the following symptoms were reported in anamnesis: difficulty in opening the mouth widely, locking, subluxation, pain on movement of the mandible, facial and jaw pain, pain and tiredness on chewing.

For evaluating the signs of TMD the masticatory system was examined in the following systematic way according to Helkimo.

Clinical examination include Measurements of maximal opening capacity, overbite and over jet, examination of occlusion, examination of impaired TMJ function which include clicking, crepitation, deviation, locking, luxation, examination of masticatory muscle pain or tenderness. The severity of the clinical signs was determined according to clinical dysfunction index by Helkimo. The severity of the clinical signs according to the scores was classified into four dysfunction groups; each group was given an index value as follows: (Di0) = Dysfunction group 0 = 0 point = clinically free. (DiI) = Dysfunction group 1 = 1 - 4 points = mild (DiII) = Dysfunction group 2 = 5 - 9 points = moderated. (DiIII) = Dysfunction group 3 = 10 - 25 points =sever dysfunction.

HAD scale was used to identify and measure the intensity of anxiety and depression in non psychiatric environments, as in the present population, and has been applied to this type of population in several previous studies [15]. The scale consists of 14 items divided into two scales. Seven items measure anxiety (HADS-A), and seven measure depression (HADS-D). Thus, the concepts of anxiety and depression are separated [16].

To complete the questionnaire, the participant selects the answer choice that is closest to what he/she felt during the previous week. Each item is scored from 0 to 3, depending on the response, and the maximum score is 21 points for each scale. In both scales a score of 0 - 7 indicates absence of anxiety or depression, a score of 8 - 10 indicates possible anxiety or depression, and a score of 11 or higher indicates presence of anxiety or depression [15] [16]. Thus, an individual could have no, either, or both anxiety and depression. Several studies, in a wide variety of clinical populations, found that HAD had good sensitivity, specificity, and internal consistency in assessing anxiety and depression symptoms [16].

2.3. Statistics

The chi-square test of independence was used to evaluate prevalence of TMD with sex and its association with anxiety and depression. To ensure the applicability of the chi-square test of independence, TMD was classified as absent and present (which included mild, moderate, and severe TMD). For presence of anxiety or depression, only two groups were considered: absence of anxiety and depression versus presence of anxiety or depression (which included individuals classified as having anxiety or depression and those with possible anxiety or depression).

3. Results

The distribution of symptoms of TMD among the investigated students had been shown in **Table 1**. 27.7% of the studied group had one or more symptoms of the TMD. The most common symptom was TMJ sounds (26% of the total sample) followed by difficulty in wide opening. There was significant gender difference according to one or more symptom, with males being significantly higher than females (P < 0.05) while insignificant gender differences were found for other symptoms of TMD (**Table 1**).

Table 2 shows the distribution of the young adults according to the anamnestic dysfunction index (Ai). Although mild and severe symptoms were more frequent in males 23.4% and 8% respectively than in females 16.9% and 7.4% respectively, there were insignificant gender differences in relation to anamnestic dysfunction index.

The distribution of signs of TMD among the investigated students had been shown in **Table 3**. 64.4% of the studied group had one or more signs of the TMD. The most common sign was pain on movement (41.9%) followed by clicking. There was significant gender difference according to one or more sign, with females being significantly higher than males (P < 0.05). For different signs only clicking was having significant gender differences (**Table 3**).

Table 4 shows the distribution of the students according to the clinical dysfunction index (Di). According to this index the percentage of the subjects decreased with increasing severity and there was no significant gender difference.

Table 1. Frequency and relative distribution of symptoms of the TMD according to sex.

Symptoms		Gender						Total		X^2
		Female			Males					
		No.	%	No.	%	No.	%			
TMJ sound	No	418	76	322	71.5	740	74			$X^2 = 2.762$ df = 1 P > 0.05
	Yes	132	24	128	28.5	260	26			
Feeling of stiffness	No	529	96.2	423	94	952	95.2			$X^2 = 0.421$ df = 1 P > 0.05
	Yes	21	3.8	27	6	48	4.8			
Difficulty in mouth opening	No	517	94	421	93.5	938	93.8			$X^2 = 0.532$ df = 1 P > 0.05
	Yes	33	6	29	6.5	62	6.2			
Pain on movement	No	531	96.5	429	95.3	960	96			$X^2 = 0.316$ df = 1 P > 0.05
	Yes	19	3.5	21	4.7	40	4			
Pain or tenderness on chewing	No	537	97.6	434	96.4	971	97.1			$X^2 = 0.212$ df = 1 P > 0.05
	Yes	13	2.4	16	3.6	29	2.9			
one or more symptoms	No	417	75.8	306	68	723	72.3			$X^2 = 4.612$ df = 1 P < 0.05**
	Yes	133	24.2	144	32	277	27.7			

** = Significant.

Table 2. Frequency and relative distribution of students according to sex and symptoms (Ai).

Gender		Symptom code (Ai)					X^2
		Total					
		Ai0	AiI	AiII			
Females	No.	417	93	40	550		$X^2 = 3.172$
	%	75.7	16.9	7.4	100		
Males	No.	309	10.5	36	450		df = 2 P > 0.05*
	%	68.6	23.4	8	100		
Total	No.	726	198	76	1000		
	%	72.6	19.8	7.6	100		

* = Not significant; Ai0—Complete absence of subjective symptoms; AiI—Mild symptoms; AiII—Severe symptoms of dysfunction.

The relationship between the anamnestic (Ai) and clinical dysfunction index (Di) (**Table 5**) shows that students who were symptom free (Ai0, 72.3%) were found in those who had mild signs (DiI, 50.07%) and the highest percentage of the students with mild and severe symptoms (AiI 16.3%, AiII 11.4%) were also found in those who had mild signs (DiI 51.53% and 50.87%).

Table 6 shows the association of sex and course of study with anxiety and depression as determined by HAD scale. All variants were associated significantly with the anxiety and depression.

Table 7 shows association between TMD with anxiety/depression. Out of 311 students with TMD symptoms, 206 (66.23%) had signs of anxiety and depression which was statistically significant.

4. Discussion

TMD causes are complex and multifactorial. Numerous factors may lead to TMD. Those that may increase the risk of TMD are referred to as predispositions. Those that may lead to an onset of TMD are the initiatory, and

Table 3. Frequency and relative distribution of the signs of the TMD according to sex.

Signs		Gender				Total		X^2
		Female		Males				
		No.	%	No.	%	No.	%	
Clicking	No	427	77.6	346	76.9	773	77.3	$X^2 = 0.023$ df = 1 P > 0.05
	Yes	123	22.4	104	23.1	227	22.7	
Deviation	No	398	72.4	333	74	731	73.1	$X^2 = 2.986$ df = 1 P > 0.05
	Yes	152	27.6	117	26	269	26.9	
Pain or tenderness	No	493	89.7	406	91	899	89.9	$X^2 = 0.063$ df = 1 P > 0.05
	Yes	57	10.3	44	9	101	10.1	
Pain on movement	No	318	57.8	263	58.5	581	58.1	$X^2 = 0.412$ df = 1 P > 0.05
	Yes	232	42.28	187	41.5	419	41.9	
Restricted mouth opening	No	413	75.1	407	90.5	820	82.0	$X^2 = 13.63$ df = 1 P < 0.001***
	Yes	137	24.9	43	9.5	180	18.0	
one or more signs	No	169	30.7	187	41.6	356	35.6	$X^2 = 4.612$ df = 1 P < 0.05**
	Yes	381	69.3	263	58.4	644	64.4	

** = Significant, *** = Highly significant.

Table 4. Frequency and relative distribution of the students according to sex and sign (Di) codes.

Gender		Severity of signs (Di)						X^2
		Total						
		Di0	DiI	DiII	DiIII			
Females	No.	168	301	68	13	550		$X^2 = 4.982$
	%	30.5	54.7	12.3	2.5	100		
Males	No.	189	196	54	11			df = 3 P > 0.05*
	%	42	43.5	12	2.5	100		
Total	No.	357	497	122	24	1000		
	%	35.7	49.7	12.2	2.4	100		

* = Not significant.

Table 5. Relative distribution of Ai in relation to Di among students.

Symptoms		Severity of signs (Di)						X^2
		Total						
		Di0	DiI	DiII	DiIII	No.	%	
Ai0	No.	298	362	63	00	723	72.3	$X^2 = 36.68$
	%	41.21	50.07	8.72	00			
AiI	No.	40	84	38	1	163	16.3	df = 6 P < 0.001***
	%	24.53	51.53	23.32	0.62			
AiII	No.	9	58	32	15	114	11.4	
	%	7.89	50.87	28.07	13.16			
Total	No.	347	504	133	16	1000	100	
	%	34.7	50.4	13.3	16.0			

*** = Highly significant.

Table 6. Association of study variables with anxiety or depression.

Variables		No anxiety or depression	Anxiety or depression		P value
		580 (58.0%)	420 (42%)		
Sex	Male = 450 (45%)	263 (58.4%)	187 (41.6%)		P < 0.01***
	Female = 550 (55%)	317 (57.6%)	233 (42.3%)		
	Medical = 178 (17.8%)	126 (70.7%)	52 (29.3%)		
	Dental = 310 (31.0%)	257 (82.90%)	53 (17.1%)		
Course	Physiotherapy = 165 (16.5%)	110 (66.66%)	55 (33.34%)		P < 0.01***
	Pharmacy = 170 (17.0%)	105 (61.76%)	65 (38.24%)		
	Nursing = 177 (17.7%)	63 (35.59%)	114 (64.41%)		

*** = Highly significant.

Table 7. Association between anxiety/depression and TMD.

Anxiety or depression	No TMD	TMD	P value
	689 (68.9%)	311 (31.1%)	
No anxiety/depression (580)	475 (81.9%)	105 (18.1%)	P < 0.01***
Anxiety/depression (420)	214 (51%)	206 (49%)	

*** = Highly significant.

those that affect the possibility of treatment or increase its progression are referred to as prolonging factors. In some cases one and the same factor may be a predisposition, an initiating and a prolonging factor at the same time [17] [18].

The role of psychological stressors, parafunctions and behavioral processes in TMD pain has been examined in a number of studies [19].

Excessive tension can lead to constant dental clamping, which alters local circulation in muscles and ion exchange in cell membranes. These lead to accumulation of lactic and pyruvic acids, which contributes to stimulation of pain receptors [20]. A possible explanation for the association between TMD and headache is that headaches are related to muscle activity, so activity involving the head and neck is probably important in the etiology of many headaches. The presence of noise in TMJ may be due to incorrect positioning of the articular cartilage, which displaces the mandibular condyle superiorly when the mouth is opened, resulting in a click [20].

Individuals subject to stress may develop parafunctional habits and muscle tension, which lead to development of TMD [20]. Thus, parafunctional components, especially those that increase muscle tension, and changes in emotional states are good indicators of jaw pain in people with TMD, which suggests that anxiety and depression are etiological factors in TMD.

In this study the prevalence of TMD was found to be 31.1%. There were studies in the literature which had found the same prevalence [21]. However, there were other studies in the literature which found high prevalence rate in same type of population [15] [22] [23]. These differences in reported TMD prevalances may be due to the characteristics of the course of study, the time when the questionnaire was administered and the characteristics of the population.

In this study there was significant sex difference concerning one symptom or more, males 32% being significantly higher than females 24.2%, and female to male ratio were 1:1.2. These results were not consistent with the findings of earlier studies who suggest the same frequency in males and females [15] [22] [23]. Lower percentage in females comparing to males may be due to embarrassment to answer yes comparing to males because of environments in which the questions were asked without privacy.

In this study the most common self reported TMD symptom was TMJ sound (26%) while Nomura *et al.* [22]

found 65.5% patients with TMJ sound in their study.

In this study according to anamnestic index mild symptom AiI found in 23.4% of cases which was higher to the previous studies in the literature [2] [4]. our study reveals that mild symptoms 23.4% were more frequent than severe symptoms 8%, this finding is consistent with other studies in the literature [21] [24] [25].

In this study there was no sex difference concerning anamnestic dysfunction index. This result is consistent with other studies [2] [23] [24]. However there are some studies in literature which found a higher incidence in females [25]. This can be explained by the reason that more females seek treatment for TMD than males [26].

In this study there was significant sex difference concerning one sign or more, females 69.3% being significantly higher than females 58.4%. These results are consistent with the previous studies in the literature [5] [22] [24] [25]. The most common sign in this study was pain on movement (41.9%) while in other similar studies in literature clicking was the most common sign [27].

In this study according to this clinical dysfunction index the percentage of the subjects decreased with increasing severity and there was no significant gender difference. These results tend to be close to other studies. [14] [28]

A highly significant relationship between anamnestic and clinical dysfunction index was found in this study. The majority of subjects with symptom free, mild and severe symptoms had mild clinical signs.

In this study HAD showed that 42% of the students had anxiety or depression. There are other studies in the literature which are comparable to our study [29], but Inam *et al.* found a higher prevalence of anxiety and depression in their study (60%) [30].

In this study we found that TMD was significantly associated with anxiety and depression (66.2%) which is in consistent with other studies in literature [15] [30] [31].

5. Conclusion

Our study shows significant association between emotional stress and symptoms of TMD but not clinical sign and this will support many theories of relating this to psychological cause. Thus, greater understanding of this condition among populations exposed to high levels of emotional stress such as students is of considerable importance so that we can motivate the affected students to seek proper treatment.

References

[1]   Okeson, J.P. (2003) Treatment of Temporomandibular Joint Disorders. In: *Management of Temporomandibular Disorders and Occlusion*, 5th Edition, Mosby, St. Louis, 413-435.

[2]   Kalanzi, D., Osman, Y.I. and Shaikh, A. (2005) Prevalence of Sign and Symptoms of the Temporomandibular Join Dysfunctions in Subjects with Different Occlusion Using Helkimo Index. Thesis for Degree of Masterscience in Restorative Dentistry, University of Western Cape, Cape Town.

[3]   De Boever, J.A. and Adriaens, P.A. (1983) Occlusal Relationship in Patients with Pain-Dysfunction Symptoms in the Temporomandibular Joints. *Journal of Oral Rehabilitation*, **10**, 1-7.
http://dx.doi.org/10.1111/j.1365-2842.1983.tb00093.x

[4]   Hiltunen, K., Schmidt-Kaunisaho, K., Nevalainen, J., Närhi, T. and Ainamo, A. (1995) Prevalence of Signs of Temporomandibular Disorders among Elderly Inhabitants of Helsinki, Finland. *Acta Odontologica Scandinavica*, **53**, 20-23.
http://dx.doi.org/10.3109/00016359509005939

[5]   Magnusson, T., Egermarki, I. and Carlsson, G.E. (2005) A Prospective Investigation over Two Decades on Signs and Symptoms of Temporomandibular Disorders and Associated Variables. A Final Summary. *Acta Odontologica Scandinavica*, **63**, 99-109.

[6]   Helkimo, M. (1976) Epidemiological Surveys of Dysfunction of the Masticatory System. *Oral Science Review*, **7**, 54-69.

[7]   Suma, S. and Veerendra Kumar, B. (2012) Temporomandibular Disorders and Functional Somatic Syndromes: Deliberations for the Dentist. *Indian Journal of Dental Research*, **23**, 529-536. http://dx.doi.org/10.4103/0970-9290.104965

[8]   Graber, T.M., Rakosi, T. and Petrovic, A.G. (2009) Functional Analysis—Examination of Temporomandibular Joint and Condylar Movement. In: *Dentofacial Orthopedics with Functional Appliances*, 2nd Edition, Mosby, St. Louis, 135-140.

[9]   Athanasiou, A.E. (2003) Orthodontics and Craniomandibular Disorders. In: Samire, B., Ed., *Textbook of Orthodontics*, 2nd Edition, Saunders, Philadelphia, 478-493.

[10]   Egermark-Eriksson, I., Carlsson, G.E. and Magnusson, T. (1987) A Long-Term Epidemiologic Study of the Relation-

ship between Occlusal Factors and Mandibular Dysfunction in Children and Adolescents. *Journal of Dental Research*, **66**, 67-71. http://dx.doi.org/10.1177/00220345870660011501

[11] Shiau, Y.Y. and Chang, C. (1992) An Epidemiological Study of Temporomandibular Disorders in University Students of Taiwan. *Community Dentistry and Oral Epidemiology*, **20**, 43-47. http://dx.doi.org/10.1111/j.1600-0528.1992.tb00672.x

[12] Jagger, R.G. and Wood, C. (1992) Signs and Symptoms of Temporomandibular Joint Dysfunction in a Saudi Arabian Population. *Journal of Oral Rehabilitation*, **19**, 353-359. http://dx.doi.org/10.1111/j.1365-2842.1992.tb01577.x

[13] Droukas, B., Lindée, C. and Carlsson, G.E. (1984) Relationship between Occlusal Factors and Signs and Symptoms of Mandibular Dysfunction: A Clinical Study of 48 Dental Students. *Acta Odontologica Scandinavica*, **42**, 277-283. http://dx.doi.org/10.3109/00016358408993881

[14] Helkimo, M. (1974) Studies on Function and Dysfunction of the Masticatory System, II: Index for Anamnestic and Clinical Dysfunction and Occlusal State. *Svensk Tandlakare Tidskrift*, **67**, 101-121.

[15] Bonjardim, L.R., Lopes-Filho, R.J., Amado, G., Albuquerque Jr., R.L. and Goncalves, S.R. (2009) Association between Symptoms of Temporomandibular Disorders and Gender, Morphological Occlusion, and Psychological Factors in a Group of University Students. *Indian Journal of Dental Research*, **20**, 190-194. http://dx.doi.org/10.4103/0970-9290.52901

[16] Mykletun, A., Stordal, E. and Dahl, A.A. (2001) Hospital Anxiety and Depression (HAD) Scale: Factor Structure, Item Analyses and Internal Consistency in a Large Population. *The British Journal of Psychiatry*, **179**, 540-544. http://dx.doi.org/10.1192/bjp.179.6.540

[17] McNaill, C., Danzing, D., Farrar, W., Gelb, H., Lerman, M.D., Moffett, B.C., Pertes, R., Solberg, W.K. and Weinberg, L.A. (1980) Craniomandibular (TMJ) Disorders—The State of the Art. *Journal of Prosthetic Dentistry*, **44**, 434-437. http://dx.doi.org/10.1016/0022-3913(80)90104-3

[18] Okeson, J. (1996) Orofacial Pain: Guidelines for Classification, Assessment, and Management. 3rd Edition, Quintessence Publishing, Chicago, 119-120.

[19] Uhac, I., Kovac, Z., Valentic-Peruzovic, M., Juretic, M., Moro, L.J. and Grzic, R. (2003) The Influence of War Stress on the Prevalence of Signs and Symptoms of Temporomandibular Disorders. *Journal of Oral Rehabilitation*, **30**, 211-217. http://dx.doi.org/10.1046/j.1365-2842.2003.01030.x

[20] Poveda-Roda, R., Bagán, J.V., Díaz Fernández, J.M., Bazán, S.H. and Soriano, Y.J. (2007) Review of Temporomandibular Joint Pathology. Part I: Classification, Epidemiology and Risk Factors. *Medicina Oral Patologia Oral y Cirugia Bucal*, **12**, E292-E298.

[21] Otuyemi, O.D., Owotade, F.J., Ugboko, V.I., Ndukwe, K.C. and Olusile, O.A. (2000) Prevalence of Signs and Symptoms of Temporomandibular Disorders in Young Nigerian Adults. *Journal of Orthodontics*, **27**, 61-65. http://dx.doi.org/10.1093/ortho/27.1.61

[22] Nomura, K., Vitti, M., Oliveira, A.S., Chaves, T.C., Semprini, M., Siéssere, S., *et al.* (2007) Use of the Fonseca's Questionnaire to Assess the Prevalence and Severity of Temporomandibular Disorders in Brazilian Dental Undergraduates. *Brazilian Dental Journal*, **18**, 163-167. http://dx.doi.org/10.1590/S0103-64402007000200015

[23] De Oliveira, A.S., Dias, E.M., Contato, R.G. and Berzin, F. (2006) Prevalence Study of Signs and Symptoms of Temporomandibular Disorder in Brazilian College Students. *Brazilian Oral Research*, **20**, 3-7. http://dx.doi.org/10.1590/S1806-83242006000100002

[24] Abdulla, B.A. and Hussein, S.M. (1992) Temporomandibular Disorders among a Sample of Mosul University Students. Master's Thesis, College of Dentistry, University of Baghdad, Baghdad.

[25] De Kanter, R.J., Truin, G.J., Burgersdijk, R.C., Van't Hop, M.A., Battistuzzi, P.G., Kalsbeek, H. and Käyser, A.F. (1993) Prevalence in the Dutch Adult Population and a Meta-Analysis of Signs and Symptoms of Temporomandibular Disorder. *Journal of Dental Research*, **72**, 1509-1518. http://dx.doi.org/10.1177/00220345930720110901

[26] McNeill, C. (1997) Management of Temporomandibular Disorders: Concept and Controversies. *The Journal of Prosthetic Dentistry*, **77**, 510-522. http://dx.doi.org/10.1016/S0022-3913(97)70145-8

[27] Elfving, L., Helkimo, M. and Magnusson, T. (2002) Prevalence of Different Temporomandibular Joint Sounds, with Emphasis on Disc-Displacement, in Patients with Temporomandibular Disorders and Controls. *Swedish Dental Journal*, **26**, 9-19.

[28] Pow, E.H., Leung, K.C. and McMillan, A.S. (2001) Prevalence of Symptoms Associated with Temporomandibular Disorders in Hong Kong Chinese. *Journal of Orofacial Pain*, **5**, 228-234.

[29] Jadoon, N.A., Yaqoob, R., Raza, A., Shehzad, M.A. and Zeshan, S.C. (2010) Anxiety and Depression among Medical Students: A Cross-Sectional Study. *Journal of Pakistan Medical Association*, **60**, 699-702.

[30] Inam, S.N., Saqib, A. and Alam, E. (2003) Prevalence of Anxiety and Depression among Medical Students of Private

University. *Journal of Pakistan Medical Association*, **53**, 44-47.

[31] Minghelli, B., Morgado, M. and Caro, T. (2014) Association of Temporomandibular Disorder Symptoms with Anxiety and Depression in Portuguese College Students. *Journal of Oral Science*, **56**, 127-133.
http://dx.doi.org/10.2334/josnusd.56.127

21

Effectiveness of Cognitive Therapy and Mindfulness Tools in Reducing Depression and Anxiety: A Mixed Method Study

Valerie L. Alexander*, B. Charles Tatum

Department of Psychology, National University, San Diego, USA
Email: *valexand@nu.edu

Abstract

Depression and anxiety continue to be among the most common mental disorders. This study looked at three tracks of participants diagnosed with a mood disorder. The three tracks were Cognitive Therapy (CT), Mindfulness Training (MT), and Treatment As Usual (TAU). All participants had been trained in CT and then randomly separated into three groups. These three tracks were assessed at 3, 6, and 12 months in terms of their stated level of depression (measured on the Beck Depression Inventory) and anxiety (measured by the Beck Anxiety Inventory). This study was a follow-up to two previous studies (Alexander et al., 2012; Alexander & Tatum, 2013). In the current study, the participants reported the tools and skills they used to manage their mood and anxiety and then the effectiveness of these tools/skills was examined. Two tools were identified by three independent coders as the most frequently used by the participants. Both of these tools related to thought management ("thought records" and "thought distortions"). The two tools were combined into a single category ("thought tools") and the frequency of their use was examined in relation to reductions in depression and anxiety. The results showed that a high use of these tools was connected to a significant reduction in reported depression. There was also a reduction in reported anxiety, but this effect was not statistically significant. Other tools that were reported (e.g., mood tracking, relaxation) showed no significant effects on depression and anxiety. Future research will now focus not on reported tool use, but rather on manipulating the incidence of tool use and determine the direct causal path between using a thought tool and reductions in negative moods.

Keywords

Depression, Cognitive Therapy, Mindfulness, Therapy Tools

---

*Corresponding author.

1. Introduction

Depression and anxiety are worldwide health problems. Recent statistics from the World Health Organization (2012) place depression as the leading cause of disability worldwide and affecting 350 million people of all ages and refers to depression and anxiety as two of the most prevalent non-communicable disorders. The Anxiety and Depression Association of America (2014) identify anxiety disorders as the most common disorder in the United States, affecting 40 million adults 18 and older and major depression affecting 14.8 million American adults.

1.1. Depression, Anxiety, and Cognitive Therapy

Studies on depression identify this mental disorder as treatable and research on Cognitive Therapy (CT) reveals a reduction in relapse and reoccurrence (Bockting et al., 2005; Fava, Grandi, Zielezny, Canestari, & Morphy, 1996; Jarrett et al., 2001; Paykel et al., 1999). A complicating factor is the repeated relapse rates of 80% - 90% (Chen, Jordan, & Thompson, 2006; Judd, 1997) with the risk of chronic incapacity (Kennedy, Abbott, & Paykel, 2003). The theory around CT is that the more the patients identify the relationship between their thoughts, feelings, and behavior, the better they will be able to modulate their emotional distress. Skills are taught with the supposition that if they acquire, comprehend, and practice these skills, they will have a reduction in symptoms. Although patients are taught CT skills, there are few measures available that assess how these tools promote cognitive and behavioral change. Some studies have identified measures to recognize the patients' awareness of automatic thoughts (Wright et al., 2002) or the comprehension and usage of the CT skills (Strunk, DeRubeis, Chiu, & Alvarez, 2007). One group of researchers (Jarrett, Vittengl, Clark, & Thase, 2011) developed their own measure to assess patients understanding and use of CT skills. Their findings supported their hypothesis that CT skills acquisition predicted a reduction in depressive symptoms.

Other research has demonstrated the efficacy of CT in reducing anxiety. For example, Wells (2002) viewed rumination as leading to avoidant behaviors and anxious thoughts. Matthew & MacLeod (2005) associated anxiety with automatic thoughts that the individual feels is out of their control. The relationship between negative interpretation and a vulnerability toward developing an anxious mood was supported by Salemink, van den Hout, and Kindt (2010).

1.2. Mindfulness

The introduction of mindfulness into the CT model in prevention of relapse from depression was explored by Segal, Williams, & Teasdale (2002). Clinical applications of mindfulness had already been adopted into therapeutic approaches such as Dialectical Behavioral Therapy (Linehan, 1993) and Acceptance and Commitment Therapy (Hayes, Strosahl, & Wilson, 1999). Kabat-Zinn (1994) developed Mindfulness-Based Stress Reduction (MBSR) for pain management, yet MBSR began to be used for multiple chronic illnesses. Examples include eating disorders (Courbasson, Nishikawa, & Shapira, 2011; Trapper et al., 2009), anxiety disorders (Roemer, Orstillo, & Salters-Pedneault, 2008), posttraumatic stress disorder (Owen, Walter, Chard, & Davis, 2012; Wolfsdorf & Zlotnick, 2001), and substance abuse (Courbasson, Nishikawa, & Shapiro, 2011). Deyo, Wilson, Ong, & Koopman (2009) also found MBSR to have a decrease in rumination in individuals with depressive symptoms. Hofman, Sawyer, Witt, & Oh (2010) reviewed studies of participants receiving mindfulness based treatment for a range of conditions. Their finding found a significant anxiety reduction and mood symptom improvement. Keng, Smoski, & Robins (2011) also demonstrated mindfulness in managing depression and anxiety by identifying ruminations and other cognitive processes which exacerbate and maintain the symptoms.

Mindfulness awareness has been shown to enhance one's sense of well-being by learning to modulate emotions effectively (Lau et al., 2006). The principles of mindfulness have enjoyed increased attention in the psychological literature and psychotherapy practice, moving from a Buddhist concept of understanding mental processes of impermanence, non-attachment, and letting go (Khong, 2009) to a mainstream construct in therapy viewing the subjective, fluid, and temporary nature of mental states that impact emotional regulation and cognitive flexibility (Wallin, 2007).

The purpose of this study was to identify if there were specific tools that the patients learned that they continued to use to manage their depression and anxiety to prevent relapse. This is an exploratory sequential mixed (qualitative and quantitative) method approach (Creswell, 2014) designed as a follow-up investigation of two previously published studies (Alexander et al., 2012; Alexander & Tatum, 2013). In Alexander et al., 2012, mindfulness practices and cognitive therapy were found to reduce depression and increase mindful and generalized self-efficacy in two tracks which continued to be trained in these tools post discharge from an outpatient program for depression. In Alexander & Tatum, 2013, the study utilized qualitative statements from participants on which of the cognitive therapy and/or mindfulness tools they consistently used to manage their symptoms of depression. From 17 tools/skills identified, three sets of tools were used consistently and significantly across all three tracks. These were a) catching and refuting thought distortions; b) examining thought records; and c) an activity schedule (GRAPES).

2. Method

2.1. Research Setting and Design

This study originated at a West Coast psychiatric hospital outpatient program in a large urban city. Patients were assigned to three treatment tracks and followed at regular intervals for up to one year after discharge from the Cognitive Intensive Outpatient program (COGIOP). The COGIOP was attended by adults whose primary diagnosis was a Mood Disorder and often a step down from inpatient hospitalization. The primary treatment modality for the COGIOP was CT and patients typically attended the five day a week program for six weeks. The three treatment tracks that followed the COGIOP were a) a continuation of CT; b) Mindfulness Training (MT); and c) Treatment as Usual (TAU). Patients were administered two questionnaires (for reported depression and anxiety) and asked two open-ended questions (about the use of cognitive tools) at 3, 6, and 12 months.

2.2. Participants

The participants were 201 patients who attended the COGIOP for at least 20 sessions. All were diagnosed with at least one episode of Major Depression or Bipolar Disorder, Currently Depressed, as defined by the Diagnostic and Statistical Manual of Mental Disorder-IV-TR (American Psychological Association, 2000). Current levels of depression were less than 20 on the Beck Depression Inventory (Beck, Steer, & Brown, 1996). This cut-off score was seen as an indication of the participants' capacity to concentrate and be able to focus on mindful exercises. The demographic information was collected separately and only 82 of the 201 responded. Of these individuals, forty-five percent were between 38 and 52 years of age, 72% were female, 40% married, 83% Caucasian, and 54% Christian. All had at least a high school education and 66% had a bachelor's degree or higher. One hundred percent were diagnosed with a Mood Disorder (80% Major Depression and 20% Bipolar, Currently Depressed). Fifty-two reported an additional diagnosis of an Anxiety Disorder, 52% had had seven or more bouts of depression prior to the COGIOP, 89% were still on antidepressant medication, and 9% had been hospitalized since they left the program.

2.3. Measures

Beck Depression Inventory (BDI). The BDI (Beck et al., 1996) is a 21-item self-report questionnaire that measures attitudes and symptom characteristics of the diagnosis of depression. Patients rated these symptoms such as "I don't sleep as well as I used to" or "I cry all the time now" on a scale of 0 (not at all) to 3 (all the time). Patients can score between 0 - 63. Participants in the aftercare tracks were required to have a BDI less than 20 at the day of discharge to be in the study. Scores ranged from zero (0) to three (3) when averaged across all 21 items. The BDI was completed at discharge from the COGIOP and at 3, 6, and 12 months.

Burns Anxiety Inventory (BAI). The BAI (Burns, 1999) is a 33-item self-report questionnaire that measures subjective expressions of anxiety emotionally (e.g., "feeling tense, stressed, 'uptight' or on edge"), cognitively (e.g., "difficulty concentrating"), and physically (e.g., "pain, pressure or tightness in the chest"). Each item is rated on a 0 (not at all) to 3 (a lot) scale. Patients can score between 0 - 99. Scores ranged from zero (0) to three (3) when averaged across all 33 items. The BAI was also completed at discharge from the COGIOP and at 3, 6, and 12 months.

Open-Ended Questions. All of the participants were followed up with a survey mailed to them at 3, 6, and 12 months, in a return self-addressed stamped envelope. The survey consisted of two open-ended, qualitative questions:

1) Have you continued to use cognitive tools which you learned in the program and/or in the four Monday evening sessions? If so, which tools have you continued to use?

2) Are you practicing mindfulness? If so, how often and what types of practice are you using?

2.4. Procedure

Patients who attended a minimum of 20 treatment days in the COGIOP and had a BDI score less than 20 were eligible for this aftercare study. All of the patients volunteered, signed an informed consent, and were randomly assigned to one of three tracks. The first track was the CT track. Patients assigned to this track attended a three hour, once a week session for four weeks with a focus on relapse prevention. Their format was the same as the COGIOP, where the first hour was psycho-educational followed by a 15 minute break and a 1 hour 45 minute group session. Patients reviewed CT techniques and skills. This track was taught by therapists trained in the principles of CT.

The second track was the MT. Participants attended a three hour, once a week for four weeks session, where the focus was on learning mindfulness practice. All of the participants in this track engaged in three hour mindfulness education and practice and listened daily to a 30-minute CD which consisted of mindful breathing exercises and focused on sensations in various parts of their bodies with awareness and non-judgment. Patients were further educated to mindfulness principles of letting go, staying in the present, and viewing thoughts as mental events and not facts. This track was facilitated by trained therapists with their own mindfulness practice.

The third track was the TAU and was comprised of patients who were discharged from COGIOP and followed up with outpatient therapists and/or psychiatrist.

Three independent coders, who were knowledgeable in the COGIOP program, read the patients responses to the open-ended items on the survey and placed them into 17 tool categories. The inter-rater agreement for the coders was between 80% - 90%. For a complete list and description of the 17 categories, refer to Alexander and Tatum (2013) and Appendix C.

3. Results

Table 1 is based, in part, on results reported by Alexander and Tatum (2013) and displays the average BDI, average BAI, and the two most frequent tools reported by the CT, MT, and TAU study participants across 3, 6, and 12 months. The tools are listed according to the percentage of times they were reported. Two sets of tools stood out as being used consistently across all three tracks (CT, MT, and TAU). These standouts were Thought Records (named as the most frequently used tool four times) and Thought Distortion (named as the most frequently used tool three times). Direct quotations from patients' surveys are included in Appendix A and more detail on the tools are in Appendix B.

The reporting of Thought Records and Thought Distortion as frequently used tools does not mean, however, that these tools were useful in helping to reduce depression or anxiety. Therefore, we did an analysis of the effectiveness of these tools. The strategy for these analyses was to examine whether low, moderate, and high use of the thought tools (Thought Records and Thought Distortions) was related to changes in depression or anxiety. First, we combined the Thought Records and the Thought Distortions into a single tool (what we called the "Thought Tools"). Then, we divided the Thought Tools into low, moderate, and high use categories. We defined these categories such that there were roughly equal numbers of patients in each category for the CT, MT, and TAU tracks. Specifically, low use of the tools was defined as selecting the tool, on average, zero or one time only, moderate use was when the average selection of the tool was more than once but not more than two times, and high use was three or more selections on average. We then performed an analysis of covariance (ANCOVA) with the average depression (BDI) for month three as the dependent variable and the pretest for anxiety (BAI) as the covariate. (We did not analyze the 6 and 12 month BDIs because attrition reduced the sample sizes and the data became unstable.) We performed another ANCOVA with the average anxiety (BAI) for month three as the dependent variable and the pretest depression (BDI) as the covariate (again, months 6 and 12 were unstable). Both ANCOVAs (See **Table 2**) used Treatment Track (CT, MT, and TAU) and Thought Tools (low, moderate, and high) as independent variables.

The results of the two ANCOVAs showed that the use of the tools did have a significant effect on depression but not on anxiety. The first ANCOVA, using depression as the dependent variable, revealed an interaction between Treatment Track and Thought Tools ($F[4, 73] = 2.56$, $p < .05$, MSE = .196, Eta-square = .196). Close inspection of the results indicated that increasing use of the tools had a large effect on the CT patients, a somewhat smaller effect on the MT patients, and no effect at all for TAU. Specifically, the increasing use of the Thought

Table 1. Beck depression index (BDI) and Burns anxiety index (BAI) scores (averaged across items) and tool use (thought records and thought distortions) across tracks and months.

	Cognitive Track	Mindfulness Track	Treatment as Usual Track
3 month	BDI 1.86	BDI 1.47	BDI 1.83
	BAI 2.22	BAI 1.71	BAI 1.71
	Tool Thought Records (25%) Thought Distortions (14%)	Tool Thought Distortions (13%) Thought Records (11%)	Tool Thought Records (14%) Thought Distortions (13%)
6 month	BDI 1.59	BDI 1.41	BDI 1.50
	BAI 2.01	BAI 1.62	BAI 1.77
	Tool Thought Records (20%) Thought Distortions (6%)	Tool Thought Records (13%) Thought Distortions (12%)	Tool Thought Distortions (20%) Thought Records (10%)
12 month	BDI 1.17	BDI .99	BDI 1.47
	BAI 1.86	BAI 1.38	BAI 1.62
	Tool Thought Records (18%) Thought Distortions (9%)	Tool Thought Distortions (21%) Thought Records (15%)	Tool Thought Distortions (17%) Thought records (11%)

Note: Percentages indicate the percentage of patients reporting using that tool.

Table 2. ANCOVAs used to test the effects of thought tools (low, moderate, and high) and track (CT, MT, and TAU) on depression and anxiety.

Dependent Variable	Interaction F value	*p* value	MSE	Eta square
Depression	2.56	<.05	.196	.196
Anxiety	1.78	>.05	.264	.090

Tools lowered the reported depression for CT and MT, but had no effect for TAU.

The second ANCOVA, using anxiety as the dependent variable, did not reveal an interaction between Treatment Track and Thought Tools ($F_{(4, 73)} = 1.78$ $p > .05$, MSE = .264, Eta-square = .09). Close inspection of the results showed a pattern similar to that of depression (i.e., a larger effect for the CT track than for the MT track, but no effect for TAU), but the power of the test was insufficient to yield a statistically significant effect.

It might be argued that increasing the use of any tools might lower depression and anxiety, so we conducted two additional ANCOVAs similar to the two above. However, with these ANCOVAs we replaced the Thought Tools with low, moderate, and high use categories of all the remaining tools combined (e.g., mood tracking, anger management, relaxation). Neither of these additional ANCOVAs produced any significant effects. For depression, the interaction between Treatment Track and non-thought tools was $F_{(4, 73)} = .20$, MSE = .244, Eta-square = .01, and for anxiety the interaction was $F_{(4, 73)} = .96$, MSE = .288, Eta-square = .05.

4. Discussion

This discussion will not dwell on the average BDI and BAI results and will focus mainly on tool use and its relation to depression and anxiety. The general trend for the third month was that the CT group received the largest benefit from using the thought-related tools. There was a significant reduction in depression for the CT group when they used these tools. There was a smaller reduction in depression for the MT group, but the effect was significant. There was no effect of thought tool use for the TAU group. The effect of the thought tools on anxiety was similar to that of depression (i.e., anxiety was lowered when the thought tools were used) but the effects were not statistically significant. The use of other tools such as mood tracking and relaxation had no effect on depression and anxiety.

These findings need to be interpreted with a bit of caution due to the non-experimental nature of the study. We did not manipulate the use of the tool. Rather, we acquired self reports of the tool use. It is possible that those patients who reported more use of the tools were the same patients who experienced the lowest levels of depression and anxiety. We attempted to control for this possibility by using their pre-treatment depression and anxiety scores as covariates, but this may not have been a sufficient control. Ideally, these tools should be independently manipulated and the effects of high and low levels studied in a more control, true experimental way. Nevertheless, the study is important is showing that there is a connection between the use of these tools and the reported levels of depression and anxiety.

It was notable that of all the 17 skills/tools identified by the independent coders, Thought Records and Thought Distortions were at the top of the list of reported tools. This gave validity to the CT tools of catching and disputing thought distortions and using thought records in managing symptoms of depression and anxiety. Thought distortions that the participants were trained to identify are in Appendix B. Participants reported that they were better able to identify these distortions and take a step back without the emotional reaction.

The thought records similarly required the patient to recognize their negative distortions and examine the evidence for and against the thought creating emotional distress. Patients were trained to write down the thought that contributed to a negative shift in mood and then examine the facts that both supported and negated the thought. For example: you found out you did not get a job you interviewed for and say "I am such a loser". What are the facts that support this statement and those that negate it? CT assisted the patients in decentering from the thought and assessed the validity. The premise was to come up with a balanced thought. As in the example just stated "I am a loser" a balanced thought would be that "I don't do everything faultlessly but there is much I do well".

It is interesting that the patients in the MT group showed a high frequency of reporting thought tools characterized by CT, but did not report many tools specific to MT. Current literature has highlighted the difficulty in defining the construct of mindfulness in self-report questionnaires (Baer, Smith, & Allen, 2004) and in self-report assessment (Grossman, 2011). The understanding of a construct such as being in the moment or nonjudgmental awareness will differ from those with experience in mindfulness and those who are novices (Grossman, 2011). In the returned surveys, participants used the term mindfulness as a broader concept instead of identifying specific behaviors such as focus on the breath or awareness of body sensations. For the purpose of this study, patients in the MT had training by therapists with their own mindfulness practice and reportedly practiced the awareness of the breath and body sensations along with an understanding of mindfulness as living in the moment, without judgment. Both CT and MT have been shown to enhance emotional regulation (Corcoran, Farb, Anderson, & Segal, 2010; Farb et al., 2010) and decrease rumination via disengagement from the cognitive processes (Cambers, Lo, & Allen, 2008). In this sense it may be difficult for the patient to specifically identify which skill they are using. As one participants stated "I am not able to explain the exact tools I use but can say that the combination of the months I spent in the program learning these tools changed my life". While the participants in the MT engaged in 30 min. per day practice, researchers in both MBSR and MBCT (Mindfulness Based Cognitive Therapy) recommended that patients engaged in 45 minutes of daily mindful practice (Kabat-Zinn, 1994; Teasdale et al., 2000). Thus the reduced time of this practice for the study participants may have mitigated against a more vigorous and consistent integration of the practice into their daily lives and a lower reporting of MT-specific tools.

Appendix A includes direct statements from the participants returned surveys. While many reported the benefits of the program or the tools learned and practiced, it was also apparent that this was/is a continual process, that lapses occur, that patients may continue to benefit from medication in conjunction with CT or MT, and that tools do not eliminate life stressors. However, as one participant stated "Learning these tools saved my life. Things are still quite difficult but I am managing."

Further research should attempt to find more sensitive ways to identify tool use from patients receiving mindfulness training. These patients may be using MT-related tools, but the self-report technique does not seem to allow them to articulate what they are in a way that researchers can identify and use. Additional studies should also focus on those patients with a diagnosis of Bipolar Disorder, Currently Depressed to further research the use of CT and MT for the management of symptoms of this diagnosis. Another area of research is to assess is the level of anxiety reported by Bipolar Disorder, Currently Depressed patients and examine the relationships between anxiety and depression with this population.

5. Conclusion

Mindfulness and CT continue to be researched and utilized in treatment of depression and anxiety. While this study has brought attention to two tools and skills in CT (thought records and thought distortions) that patients reported they consistently used to manage their mood state, it was also evident that treatment is unique to each individual and that clinicians need to find not only what is most beneficial for their patients but what are the skills and tools that they will continue to use. The patients in this study continued to benefit from the use of thought records and catching and disputing thought distortions. The formats for these tools are included in Appendix B.

References

Alexander, V., & Tatum, B. C (2013). A Qualitative Analysis of Mindfulness Practice and Cognitive Therapy Tools in Preventing Relapse from Depression. *Journal of Education Research and Behavioral Sciences, 2*, 98-106.

Alexander, V., Tatum, B. C., Auth, C., Takos, D., Whittemore, S., & Fidaleo, R. (2012). A Study of Mindfulness Practices and Cognitive Therapy: Effects on Depression and Self-Efficacy. *International Journal of Psychology and Counselling, 4*, 115-122. http://dx.doi.org/10.5897/IJPC

American Psychiatric Association (2000). *Diagnostic and Statistical Manual of Mental Disorders IV-Text Revised.* Washington DC: Author.

Anxiety and Depression Association of America (2014). *Facts and Statistics.* www.adaa.org

Baer. R. A., Smith, G. T., & Allen, K. B. (2004). Assessment of Mindfulness by Self-Report: The Kentucky Inventory of Mindfulness Skills. *Assessment, 11*, 191-206. http://dx.doi.org/10.1177/1073191104268029

Beck, A. T., Steer, R. A., & Brown, G. K. (1996). *Beck Depression Inventory* (2nd ed.). San Antonio TX: The Psychological Corporation.

Bockting, C. L. H., Schene, A. H., Koeter, M., Wouters, L., Huyser, J., & Kamphuis, J. H. (2005). Preventing relapse/Reoccurrence in Recurrent Depression with Cognitive Therapy: A Randomized Controlled Trial. *Journal of Consulting and Clinical Psychology, 73*, 647-657. http://dx.doi.org/10.1037/0022-006X.73.4.647

Burns, D. (1999). *The Feeling Good Handbook* (rev. ed.). New York, NY: Plume.

Chambers, R., Lo, B. C. Y., & Allen, N. B. (2008). The Impact of Intensive Mindfulness Training on Attentional Control, Cognitive Style, and Affect. *Cognitive Therapy and Research, 32*, 303-322.

Chen, S. Y., Jordan, C., & Thompson, S. (2006). The Effect of Cognitive Behavioral Therapy on Depression: The Role of Problem-Solving Appraisal. *Research in Social Work Practice, 16*, 500-510. http://dx.doi.org/10.1177/1049731506287302

Corcoran, K. M., Farb, N., Anderson, A., & Segal, Z. V. (2010). Mindfulness and Emotion Regulation: Outcomes and Possible Mediating Mechanisms. In A. M. Kring, & D. M. Sloan (Eds.), *Emotion Regulation and Psychopathology: A Transdiagnostic Approach to Etiology and Treatment* (pp. 339-355). New York: Guilford Press.

Courbasson, C. M., Nishikawa, Y., & Shapira, L. B. (2011). Mindfulness-Action Based Cognitive Behavioral Therapy for Concurrent Binge Eating Disorder and Substance Use Disorders. *Eating Disorders, 19*, 17-33. http://dx.doi.org/10.1080/10640266.2011.533603

Creswell, J. W. (2014). *Research Design: Qualitative, Quantitative and Mixed Methods Approaches* (4th ed.). Thousand Oaks, CA: Sage.

Deyo, M., Wilson, K. A., Ong, J., & Koopman, C. (2009). Mindfulness and Rumination: Does Mindfulness Training Lead to Reductions in the Ruminative Thinking Associated with Depression? *Explore, 5*, 265-271. http://dx.doi.org/10.1016/j.explore.2009.06.005

Farb, N. A. S., Anderson, A. K., Mayberg, H., Bean, J., McKeon, D., & Segal, Z. V. (2010). Minding One's Emotions: Mindfulness Training Alters the Neural Expression of Sadness. *Emotion, 10*, 25-33. http://dx.doi.org/10.1037/a0017151.supp

Fava, G., Grandi, S., Zielezny, M., Canestari, R., & Morphy, M. A. (1996). Cognitive Behavioral Treatment of Residual Symptoms in Primary Major Depressive Disorder. *American Journal of Psychiatry, 151*, 1295-1299.

Grossman, P. (2011). Defining Mindfulness by How Poorly I Think I Pay Attention during Everyday Awareness and Other Intractable Problems in Psychology's Reinvention of Mindfulness: Comment on Brown et al. 2011. *Psychological As-*

sessment, 23, 1034-1040. http://dx.doi.org/10.1037/a0022713

Hayes, S. C., Strosahl, K. D., & Wilson, K. G. (1999). *Acceptance and Commitment Therapy: An Experiential Approach to Behavior Change.* New York: Guilford Press.

Hofman, S. G., Sawyer, A. T., Witt, A. A., & Oh, D. (2010). The Effect of Mindfulness Based Therapy on Anxiety and Depression: A Meta-Analytic Review. *Journal of Consulting and Clinical Psychology, 78,* 169-183. http://dx.doi.org/10.1037/a0018555

Jarrett, R. B., Kraft, D., Doyle, J., Foster, B. M., Eaves, G. G., & Silver, P. C. (2001). Preventing Recurrent Depression Using Cognitive Therapy with and without a Continuation Phase: A Randomized Clinical Trial. *Archives of General Psychiatry, 58,* 381-388. http://dx.doi.org/10.1001/archpsyc.58.4.381

Jarrett, R. B., Vittengl, J. R., Clark, L. A., & Thase, M. E. (2011). Skills of Cognitive Therapy (SoCT): A New Measure of Patients' Comprehension and Use. *Psychological Assessment, 23,* 578-586. http://dx.doi.org/10.1037/a0022485

Judd, L. J. (1997). The Clinical Course of Unipolar Depressive Disorders. *Archives of General Psychiatry, 54,* 989-991. http://dx.doi.org/10.1001/archpsyc.1997.01830230015002

Kabat-Zinn, J. (1994). *Wherever You Go, There You Are: Mindfulness Meditation in Everyday Life.* New York: Hyperion.

Keng, S. L., Smoski, M. J., & Robins, C. J. (2011). Effects of Mindfulness on Psychological Health: A Review of Empirical Studies. *Clinical Psychological Review, 31,* 1041-1056. http://dx.doi.org/10.1016/j.cpr.2011.04.006

Kennedy, N., Abbott, R., & Paykel, E. S. (2003). Remission and Reoccurrence of Depression in a Maintenance Era: Long-Term Outcome in a Cambridge Cohort. *Psychological Medicine, 33,* 827-838. http://dx.doi.org/10.1017/S003329170300744X

Khong, B. S. L. (2009). Expanding the Understanding of Mindfulness: Seeing the Tree and the Forest. *The Humanist Psychologist, 37,* 117-136. http://dx.doi.org/10.1080/08873260902892006

Lau, M. A., Bishop, S. R., Segal, Z. V., Buis, T., Anderson, N., Carlson, L., Shapiro, S., & Carmody, J. (2006). The Toronto Mindfulness Scale: Development and Validation. *Journal of Clinical Psychology, 62,* 1445-1467. http://dx.doi.org/10.1002/jclp.20326

Linehan, M. M. (1993). *Cognitive-Behavioral Treatment of Borderline Personality Disorder.* New York: Guilford.

Matthew, A. & MacLeod, C. (2005). Cognitive Vulnerability to Emotional Disorders. *Annual Review of Clinical Psychology, 1,* 167-195. http://dx.doi.org/10.1146/annurev.clinpsy.1.102803.143916

Owen, G. P., Walter, K. H., Chard, K. M., & Davis, P. A. (2012) Changes in Mindfulness Skills and Treatment Response among Veterans in Residential PTSD Treatment. *Psychological Trauma: Theory, Research, Practice and Policy, 4,* 221-228. http://dx.doi.org/10.1037/a0024251

Paykel, E. S., Scott, J., Teasdale, J. D., Johnson, A. L., Garland, A., & Moore, R. (1999). Prevention of Residual Depression by Cognitive Therapy: A Controlled Trial. *Archives of General Psychiatry, 56,* 829-835. http://dx.doi.org/10.1001/archpsyc.56.9.829

Roemer, L., Orsillo, S. M., & Salters-Pedneault, K. (2008). Efficacy of an Acceptance-Based Behavior Therapy for Generalized Anxiety Disorder: Evaluation in a Randomized Controlled Trial. *Journal of Consulting Clinical Psychology, 76,* 1083-1089. http://dx.doi.org/10.1037/a0012720

Salemink, E., van den Hout, M., & Kindt, M. (2010). How Does Cognitive Bias Modification Affect Anxiety? Mediation Analysis and Experimental Data. *Behavioral and Cognitive Psychotherapy, 38,* 59-66. http://dx.doi.org/10.1017/S1352465809990543

Segal, Z. V., Williams, J. M. G., & Teasdale, J. D. (2002). *Mindfulness-Based Cognitive Therapy for Depression: A New Approach to Preventing Relapse.* New York: Guilford Press.

Strunk, D. R., DeRubeis, R. J., Chiu, A. W., & Alvarez, J. (2007). Patients' Competence in the Performance of Cognitive Therapy Skills: Relation to the Reduction of Relapse Risk Following Treatment for Depression. *Journal of Consulting and Clinical Psychology, 75,* 523-530. http://dx.doi.org/10.1037/0022-006X.75.4.523

Teasdale, J. D., Williams, J. M., Soulsby, J. M., Segal, Z. V., Ridgeway, V. A., & Lau, M. A. (2000). Prevention of Relapse/Recurrence in Major Depression by Mindfulness-Based Cognitive Therapy. *Journal of Consulting and Clinical Psychology, 68,* 615-623. http://dx.doi.org/10.1037/0022-006X.68.4.615

Trapper, K., Shaw, C., Illsey, J., Hill, A. J., Bond, F. W., & Moore, L. (2009). Exploratory Randomized Controlled Trial of a Mindfulness-Based Weight Loss Prevention for Women. *Appetite, 52,* 396-404. http://dx.doi.org/10.1016/j.appet.2008.11.012

Wallin, D. J. (2007). *Attachment in Psychotherapy.* New York: Guilford Press.

Wells, A. (2002). GAD, Metacognition and Mindfulness: An Information Processing Analysis. *Clinical Psychology: Science & Practice, 9,* 95-100. http://dx.doi.org/10.1093/clipsy/9.1.95

Wolfsdorf, B. A., & Zlotnick, C. (2001). Affect Management in Group Therapy for Women with Posttaumatic Stress Disorder and Histories of Childhood Sexual Abuse. *Journal of Clinical Psychology, 57,* 169-181. http://dx.doi.org/10.1002/1097-4679(200102)57:2<169::AID-JCLP4>3.0.CO;2-0

World Health Organization (2012). Fact Sheet on Depression. www.who.int/topics/depression/en

Wright, J. H., Wright, A. S., Salmon, P., Beck, A. T., Kuykendall, J., Goldsmith, L. J., & Zickel, M. B. (2002). Development and Initial Testing of a Multimedia Program for Computer-Assisted Cognitive Therapy. *American Journal of Psychotherapy, 56, 76-86.*

Appendix A

Statements of Tool Use by Participants

CT: "I'm better able to be objective/detached about a situation I would have overreacted to in the past. Also I am better at noticing when I'm negatively judging myself and my emotions and can stop it."

CT: "I have never been happier in my life and can actually say that 'cog therapy' works; it is not the medication (although it helps) but it is the understanding of our psyche... You can use me as an example that cog works. It was very difficult to cope with life before due to my upbringing and culture. But now I am totally different person, I take responsibility for my actions, I can see clear my future."

CT: "The return to the work environment has been stressful but I manage using different COG tools. I think about my time in the program and it was the best, healthiest thing I have ever done for myself."

CT: "I'm going through a bit of a lapse right now and am trying to use the tools from COG to fight it. So far I am doing fine."

CT: "I really learned to be aware of my distorted thoughts. There's constantly an alarm going off in my head when one comes across. Before, I was completely unaware of my distorted thoughts."

MT: "Thought stopping, relaxation, mindfulness, and mental thought records. I repeat new core beliefs mentally when anxiety increases or old core beliefs raise their ugly head."

MT: "I am dealing with my anxiety in a positive way and I am going to be OK no matter what because I have come to the realization that every moment is precious and I intend to live and experience these moments as they may never come again. I want to say I lived my life and not my life happened."

MT: "Learning these tools saved my life. Things are still quite difficult but I am managing."

MT: "I believe the cognitive therapy skills and group and mindfulness meditation techniques changed my life for the better. I learned how to think and act and respond in healthy ways and how to know and respect myself and how to protect myself."

MT: "I understand the importance of...staying on top of unpleasant thoughts. I have been avoiding using some of the techniques and saw my mood drop. I feel as though they were great things to learn."

MT: "I've been feeling quite well... Anytime I feel I am slipping a bit, I just analyze things like a thought record or de-catastophizing worksheet. Bad thoughts just don't last."

MT: "Life still has some real challenges. Now I face them and deal with them. I can still improve in some areas of my life, but I no longer tear myself up for my shortcomings. I have the tools and the abilities to have a really cool life and I look forward to living it instead of fearing it all the time."

TAU: "I strongly rely on the cognitive tools. This program saved my life and made it better."

TAU: "This program really helped. I wish I had known about it before life got so bad. It is one of the main components to me dealing with depression..."

TAU: "I have had increasing success in recognizing distorted thoughts as distorted, recognizing the types of avoidant or reactionary behaviors I "automatically" adopt in response to cognitive distortions, and taking the time/energy to challenge and change thought/behavior patterns that keep me locked in cycles of distorted thinking behaviors."

TAU: "I no longer have thoughts of suicide because I now know why I was having these thoughts. I do not suffer from depression. Every day I look happily forward."

TAU: "Cognitive Therapy continues to be a big part of my life and feeling of successfully being able to function."

TAU: "Reframing my thoughts if they are negative, I am learning to be loving and compassionate with myself. This is a new way of living for me."

TAU: "I am not able to explain the exact tools I use but can say that the combination of the months I spent in the program learning these tools changed my life. I've worked pretty hard on some old issues that have been quite challenging. While going through them was quite painful it was healing and an ongoing process. I am taking it slow and can feel the progress."

Appendix B

Tools Used Most Consistently by Participants

THOUGHT DISTORTIONS: Through training in identifying thought distortions such as all or nothing thinking (see examples in Appendix A), patients were able to increase their awareness of their faulty thinking and

come up with more balanced thoughts
1. All or nothing thinking (thinking in extremes)
2. Minimizing or magnification (exaggerate negative factors and dilute positive factors)
3. Overgeneralization (sweeping judgments on a single event)
4. Filtering (focusing on one aspect of a situation, typically the negative aspect)
5. Catastrophizing (thinking that the worst case scenario will come true)
6. Personalization (taking responsibility for things that don't apply to you)
7. Jumping to conclusions (making negative assumptions without the evidence to support this)
8. Labeling (assigning labels to self or others)
9. Should statement (rigid unrealistic rules of self and others)

Participants reported that they were better able to identify these distortions and take a step back without the emotional reaction.

THOUGHT RECORD

Situation	Automatic Thought	Emotion	Rating (0% - 100%)	Rational Response	Re-rating (0% - 100%)

Test of Evidence

Evidence Thought is not 100% True

Evidence Thought is True

1. When you experience a shift in mood, what is the situation?

2. Identify the emotion you are experiencing such as depression, anger, anxiety. One emotion per thought record.

3. Rate the emotion on a scale from 0% - 100% (100 = most extreme, 0 = absence of the emotion).

4. Identify the thought that is causing this elevated rating in mood. If there are several thoughts, choose the most extreme.

5. Evidence the thought is true: Come up with as many facts as you can that support the thought.

6. Dispute the thought: What is the evidence the thought is not true.

7. After disputing the thought, identify a more rational thought.

8. Re-rate the intensity of the emotion.

Appendix C

The 17 Tools

1. Mood tracking/daily inventory: A brief inventory with ten items, measuring the patient's level of depression that day and charted to show fluctuations in daily mood.

2. Conflict resolution worksheets: Healthy and unhealthy ways of managing and resolving conflict worksheets.

3. Thought records: Examining the situation, thoughts, feelings, and behaviors. What is the evidence that the thought is true and what is the evidence the thought is not true? The goal is to come up with a more balanced thought.

4. Thought distortions: Identifying faulty thinking and changing it.

5. Activity Schedule (GRAPES): A worksheet that lists daily activities related to G (gentle with self), R (relaxation), A (accomplishments), P (pleasure), E (exercise), and S (social).

6. Assertiveness script (DEESC): Write out a script to increase assertive behavior. D (describe problem), E (express emotions), E (empathy; how does this impact the other person), S (specifics; i.e. I want ...or I need...), C (consequences; if ...then...).

7. Core belief/Schema work: Beliefs about ourselves, others, and the world from early experiences which is the way in which we interpret and process situations. Core belief work assists the patients in identifying their personal beliefs which make them vulnerable to depression.

8. Journaling: A log of our beliefs and feelings at the present moment to have a better understanding of how we are interpreting information and events.

9. Responsibility pie: To process our role in a situation. If the situation or event were a piece of pie, how big would your role be? Who else would be involved in the event and what would their roles be?

10. Boundaries: Discussing behaviors indicative of fluid, healthy, and rigid boundaries.

11. Distractions: Ways to remove ourselves from difficult emotional states such as counting backwards by 7.

12. Motivation model: Action leads to motivation which leads to more action. Examining the pros and cons of avoidance and action.

13. Pros/Cons worksheet: Problem identification, brainstorming possible solutions, and listing the pros and cons of each option.

14. Decatastrophizing worksheet: Identifying the situation creating anxiety and one's belief about the danger. The worksheet examines the evidence of support and refutes the belief about the danger (my job is at risk) and about one's control (there is nothing I can do about it).

15. Anger management: RETHINK model. R (recognize that you are feeling angry), E (empathize with the person or situation causing the anger), T (think instead of just emoting), H (hear what the other person is saying), I (integrate respect but thinking in a non-angry way), N (notice your body's reaction to anger), K (keep focused on the present event and not past grudges. Think of solutions).

16. Relaxation techniques: Imagery, diaphragmatic breathing, and progressive muscle relaxation.

17. Mindfulness: Of being in the moment, practicing letting go, increasing awareness without judgment, focus on the breath and body awareness.

22

The Role of Self-Control on Mood States and Health Anxiety in a Sample of Blind and Visually Impaired People

Pierluigi Diotaiuti, Filippo Petruccelli, Luigi Rea, Angelo Marco Zona, Valeria Verrastro

Department of Human, Social and Health Sciences, University of Cassino and South Latium, Cassino, Italy
Email: p.diotaiuti@unicas.it

Abstract

Blind people face daily a stressful condition that they seek to better manage through the control of the surrounding environment. They prefer the maintenance of routines and the contacts with familiar people and frequentation of well-known places. We hypothesize that in people with a serious visual impairment, the exercise of self-control, both as self-regulation both as coping of negative emotions, is significantly associated with the general tone of mood and can act as a protective factor with respect to the concern for their own health. The assumption underlying this study is that the levels of mood and self-rate of health concern are privileged indicators of the quality of life for blind people. 262 blind subjects were administered about personality inventory, scales for measuring resilience, the mood state, the anxiety about their health. Among the key findings, we noted that self-regulation was highly correlated to the mood of males, but only on the condition of acquired blindness, and that it could mediate anxiety levels with respect to their health. Self-esteem was not found to be a protective emotional factor for blind subjects. The study opens up the need to further investigate the capacity of self-regulation on the emotional sphere of people with disabilities in order to create more effective intervention programs to enhance the adaptive capacity of the subject.

Keywords

Self-Control, Self-Regulation, Mood States, Health Anxiety, Visually Impaired

1. Introduction

The loss of vision requires a significant psychosocial adaptation, a process with which many blind people are constantly fighting. The psycho-social impact of blindness and visual impairment is deep, as evidenced also by the high risk of depression, with high levels of emotional stress, and the negative impact on quality of life and overall health status. The visual impairment is usually associated with particular psychosocial conditions such as isolation, cognitive impairment, increased dependency on others, low self-assessment of health status, depression (Macfarland, 1966).

The visual limitation can increase the sense of vulnerability especially in the elderly, making them feel confined and imprisoned in their houses, deprived of important social interactions; this leads to some cases of depression, alcohol abuse and also of other substances (Graham & Schmidt, 1999).

Generally the blind from birth seem more adapted to their condition and they show greater confidence in their own ability in carrying out every day practices, such as the use of public transport (buses, trains and subways); they also appear further integrated within a culture blind (Heyl & Wahl, 2001).

At contrast, those who become blind as a result of a sudden event (illness or injury), become immediately aware of a rapid transition to status of an individual considered generally unable to perform even simple tasks and activities. Living with an important functional limitation such as sight, constantly imposes the task of preserving the residual skills. It also includes the exposure to risks and challenges when coping strategies cease to function, or for a deterioration of functional limitation or because of environmental barriers outside the control of the subject. The work of adaptation could be represented as a route consisting of several phases (recognition, exploration, re-acquisition, maintenance) but not necessarily a continuous process from one step to another (the length may be longer or shorter and in some cases the subject may stop and go back) (Bergeron & Wanet-Defalque, 2013; Diotaiuti, 2011).

Blind and visually impaired people live in a naturally stressful condition, which are constantly engaged in research and conservation of the control of environmental conditions, with a preference for the maintenance of routine and relations with familiar people and well known places. It is possible to find an explicit or implicit fear in front of the possibility of unexpected change of stable frames of reference. Many have learned by the time how to best manage this fear, however, that re-emerges with all its anxiety, in cases of emergency or sudden change (Verstraten et al., 2005). Blind people who are more ready often react to the frustrations with outbursts of anger; this is a positive factor because it means an orientation to the relationship that allows individual to direct the stress. Others, however, are closed in themselves, in a completely passive way, excluding the possibility of a reaction externally oriented.

The risk of depression, especially in elderly blind and visually impaired people can be reinforced by other factors, such as the negative perception of the quality of life, poverty and other health problems less important than visual impairment (Kemp, 2000). Depression is manifested by changes in mood and behavior, lack of motivation, digestive problems, weakness, persistent irritability and sadness, deficit in memory and inability to properly relate to others (De Leo et al., 1999). For some people alcohol abuse may be a form of adaptation and coping with the new disability and may provide temporary relief but actually this increases social isolation over time and weakens coping skills, influencing the onset of new health disorders.

Perceptions of self-efficacy play a key role in the management of chronic diseases. They will determine whether an individual will seek to implement new behaviors strongly oriented to health (Holman & Lorig, 1992; Clark & Dodge, 1999). Lazarus and Folkman (1984) have identified two general types of coping. The first is defined problem focused coping and can be referred to the efforts made by patients to manage stress, actively intervening to change the source of stress. This strategy includes the problem definition, generation of alternatives, evaluation of alternative situations. The second type of coping is instead focused on emotions, including attempts to reduce or manage the emotional stress associated with the situation. This strategy involves minimization, distancing, selective attention, positive comparisons, looking for positive values in negative events, self-illusions, avoidance.

The problem-focused coping strategies are used when individuals consider the event modifiable or manageable, and when individuals recognize that the situation should simply be accepted, and they are likely to use emotion-focused strategies. This approach stresses that the way in which the patient reads their condition will influence the type of coping used, which in turn will determine whether an experience of psychological stress or acceptable quality of life will take place (Lazarus & Folkman, 1984). The relationship between the evaluation of the disease, coping and adaptation is central in another model called social cognition model of self-regulation (Cameron & Leventhal, 2003). The adjustment involves a modulation of thought, affect, behavior, attention, or the intentional use of specific mechanisms or automatic supportive meta-competencies. The self-regulating processes start when the subject is prevented from routine activity or when the orientation of the object changes its salience (e.g. the occurrence of a challenge, the failure of usual action models) (de Ridder & De Wit, 2006). Various studies have emphasized the role that the subjective salience may have in the ability to exercise self-control, and identified the mechanisms and strategies through which self-control can be activated in order to protect subject's important goals (van der Pligt & de Vries, 1998; Levine, 2010).

In the light of these considerations, we hypothesize that people with a visual impairment the exercise of self-control (both as a self-regulating, both as an exercise in the management of negative emotions) is significantly associated with the general mood tone and can act as a protective factor with respect to the concern for their own health. The assumption underlying this study is that the levels of mood and their health experience are privileged indicators of the quality of life for blind and visually impaired people. A well-known risk factor for mental health disorders frequently associated with many visual slow but progressive degeneration, is the so-called syndrome of the sword of Damocles. The individual lives in a constant state of anxiety and concern for their health but the greatest anxiety is due to the idea that, sooner or later, the residual vision will fade to make the person completely blind (Hayman et al. 2007). In this sense, individuals evaluate events as uncontrollable, feeling at their mercy and become passive, resigned, anxious and depressed. A positive mood disposition, especially the optimism, produces a significant increase in subjective well-being, understood also as favorable evaluation of their own existence (Wrosch & Scheier, 2003).

According to Fredrickson (2001) the effects of positive emotions consist not only in the creation of a state of subjective well-being, safety, adaptation to their ecological niche, but would also serve to inhibit the harmful effects produced by negative emotions. They are therefore a kind of antidote to adverse outcomes generated by negative emotional experiences.

For this reason, we believe it is important to identify elements whose presence may facilitate the persistence of positive mood states. Self-control as well as to facilitate adaptation may prove to be associated with positive mood states.

Among different components of the self-control we have considered in particular the self-regulatory skills, the ability to cope with negative emotions, and resilience.

To sum up among the main goals we have set in our study is investigating relationships between personality features of blind subjects (such as self-esteem, social desirability, self-regulation, resilience and ability to cope) with the levels of mood and feelings of concern related to their health state.

2. Methodology

2.1. Participants

262 blind subjects randomly selected from the Italian centers of the "Italian Union of Blind and Visually Impaired" (Unione italiana dei Ciechi e degli Ipovedenti-UICI): 154 males and 108 females, with an average age between 46 and 60 years old.

2.2. Instruments

1) Multidimensional Personality Profile (MPP) standardized by GV Caprara et al. (2006). It is a tool that allows highlighting the skills of individual adaptation to life situations, even enabling to get any indication about future behavior in terms of psychological well-being. In particular, the key areas of personality measured by MPP are five:

a) Agency: Enforcing their views, setting itselves ambitious goals, to know how to lead and motivate others, in conducting its activities with vigor and alertness. It consists of: Identification, Ambition, Leadership, Business.

b) Social and emotional intelligence: Individual skills that manifest in empathy, emotional intelligence and a general trusting orientation toward others and relationships. The related sub-dimensions are: Empathy, pro-sociality, Sociability, Interpersonal Trust.

c) Self-regulation: Individual skills related to the planning and persistence in achieving a goal, self-discipline meaning both self-reflexive organization skill and tenacity to success. It is divided into sub-areas: Action-oriented, Tenacity, Reliability, Accuracy.

d) Coping Ability (in critical situations): Emotional balance as mood stability, the efficient management of stress, frustration and adversities, in the management of negative emotions, and the resilience and strength against events that cause discomfort and disappointment. It consists of: Emotional balance, Stress Management, Management of negative emotions, Elasticity/Resilience.

e) Innovation: This dimension is embodied in the interest and curiosity about cultural activities and individual skills such as creativity and the pleasure towards new situations and solutions. Next to the five areas above, there are four scales for examining self-presentation: Self-esteem, social desirability, "Machiavellianism", management of their thought (about the others).

2) Resilience Scale for Adults—RSA (Friborg et al., 2005) consists of 33 items distributed across six factors measured through three subscales: social skills, structured style and personal strength that is in turn made up of two factors, self-perception (how the individual perceives his current skills and strengths) and planning for the future (how the individual sees the opportunity to achieve their goals in the future). The support and family cohesion and external support are measured respectively by the family cohesion subscale and the subscale social resources.

3) To estimate the level of mood owned by individuals (humoral self appraisal) we have created a self-assessment checklist on a 6-point Likert scale in which the subject was asked to define his level of humor. The points of the scale were coded as: a) extremely low; b) low most of the time; c) more low then high; d) more high then low; e) in a good mood; f) excellent mood. It was required the subject to refer to the two weeks preceding the interview.

4) For the estimation of concern for their own health, we created a self-assessment checklist on a 6-point Likert scale in which the subject was asked to indicate how much his state of health aroused concern. Respectively, the points of the scale were coded as: a) for nothing; b) a little; c) enough; d) a lot; e) very much; f) enormously. All the instruments described above were administered orally by properly trained operators.

2.3. Procedure

The specific conditions of the protagonists of the investigation led to the administration of the instruments by interviewers specifically trained in order to don't distort detection. The meetings took place in presence, at home or in the associative structures, by appointment, in which each respondent was available for an hour, specifically and exclusively for the survey.

Participants were informed about the aims of the study and their participation was free. The questionnaires were anonymous and self-administered. The study protocol complied fully with the guidelines of the Ethics Committee of the Cassino University of South Lazio and was approved by the Institutional Review Boards in accordance with local requirements. It was conducted in accordance with the Good Clinical Practice guidelines and the Declaration of Helsinki (1964) and subsequent revisions. After receiving information about the study, all the subjects provided written informed consent.

2.4. Statistical Analysis

The analyzes were conducted with the statistical package SPSS (version 20.0). When the studied variable had a normal distribution in the population from which the sample was extracted, we used the Student's t test to compare two independent means. When the studied continuous variable had not a normal distribution non-parametric tests were used. Significance level was set at $p < 0.05$.

By subjecting all 152 items of the scale MPP to Reliability Analysis, the validity of the model used was confirmed, which has positive indices of reliability: Cronbach' alpha = 0.89. Even the RSA was confirmed to be a reliable scale with good internal consistency demonstrated by Cronbach's alpha values of 0.79, while among the six factors, the range is from 0.67 (structured style) to 0.81 (self-perception). The correlation of the 33 items of the subscales is high. In order to examine the structure of the MPP and RSA used in this study we used the Principal Components Analysis (PCA) of the correlation matrix of the questions which compose the scales. In order to identify which questions more represented by which component we used as a criterion with a factor loading greater than 0.4. For the inclusion of a question in the model to be submitted to the Principal Components Analysis we used as a criterion the coefficient of determination (R^2) greater than 0.15.

3. Results

As a first instance, we found that the overall sample of the blind compared with the normative, had high scores on the social desirability scale MPP. The scores of these subjects were all within high range. The women reported an average score of 61, the men of 60. With regard to the dimension of self-esteem, the scores of women fell within average range, while the scores of men fell within low range. With regard to the dimension of self-regulation, the scores obtained from both genders were part of the low range. With regard to the coping ability, for both males and females, scores fell within average range.

We examined then whether the condition of the onset of the disease (blind congenital or acquired), for N = 262 (Males: 154, Females: 108), average age = 54.95, born blind and blind acquired: 122 and 140, was significantly associated with levels of mood self-appraisal. Statistical analysis revealed no significant differences in the mood levels in function of the condition of onset disease. We then verified the scores of self-regulation and the coping ability, as measured by the MPP according to the condition of the subjects. For both males and females, there were no significant differences on the scale of self-regulation and the coping ability among those blind at birth and those acquired. We then compared the group of subjects with positive mood with those with negative mood. There were statistically significant differences regardless to the condition of onset of disability and gender to the scores of the scale of coping ability. Positive mood: 76.8; negative mood: 71.8 (Sig, 0.001) (See **Figure 1**). The same significant differences emerged between the group that showed high concern for their health and the group who reported low levels (high concern group with a mean 72.9 and 75.8 the mean for low concern group—Sig, 0.013) (See **Figure 2**).

Comparing male subjects with positive mood and those with negative mood, there were statistically significant differences (Sig, 0.001) in average scores on the scale of self-regulation: positive mood 77.4; negative mood 73.9 (See **Figure 3**) and on the scale of resilience (RSA) (Sig, 0.002; 132 positive mood, negative mood 115) (See **Figure 4**).

Depending on the onset disease condition, only for males with acquired blindness, there was a significant difference (Sig, 0.001) to the scales of self-regulation (78 positive mood, negative mood 73) (See **Figure 5**), resilience (131.2 positive mood, negative mood 111.2) (See **Figure 6**) and coping ability (76.9 positive mood, negative mood 72.6).

For females there was a significant difference (Sig, 0.01) to the scale of resilience (RSA): average score of 127 positive and 110 negative mood (See **Figure 7**). Depending on the onset disease condition, the differences remain unchanged.

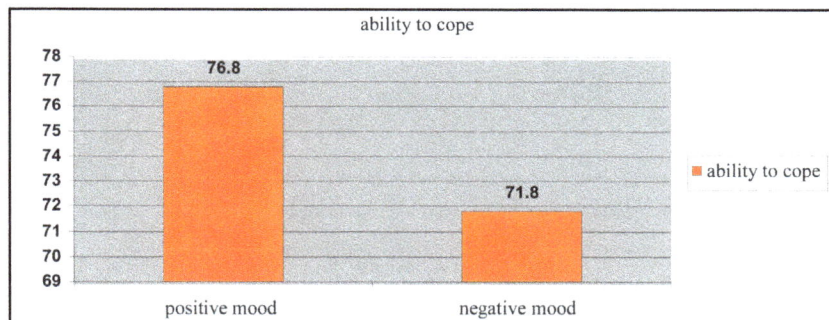

Figure 1. Ability to cope and mood.

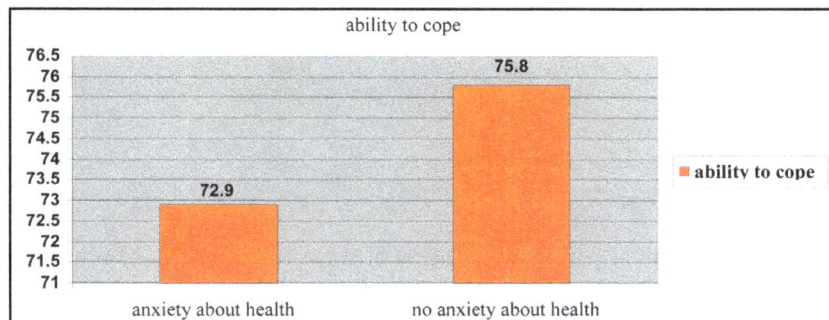

Figure 2. Ability to cope and health anxiety.

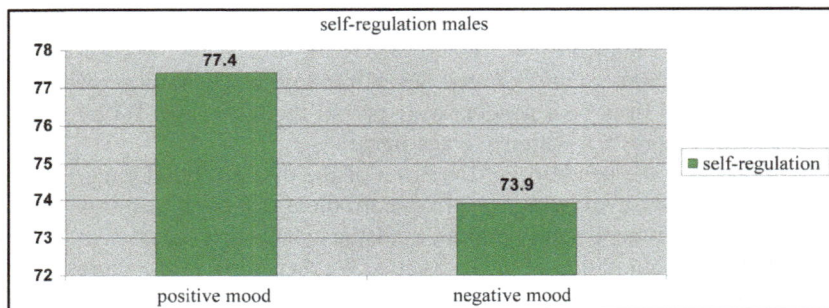

Figure 3. Self-regulation and mood in male blind.

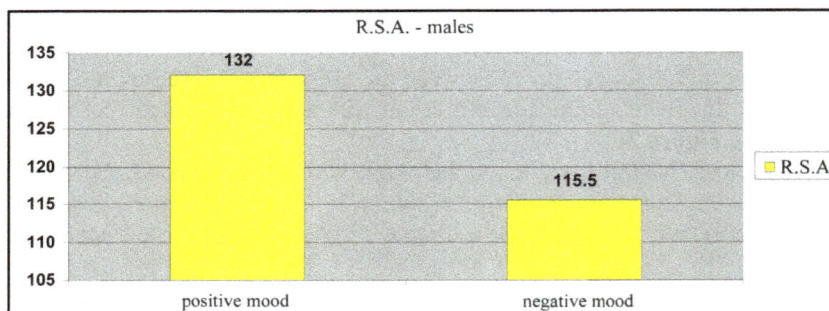

Figure 4. Resilience and mood in male blind.

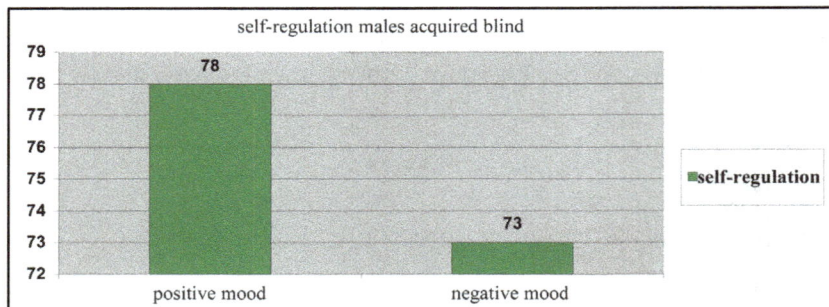

Figure 5. Self-regulation and mood in males acquired blind.

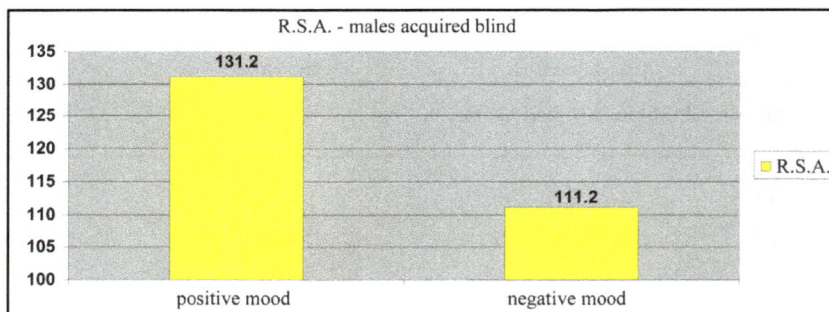

Figure 6. Resilience and mood in males acquired blind.

Another interesting information emerged by analyzing the sample of males born blind. In this group there were no significant differences to the scale of social desirability, among those who reported a positive mood than those who reported a negative mood (positive mood: mean 27.65—negative mood: mean 23.37; Sig, 0.05) (See **Figure 8**).

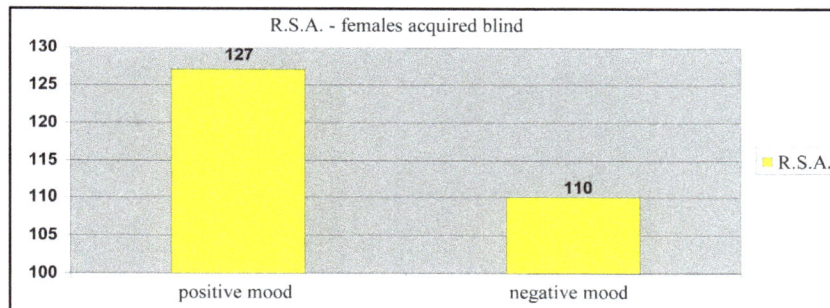

Figure 7. Resilience and mood in females acquired blind.

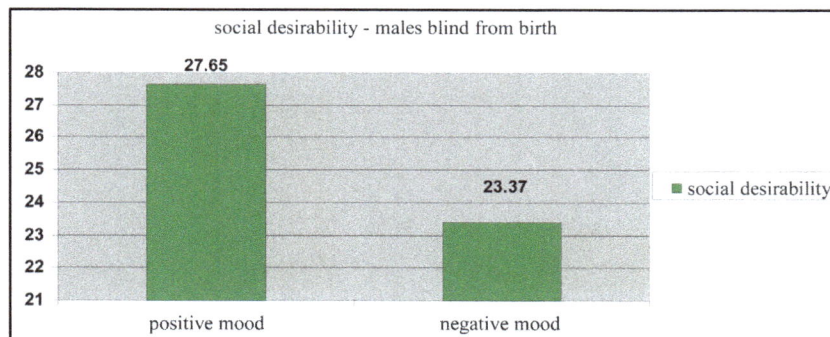

Figure 8. Social desirability and mood in males blind from birth.

By analyzing the sample in function of the concern about their health status, statistically significant differences appeared in average scores on the scale of self regulation. Those who showed high levels of concern about their own health status reported an average score to the scale of self-regulation significantly lower than those who showed low levels of concern (mean worried 74.9—not worried mean 76, 9; Sig, 0.01) (See **Figure 9**). Nevertheless, considering the variable self-esteem, there were no significant differences between those who showed high levels of concern for their health and those who showed low levels of concern (See **Figure 10**).

We then examined whether there were any significant differences in the scale of self-esteem among those who reported a positive mood and those who showed a negative mood. Considering the overall sample, according of both the gender and to the onset of disability, no statistically significant differences emerged (See **Figure 11** and **Figure 12**).

4. Discussion

In the literature, self-esteem is universally considered a factor that mediates the impact of negative events on emotional life, promoting the activation of individual resources, that are useful to the preservation of the Self (Mann et al., 2004; Cott et al., 1999). In our study however the findings suggest to reconsider this proposal. In fact, among the blind population, considered in all experimental conditions and in spite of the gender, there were no significant correlations in this regard. This leads us to reconsider the weight of the dimension of self-esteem in emotional experience for blindness.

For all subjects, coping ability and resilience emerged as the most important personality characteristics for the process of mediation of emotional states, such as mood appraisal and levels of anxiety related to health status. By contrast, the ability of self-regulation has been shown highly positively related to mood among males, but merely in the condition of acquired blindness. This condition may reflect a particular experience of loss, in which the subject is required a greater ability to adapt and emotional and cognitive restructuring. This may be the reason why the skill of self-control plays a decisive role on the mood status. Positive mood would be promoted by the skills of individual self-regulation, even in the context. On the other way, for males who born blind, mood status was found to be associated with social desirability. It is evident that those who reported high score to the scale of social desirability, also reported a positive mood.

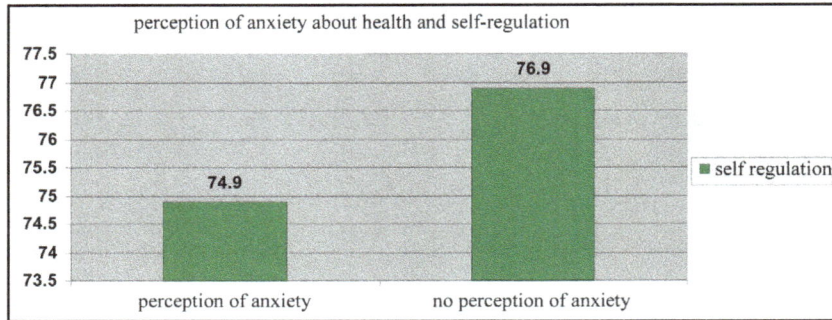

Figure 9. Self-regulation and health anxiety.

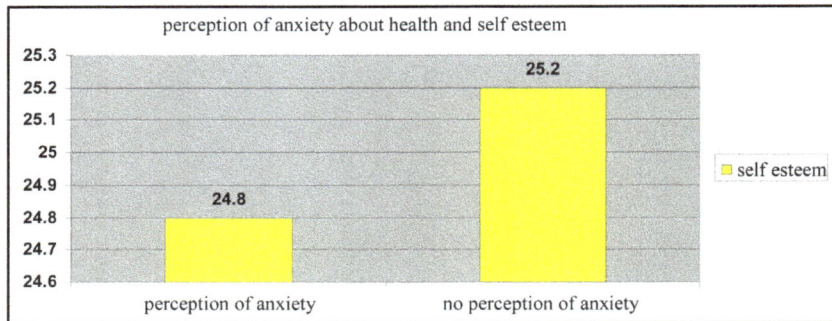

Figure 10. Self-esteem and health anxiety.

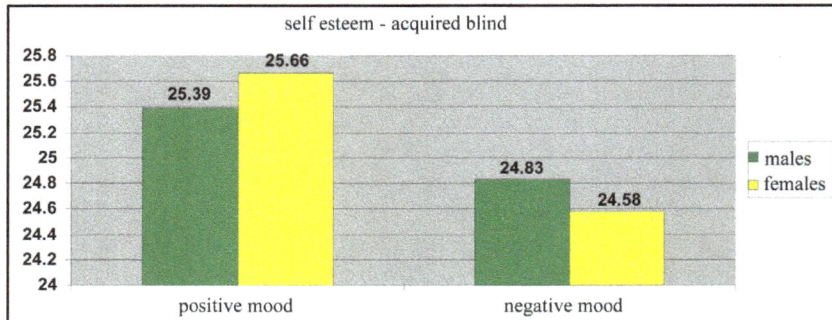

Figure 11. Self-esteem and mood in acquired blind.

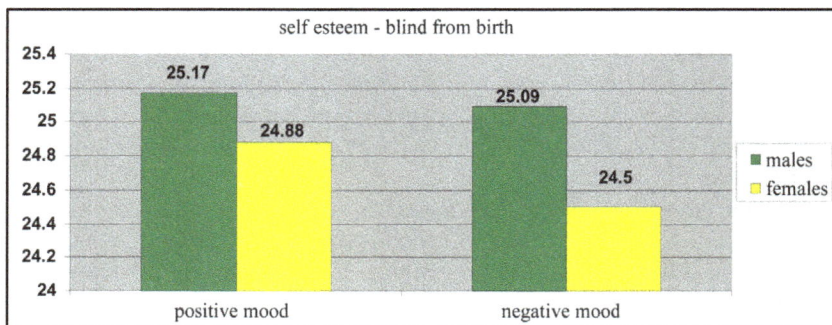

Figure 12. Self-esteem and mood in blind from birth.

The ability for self-regulation would appear to be crucial to mediate the experience of anxiety related to perception of individual health status. In this case, it is shown that those who have high ability for self-regulation, feel less concern about their state of health. Even in this case, self-esteem levels don't seem to have any influence. The study open to the need to further investigate the weight of the ability for self-regulation on emotional life in people with visual impairments, introducing also experimental conditions in which it is possible manipulate the levels of self-regulation, in order to produce intervention programs that are more effective to enhance individual ability of adapt.

5. Conclusion

The resilience and the coping ability were found to be protective emotional factors for the subjects in all experimental conditions. For males, the ability for self-regulation may be an important factor in order to protect the emotional experience among subjects in condition of acquired blindness, resulting in better levels of mood and quality of life. The ability for self-regulation may mediate anxiety levels concerning to their health. For women with acquired blindness, self control is not a factor of emotional protection. For males born blind, positive mood is associated with social desirability. In contrast to resilience, the ability for self-control is not related to mood levels in subjects with the condition of congenital blindness. In our study, self-esteem was not found to be an emotional protective factor in blind subjects. Based on the findings, we believe in agreement with Kef (2002), that a program of interventions aimed to strengthen social skills would produce significant improvements in well-being of these subjects. However, the work on social skills might not be quite enough to support the process of adaptation and well-being of the person who is blind or visually impaired. It would be appropriate to support and encourage the development of self-determined behavior, or the ability to define important goals for themselves and the ability to take the initiative to achieve those objectives. Educational and training interventions aimed at enhancing the intrinsic aspects (not just instrumental) of the motivations underlying the actions taken by individuals who are blind and visually impaired people may actively contribute to break the circuit of relational dependency and passivity that often characterize their sphere of social contact. When subjects take part in activities that they have freely chosen and over which they exercise control, intrinsic motivation increases and the level of perceived well-being with it. Through an intrinsically oriented motivation the interest among the activities, the need of competence, and the self-realization will persist even after reaching the goal (Deci & Ryan, 2002). All this can contribute to the persistence of positive mood states.

References

Bergeron, C. M., & Wanet-Defalque, M. C. (2013). Psychological Adaptation to Visual Impairment: The Traditional Grief Process Revised. *British Journal of Visual Impairment, 31,* 20-31. http://dx.doi.org/10.1177/0264619612469371

Cameron, L. D., & Leventhal, H. (2003). *The Self-Regulation of Health and Illness Behaviour.* New York: Routledge.

Caprara, G. V., Barbaranelli, C., De Carlo N., & Robusto, E. (2006). *Multidimensional Personality Profile (MPP).* Milano: FrancoAngeli. PMCid: PMC2786217.

Clark, N. M., & Dodge, J. A. (1999). Exploring Self-Efficacy as a Predictor of Disease Management. *Health Education Quarterly, 5,* 371-379.

Cott, C. A., Gignac, M. A., & Badley, E. M. (1999). Determinants of Self Rated Health for Canadians with Chronic Disease and Disability. *Journal of Epidemiology and Community Health, 53,* 731-736. http://dx.doi.org/10.1136/jech.53.11.731

De Leo, D., Hickey, P. A., Meneghel, G., & Cantor, C. H. (1999). Blindness, Fear of Sight Loss, and Suicide. *Psychosomatics, 40,* 339-344. http://dx.doi.org/10.1016/S0033-3182(99)71229-6

de Ridder, D. T. D., & De Wit, J. B. F. (2006). *Self-Regulation and Health Behavior.* Chichester: John Wiley & Sons. http://dx.doi.org/10.1002/9780470713150

Deci, E. L., & Ryan, R. M. (Eds.) (2002). *Handbook of Self-Determination Research.* Rochester, NY: University of Rochester Press.

Diotaiuti, P. (2011). *Autoregolazione. Strategie Cognitive Dell'autocontrollo.* Frosinone, FR: Teseo Editore.

Fredrickson, B. L. (2001). The Role of Positive Emotions in Positive Psychology: The Broaden-and-Build Theory of Positive Emotions. *American Psychologist, 56,* 218-226. http://dx.doi.org/10.1037/0003-066X.56.3.218

Friborg, O., Barlaug, D., Martinussen, M., Rosenvinge, J. H., & Hjemdal, O. (2005). Resilience in Relation to Personality and Intelligence. *International Journal of Methods in Psychiatric Research, 14,* 29-42. http://dx.doi.org/10.1002/mpr.15

Graham, K., & Schmidt, G. (1999). Alcohol Use and Psychosocial Well-Being among Older Adults. *Journal of Studies on Alcohol, 60,* 345-350.

Hayman, K. J., Kerse, N. M., La Grow, S. J., Wouldes, T., Robertson, M. C., & Campbell, A. J. (2007). Depression in Older People: Visual Impairment and Subjective Ratings of Health. *Optometry & Vision Science, 84,* 1024-1030. http://dx.doi.org/10.1097/OPX.0b013e318157a6b1

Heyl, V., & Wahl, H. W. (2001). Psychosocial Adaptation to Age-Related Vision Loss: A Six-Year Perspective. *Journal of Visual Impairment & Blindness, 95,* 739-748.

Holman, H. R., & Lorig, K. (1992). Perceived Self-Efficacy in Self-Management of Chronic Disease. In R. Schwarzer (Ed.), *Self-Efficacy: Thought Control of Action* (pp. 305-323). Washington DC: Hemisphere.

Kef, S. (2002). Psychosocial Adjustment and the Meaning of Social Support for Visually Impaired Adolescents. *Journal of Visual Impairment & Blindness, 96,* 22-37.

Kemp, B. J. (2000). Psychosocial Considerations in a Rehabilitation Model for Aging and Vision Services. In J. E. Crews, & F. J. Whittington (Eds.), *Vision Loss in an Aging Society: A Multidisciplinary Perspective* (pp. 133-153). New York: AFB Press.

Lazarus, R. S., & Folkman, S. (1984). *Stress, Appraisal and Coping.* New York: Springer.

Levine, R. M. (2010). Identity and Illness: The Effects of Identity Salience and Frame of Reference on Evaluation of Illness and Injury. *British Journal of Health Psychology, 4,* 63-80. http://dx.doi.org/10.1348/135910799168470

Macfarland, D. C. (1966). Social Isolation of the Blind: An Underrated Aspect of Disability and Dependency. *Journal of Rehabilitation, 32,* 32-49.

Mann, M., Hosman, C. M. H., Schaalma, H. P., & de Vries, N. K. (2004). Self-Esteem in a Broad-Spectrum Approach for Mental Health Promotion. *Health Education Research, 19,* 357-372. http://dx.doi.org/10.1093/her/cyg041

van der Pligt, J., & de Vries, N. K. (1998). Expectancy-Value Models of Health Behavior: The Role of Salience and Anticipated affect. *Psychology and Health, 13,* 289-305. http://dx.doi.org/10.1080/08870449808406752

Verstraten, P. F. J., Brinkmann, W. L. J. H., Stevens, N. L., & Schouten, J. S. A. G. (2005). Loneliness, Adaptation to Vision Impairment, Social Support and Depression among Visually Impaired Elderly. *International Congress Series, 1282,* 317-321. http://dx.doi.org/10.1016/j.ics.2005.04.017

Wrosch, C., & Schreier, M. F. (2003). Personality and Quality of Life: The Importance of Optimism and Goal Adjustment. *Quality of Life Research, 12,* 59-72. http://dx.doi.org/10.1023/A:1023529606137

The Effectiveness of Assertiveness Training on Social Anxiety of Health Volunteers of Yazd

Raziyeh Saeed Manesh[1], Sedigheh Fallahzadeh[2*], Mohammad Sadegh Eshagh Panah[2], Naser Koochehbiuki[3], Azam Arabi[1], Mohamad Ali Sahami[1]

[1]Yazd Health Network, Shahid Sadoughi University of Medical Sciences, Yazd, Iran
[2]Abarkouh Health Network, Shahid Sadoughi University of Medical Sciences, Yazd, Iran
[3]Afshar Hospitel, Shahid Sadoughi University of Medical Sciences, Yazd, Iran
Email: *sfallah.eshagh@yahoo.com

Abstract

The aim of this study was to determine the effectiveness of assertiveness training on decreasing social anxiety of health volunteers in Yazd Health Center. Research method was quasi-experimental with pre-test, post-test design by placebo and control groups, in order to measure the dependent variable used with Social Phobia Inventory (SPI). The population of this study was volunteers of Yazd city, 90 subjects were selected by simple random sampling, and then randomly assigned to three groups (experimental, control and placebo) and pre-test was conducted on them. Then, experimental group received assertiveness training in 8 sessions of at most 60 minutes. Placebo group was trained in prevention of different diseases in 8 sessions of at most 60 minutes. After the training period, all three groups were tested (post-test). In order to analyze the data, the analysis of repeated measurements was used. Results indicated that social anxiety scores in the intervention and control groups decreased more than in the placebo group. Result of present study indicates the importance of assertiveness skill training on the social anxiety. Results of this research are convergent with other research.

Keywords

Assertiveness, Social Anxiety, Training, Health Volunteers, Yazd City,
Quasi-Experimental

---

*Corresponding author.

1. Introduction

Today, despite deep cultural changes and changes in lifestyle, many people lack the essential ability in dealing with life issues. This makes them vulnerable in facing the problems of everyday life and its requirements. Many of the health problems as well as mental and emotional disorders have social origins. One way to enhance the psychosocial abilities of individuals is life skills training. The term "life skills" means stabilizing an appropriate and effective interpersonal relationship for doing social responsibility, making right decisions and solving the conflicts without resorting to actions that harm us or others (Rafiee et al., 2009).

On the other hand, assertiveness is the heart of interpersonal behavior and the key of human relations (Lin et al., 2004). Assertiveness (certainty) means that people express their positive and negative emotions without violating the rights of others (Paterson et al., 2002). Assertive people are not afraid of speech. They express their feelings and take the first step. Assertive people have social influences (Powell & Newgent, 2011). Wolpe (1958) was the first one who used the term assertiveness and proposed the principle of mutual inhibition. Assertiveness training aim is to help people change their view about themselves, expressing their beings, moods and thoughts reasonably and improving their self-confidence.

Social anxiety (social phobia) is a prevalent mental disorder with the outbreak rate of 3% - 13% during the lifetime (Mahmoudi et al., 2010). The outbreak rate of 13% of this disorder in society placed it in the third rank of psychiatric disorder after major depression and alcohol dependence (Kessler, Berglund, & Demler, 2005). Patients with this disorder suffer from considerable damages in daily activities, social relationships and work (Reich & Hofmann, 2004). Hertel & Garner (2005) stated that people with social anxiety examined the condition repeatedly and mentally .They imagine the worst and the most negative position before encountering with social situations. First, Salter (1991) tried to treat anxiety using the assertiveness training.

Volunteer health workers are the leaders of public assistance who help people voluntarily in health provision and promotion. Volunteer health workers consider themselves responsible for the problems in their neighborhood. They state the problems to administrate staff and their colleagues and try to solve them. They try to learn the basic facts required for the health of individual, family and community and to have active participation in the learning. Who is better than volunteer health workers for transferring this vital knowledge to the public? After learning the true and profounding health implications, they transfer them to their neighbors in their own language (Fatehi, 2009).

A preventive program which is regarded globally is the assertiveness skill training. Many studies have been conducted about the effect of assertiveness training on social anxiety. Orenstein & his collogues (1975) showed that there was an inverse relationship between assertive behavior and anxiety. Gharib (1992) indicated that assertiveness has an inverse association with anxiety. In association with this research, Vakiliyan et al. (2008) investigated the effects of social skills training on group cognitive-behavioral therapy in the treatment of students' social anxiety. The statistical analysis showed that adding this social skills training to group cognitive-behavioral therapy group decreased the students' social anxiety significantly. Sharifi Rad et al. (2011) showed that there was a significant and inverse relationship between these two factors of academic anxiety and determination.

Therefore, by empowering the individuals with assertiveness skills training, this study is concerned with this question: Is the assertiveness skills training effective for improving the social anxiety of trained volunteer health workers?

2. Materials and Methods

This is a quasi-experimental research with pre-test and post-test of control group and the placebo group. The population in this study consists of all volunteer health workers of Yazd health center in 2011-2012. The sample includes 90 volunteer health workers who were selected by simple random sampling method and divided randomly into three groups (experimental and placebo control) of 30 health workers. Based on researching the objectives, the pre-test was performed for all three groups. Then, the subjects of the study were exposed to the independent variable (assertiveness training). At the end, the effects of assertiveness training on the dependent variables (social anxiety) were measured by the post-test. The experimental group received eight one-hour sessions of assertiveness training. First, each subject was taught by the method of question and answer. Then, some groups were asked to make a story out of the trained issues and play a role in it.

After watching, the rest of the participants examined it critically. At the end, while summarizing the contents of the session, an assignment has been given for the next session. In some cases, the subjects were not regularly attend the sessions. Therefore, the researcher and trainer held the make-up sessions in that week, before the next session to prevent any problem in the process of learning. There was no training for the control group. For the placebo group, 75-minute training was presented on disease prevention by experts fighting against diseases of Health Center of Yazd to neutralize the effect of the experimenter. There was no training for the control group. Immediately after the training sessions, the post-test was performed for all three groups to quantify the impact of training.

The tools that have been used in this study include: the Assertiveness Inventory of Gambrill & Richy (1975) and the Social Phobia Inventory (SPI) (2002).

1) The Assertiveness Inventory of Gambrill & Richy: This questionnaire consists of 40 test items. Each item shows a special occasion that requires assertive behavior .This assertiveness questionnaire has two parts. One section is devoted to measuring the degree or extent of the discomfort. Another part examines the probability of the assertive behavior. In this questionnaire, the respondents were asked to express the extent and severity of their discomfort when they are faced with situations that require assertiveness, based on a rating scale of 5 Choices. The reliability and validity of this scale were reported favorable in several studies (Rahimi et al., 2006). In the present study, the reliability of Assertiveness Inventory of Gambrill & Richy was calculated 0.78 by Cronbach's alpha.

2) The Social Phobia Inventory (SPI): This questionnaire has 38 questions constructed by Mashavi (2002). Some of the questions have been constructed using valid diagnostic criteria and studying the literature on social phobia. Another part of the questions in this questionnaire (15 questions) have been constructed using the Social Phobia Inventory of Jonathan Davidson (Davidson et al., 1997) quoted by Moshaveri (2002). The reliability of the Social Phobia Inventory was calculated 0.69 by Cronbach's alpha.

Trainings were provided as follows:

The topics discussed in the sessions are adapted from "behavior skills" of Mutabi and Otoufi (for adult) (2012) and the training PowerPoint of life skills training workshops for Ph.D. students by Ladan Fanni, Dr. F. Mutabi and M. Kazem Zade Otoufi (2011).

First session: Defining and articulating the need for assertiveness and its benefits in life; Expressing the important aspect of goal setting (for example, the capacity of a person to show an assertive behavior in a special situation).

Second session: Behavioral styles (aggressive, assertive and passive behavior).

Third session: Training the components of each communication style (beliefs, behavior, nonverbal behavior, confrontation and problem solving, emotion and impact that each of these three styles has on others).

Fourth session: Training the importance of assertive behavior.

Fifth session: Training the individual rights.

Sixth session: Training the all kinds of assertive behaviors and how to behave assertively.

Seventh session: Training some recommendations for telling "no" and refusing the unreasonable demands of others. Training specific techniques for difficult situations (strikethrough and disarmament).

Eighth session: Training the negative consequences of assertiveness and increasing assertiveness, discussion and conclusion.

3. Findings

Descriptive findings, regarding the participants, indicated that most of the participants were in the age range of 30 to 39 years and all participants were housewives.

Comparing the three groups scores in the pre-test and post-test, the results is presented in **Table 1**.

The comparison of anxiety mean of groups in pre-test and post-test (**Table 1**) shows the great reduction in the experimental group's mean in post-test. The experimental group's mean was 110.93 at pre-test and 68.50 in post-test. The placebo group's mean was 107.30 at pre-test and 105.26 in post-test. The control group's mean was 106.50 at pre-test and 109.06 in post-test.

The results of the Levine's test for homogeneity of variance assumption were confirmed in two stages: pre-test and post-test (the variances of the dependent variables are equal in two groups). The results of this test showed that the groups were not significantly different. Therefore, to analyze the current hypothesis, the analysis of repeated measurements can be applied. Since the test of homogeneity of covariance matrices was signify-

Table 1. Mean and standard deviation of groups scores in pre-test and post-test on social anxiety.

	Number	Pre-Test		Post-Test	
		Mean	Standard Deviation	Mean	Standard Deviation
Experimental Group	30	110.93	17.36	68.5	16.75
Placebo Group	30	107.3	26.58	105.26	22.56
Control Group	30	106.5	22.79	109.6	22.44
Total	90	108.24	22.39	94.28	27.57

cant, this assumption is confirmed. This result suggests that the analysis of repeated measurements can be applied for analyzing the present hypothesis.

Results of **Table 2** show the difference between steroids ($p < 0.0001$).

There is a significant interaction between time and social anxiety ($p < 0.0001$). The results show that the impact of time on groups' social anxiety is significant. The difference between the scores of social anxiety in both tests is significant. The test power is about 100 percent. The Type II Error is equal to zero.

The findings of **Table 3** show that the tests (pre-test and post-test) had a significant effect on intra-group social anxiety scores. The difference of scores over time is significant. It means that there is some difference between pre-test and post-test. The difference between scores is 20% over time. It means that 20% of the variance in social anxiety scores is related to the difference between the times. There is a significant interaction between time and social anxiety ($p < 0.0001$). The differences between the groups are also significant ($p < 0.0001$). It means that, in some groups, group membership had a significant effect on the results of the test. The effect of group membership (The effect of assertiveness training) by controlling the test with F = 11/13 is significant at $p < 0.0001$. This means that the difference between the three groups; experimental, control and placebo, was significant.

Tukey test was used to determine the significant difference between comparing groups which had a significant F. **Table 4** presented the results of those groups which had a significant difference between their means.

The results show that, in social anxiety scores, there is a significant different between the experimental, placebo and control groups in the level of 0.05. Based on the groups Mean at the post-test, the experimental group social anxiety scores declined compared to two other groups. Therefore, this result shows the effectiveness of the Assertiveness Skills Training on reducing the social anxiety of volunteer health workers.

4. Discussion

The aim of present study is to investigate the effectiveness of assertiveness training on social anxiety of volunteer health workers. Finally, it was shown that the assertiveness training decreases the social anxiety. This finding is compatible with the findings of Ornstin et al., Ghareeb & Ghareeb. (1992), Neisi & Shahni Yeylagh (2001), Mahmoudi Alami et al. (2004), Vakiliyan et al. (2008), Haivand et al. (2009), Kaivand et al. (2009), Sharifi Rad et al. (2011) and Farzaneh & Mojtaba (2011). Thus, studies have shown that the assertiveness training is an efficient method for reducing social anxiety. Changing expectations, beliefs, attitudes, and positive evaluation rather negative assessment, it can provide the causes of social anxiety reduction. People with social anxiety have social avoidance and distress. Social avoidance and distress means abdication of people and having negative feeling in social interactions. Relying on Bandura's social learning theory (Bandura, Adam, & Beyer, 1977), the findings of this hypothesis indicate that human learning is achieved through observation of others' behavior and its consequences. The self-efficacy, as a function of the individual's role, can be strengthened in this way.

Observing the pattern is an obvious issue in observational learning. Without observing the pattern behavior, there will be no acquisition. The pattern can be present in its living form, non-living form, as a film, video or graphic novel. Since the assertiveness skills training methods are based on objective and visual observation, it is a kind of observational learning which is among the most effective methods in behavior learning. It also increases the resistance and struggle against problems and decreases anxiety and psychological problems. One of the reasons of non-assertive problems is the lack of familiarity with individual rights. In other words, if people enjoy the assertiveness skills, they will have better mental health. The consequence of better mental health is

Table 2. MANOVA about the effects of time on social anxiety.

Resources	Effect	Value	F	Significant Level	The Effectiveness	Statistical Power
Time	Follow-Up Effects Wilks Lambda Hotelling Effects Root	0.202	22.03	0	0.2	0.99
		0.798	22.03	0	0.2	0.99
		0.253	22.03	0	0.2	0.99
		0.253	22.03	0	0.2	0.99
Time and Group Membership	Follow-Up Effects Wilks Lambda Hotelling Effects Root	0.347	23.08	0	0.35	1
		0.653	23.08	0	0.35	1
		0.531	23.08	0	0.35	1
		0.531	23.08	0	0.35	1

Table 3. Intra-group and inter-group variance analysis using the repeated measurement for studied groups' social anxiety scores.

Sources of Changes	Effects	Sum of Squares	df	Mean Square	F	Significant Level	The Effectiveness
Inter-Group	The Effect of Test	8778.05	1	8778.05	22.03	0	0.20
	The Effect of Interaction	18391.6	2	9195.08	23.08	0	0.35
	Error	34653.85	87	398.32	-	-	-
Inter-Group	The Effect of Group Membership	12062.18	2	6031.09	11.132	0	0.20
	Error	47133.05	87	541.76	-	-	-

Table 4. Tukey test to determine the significant relationship between the compared groups in social anxiety

Cases of Comparison	Mean	Mean Difference	SD Error	Significant Level
Experimental				
Placebo	68.50105.26	*−16.5667	4.250	0.001
Control	109.06	*−18.0667	4.250	0.001

*$p < 0.05$.

moving toward personal goals and objectives without damaging the other people rights. This reduces social anxiety.

According to Bandura's social learning theory, self-regulation has caused the volunteer health workers to believe themselves and their efficiency. This reduces their social anxiety in social situations. Wilson & Rapee (2006) indicated that people with social anxiety have irrational beliefs such as doing everything perfectly. They think that their minds will be read by others and all people are looking at them. Because of these beliefs, they become nervous and uneasy when they are in social situations. These people, in these sessions, find a sense of competency with the purpose of changing the assessment. Through this experience, their social anxiety will be decreased.

5. Conclusion

The main limitation of this study, which leads to be cautious in generalizing the results, is the fact that the results of this study are related to volunteer health workers of Yazd Health Center. These results cannot be generalized to the entire population. So, it needs to be replicated in other communities. It is worth noting that this study can be used practically such as the use of this program as a non-medical method for the treatment of social anxiety.

References

Bandura, A., Adam, N., & Beyer, J. (1977). Cognitive Processes Mediating Behavioral Change. *Journal of Personality and*

Social Psychology, 35, 125-139. http://dx.doi.org/10.1037/0022-3514.35.3.125

Davidson, J. R. T., Miner, C. M., De Veaugh-Geiss, J., Tupler, L. A., Colket, J. T., & Potts, N. L. (1997). The Brief Social Phobia Scale: A Psychometric Evaluation. *Psychological Medicine, 27,* 161-166. http://dx.doi.org/10.1017/S0033291796004217

Farzaneh, K., & Mojtaba, M. (2011). The Effectiveness of Assertiveness Training on Social Anxiety, Academic Achievement and Social Skills of Students. *Journal of Educational Psychology, Islamic Azad University Tonkabon, 5,* 116-103.

Fatehi, M. (2009). *Training of Health Volunteers for Coaches.* Tehran: Resalat, Ministry of Health and Medical Education.

Ghareeb, A., & Ghareeb, F. (1992). The Relationship between Assertiveness and Anxiety in Emirates (Male/Female) Sample. *Journal of Education, 27,* 1-21.

Haivand, F., Shafi Abadi, A., & Sodani, M. (2009). The Effectiveness of Communication Skills Training on Social Anxiety in First Year High School Male Students in Ahwaz Education District 4. Knowledge and Research in Applied Psychology. Islamic Azad University (Isfahan), 24-1.

Hertel, E., & Garner, J. (2005). Stress Inoculation Training for Social Phobia. New York: Gilford Press.

Kessler, R. C., Berglund, P., & Demler, O. (2005). Lifetime Prevalence and Age-of-Onset Distribution of DSMIV Disorders in the National Comorbidity Survey Replication. *Archives of General Psychiatry, 62,* 593-602. http://dx.doi.org/10.1001/archpsyc.62.6.593

Lin, Y. R., Shiah, I. S., Chang, Y. C., Lai, T. J., Wang, K. Y., & Chou, K. R. (2004). Evaluation of an Assertiveness Training Program on Nursing and Medical Students Assertiveness, Self-Esteem, and Interpersonal Communication Satisfaction. *Nurse Education Today, 24,* 656-665. http://dx.doi.org/10.1016/j.nedt.2004.09.004

Mahmoudi Alami, G., Azimi, H., & Zarghami, M. (2004). The Effectiveness of Assertiveness Training on Anxiety and Assertiveness of Nursing Students. *Journal of Gorgan University of Medical Sciences, 4,* 72-66.

Mahmoudi, M., Gudarzi, M. A., Taghavi, S. M. R., & Rahimi, C. (2010). The Investigation of the Effectiveness of Short-Term Treatment Focusing on Metacognition on the Symptoms of Social Anxiety Disorder. Study of a Single Subject. *Journal of Mental Health, 12,* 41-63.

Moshaveri, A. H. (2002). *The Investigation of the Effectiveness of Group Cognitive-Behavioral Therapy on Symptoms of Social Phobia in a University Freshman Students.* Master's Thesis, University of Esfehan, Esfehan.

Neisi, A. K., & Shahni Yeylagh, M. (2001). The Effectiveness of Assertiveness Training on Self-Esteem, Social Anxiety, and Mental Health of Male High School Students in Ahvaz City. *Journal of Educational Science and Psychology, Martyr Chamran University of Ahvaz, 8,* 11-30.

Orenstein, H., Orenstein, E., & Carr, J. E. (1975). Assertiveness and Anxiety: A Correlational Study. *Journal of Behavior Therapy and Experimental Psychiatry, 6,* 203-207. http://dx.doi.org/10.1016/0005-7916(75)90100-7

Paterson, M., Green, J. M., Basson, C. J., & Ross, F. (2002). Probability of Assertive Behaviour, Interpersonal Anxiety and Self-Efficacy of South African Registered Dietitians. *Journal of Human Nutrition and Dietetics, 15,* 9-17. http://dx.doi.org/10.1046/j.1365-277X.2002.00326.x

Powell, M. L., & Newgent, R. A. (2011). Assertiveness in Mental Health Professionals: Differences between Insight-Oriented and Action-Oriented Clinicians. *The Professional Counselor, 1,* 92-98.

Rafiee, H., Jafari Zadeh, H., Khalil Zadeh, H., Ashraf Rezayi, N., & Mohammadi, B. (2009). The Investigation of the Effectiveness of Life Skills Training on Young Couples Understanding Rate Who Refer to Orumiye Health Center for Marriage Counseling. *Journal of Nursing and Midwifery, 7,* 21-26.

Rahimi, J., Haghighi, J., Mehrabi Zadeh Honarmand, M., & Beshlideh, K. (2006). The Investigation of the Effectiveness of Assertiveness Training on Social Skills, Social Anxiety and Assertiveness in High School Boys. *Journal of Educational Psychology, 13,* 111-124.

Reich, J., & Hofmann, S. G. (2004). State Personality Disorder in Social Phobia. *Annals of Clinical Psychiatry, 16,* 139-144. http://dx.doi.org/10.1080/10401230490486936

Salter, S. (1991). *Conditioned Reflex Therapy.* New York: Farrar, Straus and Giroux.

Sharifi Rad, G., Mohebbi, S., Mottalebi, M., Shah Siyah, M., & Nabrayee, Y. (2011). The Impact of Assertive Training on Students' Academic Anxiety. *Journal of Medical Science, University of Sabzevar, 18,* 82-90.

Vakiliyan, S., Ali Ghanbari Hashem Abadi, B., & Tabatabayi, S. M. (2008). The Effectiveness of Life Skills Training on Group Cognitive-Behavioral Therapy in the Treatment of Social Anxiety in Students. *Journal of Mental Health, 10,* 87-97.

Wilson, J., & Rapee, R. (2006). The Interpretation of Negative Social Events in Social Phobia: Changes during Treatment and Relationship to Outcome. *Behaviour Research and Therapy, 43,* 373-389. http://dx.doi.org/10.1016/j.brat.2004.02.006

Wolpe, J. (1958). *Psychotherapy by Reciprocal Inhibition.* Palo Alto, CA: Stanford University Press.

A One-Session Treatment Protocol for Panic Attacks

Ron Robbins, Jan Parker, Charles Tatum

National University, San Diego, CA, USA
Email: jparker@nu.edu

Abstract

This article describes in detail a one-session treatment protocol for panic attacks as well as the results of two small studies of its efficacy. The treatment protocol, typically completed in 75 - 120 minutes, uses an innovative approach that combines the identification of bodily sensations and specific thoughts as the precursor or "starter" of the panic attack process. The exact treatment approach is described in detail. The results of two small studies using the protocol are analyzed. The results showed that a single session using the treatment approach produced a statistically significant, immediate decline in the reported number of panic attacks that were sustained over time. These results were achieved in two separate sets of subjects utilizing different facilitators. Descriptive information regarding the sample is also provided.

Keywords

Panic Attacks, Treatment, Anxiety Disorders

1. Introduction

This article discusses an innovative treatment approach that utilizes the identification of bodily sensations and specific thoughts to treat panic attacks in one session. The emergence of new treatments for panic attacks has been negligible in recent years (Stirman, Toder, & Crits-Cristoph, 2010). As studies of multiple methods of the treatment of panic attacks all report a significant number of subjects, 29% - 48%, who do not experience a lessening of symptoms, the need for an approach such as the one described in this article is clear (Milrod et al., 2007).

There were two major questions asked in this research project. The first was would the intervention result in a decrease in panic attack frequency? The second question was whether a study with a new facilitator with differences in age, gender and personality style would yield similar results?

Treatment for panic attacks that meets the requirements for Panic Disorder is usually based on Cognitive-Behavioral Treatment (CBT) approaches (Gloucester et al., 2014). The other most common treatment approach is biologic which is comprised of medications designed to lower anxiety. With CBT, the clients' exaggerated thought responses related to bodily experiences that are interpreted inaccurately have been shown to precede a panic attack. Fear of triggering anxiety has also been associated with the onset of a panic attack. Therefore CBT addresses the distorted reactions, beliefs, and sensitivity to the onset of a panic attack. Treatment is usually short-term, comprised of 20 - 24 sessions. Gloucester et al. cite several CBT studies which show that 50% - 80% of clients with Panic Disorder, with or without Agoraphobia, demonstrated improvement. But 5% - 30% of the subjects had a recurrence of symptoms within 12 - 24 months after ending treatment, and the great majority of the subjects had a reduction in panic attacks, without complete remission of the symptoms (White et al., 2012). In the White et al. study, half of the subjects received follow-up CBT for a minimum of 28 - 31 weeks and a maximum of 60 weeks. The subjects who were in the treatment group had a 5.2% relapse rate in comparison to the control group which had an 18.4% relapse rate.

Teachman, Marker, and Clerkin (2010) studied how clients with Panic Disorder attributed physical sensations to mean the onset of a serious medical condition such as a myocardial infarction. They stated that it is the thought process that leads to a panic attack rather than the physical sensation itself that can create panic attacks. This was seen as supporting the efficacy of the CBT approach to Panic Disorder. They assessed four CBT models: "1) Catastrophic misinterpretations and overall panic symptoms...; 2) Catastrophic misinterpretations and panic attack frequency...; 3) Catastrophic misinterpretations and panic-related distress/apprehension...; and 4) Catastrophic misinterpretations and panic-related avoidance" (p. 967). As expected a reduction in catastrophic misinterpretations led to a reduction of symptoms in all four models; however this study did not include long-term follow-up to examine whether the initial results held up over a significant period of time.

Relaxation training, including meditation, has also been studied as an alternative to medication in the treatment of anxiety in both the clinical and non-clinical population (Pagnini, Manzoni, Castelnuovo, & Molinari, 2009). This approach has shown initial positive results and is currently being researched in more detail; however the initial results seem more effective with subjects who do not qualify for a diagnosis of panic disorder. Additionally, Strohle et al. (2005) found that aerobic exercise reduced the number of panic attacks in healthy adults.

The approaches discussed above require multiple therapy sessions to achieve results, and some regression was noted in many subjects (citations). The treatment method described in this article, the Rhythmic Integration Panic Protocol (RIPP), achieved sustainable results in one to two sessions.

A chance occurrence led to the development of the RIPP Project. The first author of this article observed a woman on an airplane beginning to have a panic attack and intervened. He utilized a theory of the process of change he had developed called Rhythmic Integration (Robbins, 1990) and combined this with his knowledge of the meaning of body movements acquired in his training as a somatic bioenergetic psychotherapist. He employed techniques developed out of this background. Specifically, he observed the confluence of the utterance of an emotionally charged statement and the display of unusual body movements that coincided with the utterance. This confluence was described as the "starter" and became a central component of the protocol described below. The woman's panic symptoms subsided and there was no return of them during the balance of the trip. Sometime later he began the RIPP Project, a qualitative study that replicated the results with multiple subjects. This article is a reporting of that study.

2. Method

2.1. Overview of Project

The above protocol was studied utilizing two separate groups of subjects. Group I was facilitated by the first author, the developer of the protocol. Positive results with this group led to the formation of Group II. This second group was facilitated by a different clinician to determine if the initial findings were replicable and not tied to a particular facilitator. The design for both studies used a before and after small n model where repeated measures of panic frequency were gathered.

2.2. Participant Screening

The determination of whether subjects met the DSM-IV diagnostic criteria for panic attacks (American Psychiatric Association [APA], 1994) was done by licensed master's level clinicians using a screening instrument developed by the first author. To qualify for a panic attack the individual had to have at least four symptoms. The range of symptoms comprising the participant's panic attack was from 4 to 20.

Group I consisted of five subjects, three of whom were female and two were male. Group II consisted of eight subjects, seven of whom were female and one male. The age range for all subjects was from 20 - 45. All but one of the subjects had had some form of therapy prior to entering the study.

The majority of the subjects called for treatment based on having read articles or heard radio interviews about the panic project. Subjects also were referred by clinicians who had unsuccessfully tried more traditional forms of treatment with their clients.

In the initial telephone interview the interviewer obtained demographic and information from the client and provided a summary and rationale of the intervention's background, direction, and goals. If the subject seemed interested, a following telephone call done by master's level clinicians would obtain information to determine if the subject met the criteria for the study. These criteria included information about symptomotolgy and frequency of panic attacks, previous therapeutic experience, etc.

2.3. Procedure

The subjects each attended one treatment session which was set in the first author's office for both groups. For both studies the data were gathered over several months. The first study was facilitated by Ronald Robbins, PhD, clinical psychologist and the second study was facilitated by Ann-Marie Jensen, LCSW Licensed Clinical Social Worker. Both facilitators were trained in body-oriented psychotherapy techniques. The facilitators were of different ages, gender, and personality style.

If the client was deemed to have multiple panic attacks, as defined by the RIPP project screening instrument, they were asked if they had any questions. Questions were answered, and if agreement to follow directions was obtained, the first session was scheduled. The typical session was from 75 to 120 minutes, with most lasting less than 90 minutes, and moved through the following steps:

2.4. Treatment Protocol

1) Greeting and Contract: In the first step the client and the facilitator greet each other as equals. The rationale for the intervention being based in the body is explained. The subject is then asked again: "Do you want to have markedly fewer panic attacks, perhaps no more panic attacks?" If the subject answers affirmatively, he is told "For that to happen now, all you need to do is follow the directions given. They will be respectful, safe, and not against any fundamental values you hold. Will you commit to that?" They were also told that "Our method does not induce panic attacks, and to date no one has had one in a session." Once a clear commitment has been given then the next step of the process begins. If the commitment is not made, the reasons for it are discussed in an attempt to allow agreement. If this is unsuccessful, the protocol may not be followed and the subject no longer qualifies to be part of the study.

2) Therapist's Identification of the Starter: Once the commitment is made, the relationship changes in that the facilitator is now giving directions which the client has agreed to follow. The facilitator leads a relaxation process aimed at assisting the client to ease muscular tension, enter a dreamy state, and soften the critical aspect of the ego to allow her to experience a memory. Once this state is achieved, the facilitator asks the subject to imagine the memory of a specific panic attack and to talk about it as if it is happening now. The facilitator listens to the description and looks for the starter which is a combination of an emotionally charged sentence accompanied by a particular kind of unusual body movement (see below).

3) Starter Characteristics and Further Identification: Starters reveal body movements that would be seemingly dangerous if allowed to continue and/or done more extremely. Examples of these types of movements include rolling the eyes up so that the pupils are no longer visible which cuts off vision, and holding the chest in a frozen position which cuts off breathing. In clients with a history of panic attacks, the researchers found that these body movements and an emotionally charged statement or reaction had already been paired. Therefore the facilitator can ask the person to repeat the charged statement as many times as necessary, and each time it will automatically result in the movement. The facilitator can use this pairing to assist the subject in becoming aware of this unconscious body movement. This stage ends when the facilitator has clearly identified the unconscious body movement and the associated sentence.

4) Subject's Identification of the Starter: Once the starter is identified by the facilitator, then the subject is asked to say the charged sentence and the facilitator interrupts the process by asking what the person just did with his body. This leads to some disorganization so that the subject is no longer in the relaxed state and is being asked to do two things that do not fit together naturally. This is repeated as many times as is necessary for the subject to become consciously aware of the body movement. This stage ends once a repeated awareness of the presence of the starter is reported by the subject.

5) Strengthening Awareness of the Starter: The next stage is designed to strengthen the conscious awareness of the starter by the facilitator and subject experimenting with the movement. They may exaggerate the movement, name the movement, or do the movement rapidly or in slow motion, etc. The purpose is to allow the subject and the facilitator to heighten awareness of the movement whenever it happens.

6) Topics of Psycho-education: The subject now becomes excited about the ability to notice the movement and is more open to taking in more information about the process. The facilitator becomes inspired to learn more about the subject's full panic picture. Several types of psycho-education take place during this phase. The subject learns how the fight, flight, or freeze response can be triggered without thought (i.e., physiological responses designed to help with survival are set off without the presence of actual danger). Therefore, the situation is misread by the primitive areas of the brain which react with a host of emergency responses that are intended to support survival. However, there is no real danger present. The emergency responses become symptoms of panic. For example, readiness to run from danger becomes rapid breathing and increased heart rate. In light of this, it's reasonable that one of the symptoms of the panic attack is to think: "I'm going crazy!" It's reasonable, too, that in response to a rapid heartbeat, feelings of choking, and detachment from oneself, fears, and thoughts of dying occur in many subjects.

Other topics often considered during this phase of the session are: How can panic attacks occur while sleeping? How can a panic experience become tied to the environment in which it first occurred leading a sufferer to phobically avoid returning to the setting?

Classical conditioning is explained to the subjects. This stage ends when the subjects begin to reflect on what this means especially to their situation. Inspired, the subject asks: "How can this information help me to change my suffering from frequent panic attacks?" One question leads to others. The doorway opens to a period of analysis.

7) Analyzing: Once the subject begins to analyze his or her own situation, other questions arise. Some typical ones are presented along with their answers.

Question: Are the feelings that come with the starter like the feelings of a panic attack?

Answer: Yes, you notice that they are but with markedly less intensity. The feelings are a shadow of the feelings of panic.

Question: Does the starter's appearance mean an attack will necessarily come?

Answer: No, often the starter will resolve itself on its own. Later in the session specific ways to resolve the starter before an attack occurs will be given.

Questions: Will I always have to be conscious of the starter when it happens?

Answer: No, we will work together to weaken or eliminate the link so that the starter either does not occur at all, or if it happens it is less likely to lead to a panic attack. If it does you will experience that attack differently due to your understanding of what is happening and your ability to stop it using the tools we will give you later in the session.

Question: So what do I do next?

Answer: This is what we will work on now.

8) Solidifying Work: The facilitator advises that change can occur. It will take solid hard work but it can be done. The subject is asked to tell a memory of another panic attack, again "as if it is happening now". This time when the subject catches the starter he or she is to keep repeating it until *on its own* the sentence loses its charge and is no longer accompanied by the starter.

After a few repetitions there is invariably resistance. For example, subjects may consciously suppress the body movement, or they may focus on the reactions of the facilitator rather than on their own. They may say they want to stop because the repetitions are boring. They may say they feel a change in the charge before they actually do.

If they do or say any of these things subjects are informed that some people may need to repeat the charged sentence up to 100 times in order to achieve the result. This, although factious, puts the process in perspective.

Indeed the whole session only lasts 120 minutes. It is hard but not that hard. This reality usually dissolves the resistance with all subjects. They resumed the task and a fuller level of involvement is clearly seen. When necessary for clarity, subjects may be asked to rate the strength of the charge that accompanies the body movement on a scale of 1 to 10, 1 being no charge and 10 being the strongest charge they have had with any panic attack. Once the report of the charge has been reduced to at least a 1 or 2 the facilitator acknowledges the subject's progress. At this point subjects are typically excited about their ability to do something to change the effect of the starter. To further understanding a metaphor of the starter being similar to the starter of a car is used. The starter starts the car but it needs more to move. Similarly with panic attacks the starter readies the subjects for panic to develop but more is needed in the form of catastrophizing sentences or images, or hyper-excited emotionality. If the subjects are able to catch the starter, they can stop the process before the panic attack erupts. Therefore, the subjects are able to see that if the starter can be identified the panic can be avoided.

9) Achieving a Difference: Once the subject obtains the awareness that the starter can be interrupted to prevent a panic attack from occurring, work begins to make this a reality. In this stage clients learn techniques to utilize in the real world that allows them to identify and interrupt the starter even when experiencing a high level of emotion.

In modern society, most people have tension in the head and neck area. The first step in the process is to teach clients images that relax these body zones. It is essential to relax these areas first in order for the subject to make effective use of subsequent images that will be given to effect the tensions related to their starter.

The client is asked to sit upright in a straight backed chair. The facilitator then asks permission from the client to touch the client's head. After permission is granted the facilitator puts one hand on the client's forehead and cups the back of the skull with the other hand and gently rotates the head in all directions. When areas of tension or jerky movements occur, the facilitator repeats the movement that causes it, and asks the client to be aware of what they are sensing. This raises the client's awareness of their tension. Then the facilitator tells the client, "we are going to now work with your imagination in a different way." The facilitator asks the client to close his or her eyes and imagine a horse. The client is asked to tell the facilitator about the horse. This intervention identifies any difficulties the client has working with images, and helps those who protest saying they do not visualize, accept the fact that they imagine even if they do not see anything in their mind's eye.

Once the client is comfortable using the imagination, the facilitator works successively with three images adapted from the work of Todd (1937) and Sweigard (1974) which is designed to relax the tension in the head and neck. The first image asks the client to imagine the neck lengthening upwards. The second image is imagining a cap or shawl sliding smoothly in a continuous movement over the top of the head and down to the eyebrow. The third image is imagining the head as a helium balloon floating straight upwards.

After the client completes the work with the three images, the facilitator asks for permission to again touch the head, moves it in the manner previously described, and asks the client how what is now being experienced is different from what was felt before. The result of this entire process should be an awareness of less constriction, greater ease, and freedom of movement. When the easing of tension does not occur it is invariably because the client rejects the image for some idiosyncratic reason (i.e. "I am not sure what a 'shawl' is"). In such cases, a new image is given, one that suggests the same line of movement. When this is accepted, the desired easing occurs.

The client is now ready to address the specific body tension that activates the starter which has led to the beginning of a panic attack. For example, the eyes roll up into the head. The image could be of the muscles in and around the eyes melting like butter. A different starter might be the chest held in a locked position interfering with the ability to breathe. With this the client might be asked to imagine the ribcage collapsing towards the center of the chest cavity. The use of these images leads to an immediate change in how the client is feeling. When asked to describe the change, the client will report an easing of the tension. With the ability to imagine, the image comes an awareness that the client can now respond in a way that prevents the starter from moving into panic. The client has now achieved choice and autonomy. They can choose whether to have a panic attack or not.

10) Final Phase: The final phase of the protocol calls for a review of the entire session. The facilitator asks the client to describe what has happened. Following this the facilitator provides a review. During this review the facilitator ensures that the client remembers how to identify the starter, how to use the images to ameliorate the starter, and reminds the client of the necessity to practice this for several days until he or she becomes adept at using it whenever it is needed.

3. Results

Two separate studies were conducted. Study 1 had five subjects and Study 2 had eight subjects for a total sample size of 13. **Figure 1** shows the results of reported panic attacks for both studies. **Figure 1** shows that the month prior to the intervention the number of panic attacks ranged from 5 to 26 and the average was quite high (9.6 for Study 1 and 17.6 for Study 2). Following the intervention, the number of panic attacks dropped off precipitously for both study groups (less than one on average for both groups). No matter how many symptoms the participant had the results were the same: large drops in panic attack frequency. The one exception was a participant who had a history of only three panic attacks prior to the intervention. In this case, the number of panic attacks dropped to zero. Despite the small sample size, the statistical analysis was quite robust. Overall, the decline in panic attacks was statistically significant: $F(4, 40) = 35.52$, $p < .001$, MSE = 39.26, eta square = .75. The main effect for the comparison between the different study groups was not significant [$F(1, 10) = 1.93$, $p > .20$, MSE = 3.14, eta square = .16] and the interaction between time and study group was not significant [$F(4, 40) = 3.25$, $p > .08$, MSE = 39.26, eta square = .25]. When contrasting the number of reported panic attacks one-week prior to the intervention with the number of attacks one week after the intervention, the difference was highly significant [$F(1, 10) = 32.89$, $p < .001$, MSE = 59.29, eta square = .77]. All contrasts between the other post-intervention reports (one month, six months, and one year) were not statistically significant ($p > .5$).

Both study groups reported the number of symptoms they experienced prior to the start of the intervention. The first study group reported 12.6 (SD = 4.4) prior symptoms and the second group reported 11.9 (SD = 2.4). The difference in reported symptoms between the two groups was not significant: $F(1, 11) < 1.00$. In addition, there was no significant correlation either between the number of symptoms and the number of prior panic attacks ($r = -.08$, $p > .8$) or between symptoms and number of panic attacks one year later ($r = .23$, $p > .4$).

The participants in Study 2 were also asked a series of background questions related to a) did they experience any balance problems, b) were they on any psychotropic drugs, c) were they currently in therapy, d) had they been in therapy prior to the study, and e) had any relatives experienced panic attacks? **Table 1** summarizes the results from these questions.

Table 1 indicates that all of the subjects were taking psychotropic drugs and the majority was either currently

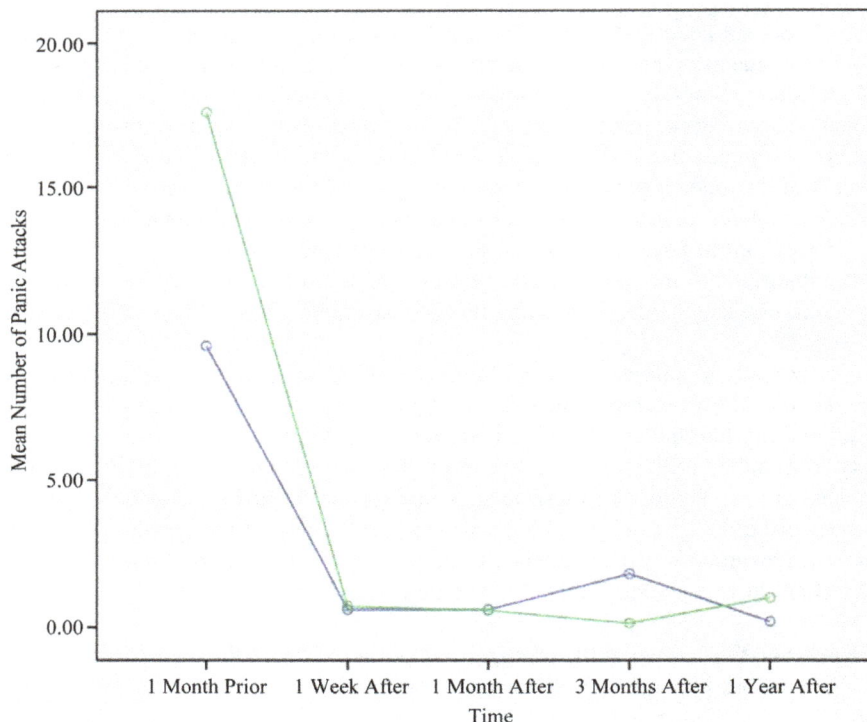

Figure 1. Mean number of reported panic attacks before (1 month prior) and after (1 week, 1 month, 3 months, and 1 year) the intervention.

Table 1. Responses from Study 2 for background questions.

Balance Problems	Psychotropics	In Therapy	Previous Therapy	Relatives with Panic Attacks
No	Yes	Yes	Yes	No
Yes	Yes	Yes	Yes	Yes
No	Yes	No	No	No
No	Yes	Yes	Yes	No
Yes	Yes	No	Yes	
No	Yes	Yes	Yes	No
No	Yes	No	Yes	Yes
Yes	Yes	No	Yes	Yes
37.5% Yes	100% Yes	50% Yes	87.5% Yes	43% Yes

in therapy or had been in therapy prior to the study. About a third had balance problems and over 40 percent of those who responded had relatives who had experienced panic attacks.

4. Discussion

The intervention described in this article clearly produced significant results. Study 1 and Study 2 both show large drops in panic frequency when the number of attacks in the month prior to the study and the number of attacks in the month after the study are compared.

The low level of attacks was maintained when follow-up data were collected during the year after the intervention.

The two major questions asked in this research project were: Would the intervention result in a decrease in panic attack frequency and would a study with a new facilitator with demographic differences yield similar results in the reduction of panic attack frequency. The answer to both of these questions was yes. This seems to indicate that the effect was created by the intervention itself.

4.1. Limitations

The small size of the sample limits the generalization of the study in ways that will be discussed below in the Implications section. Given the consistent effects observed, it is doubtful if a larger number of participants would have altered the findings in any meaningful way. If there had been more participants we could have studied multiple other aspects, such as the effect of gender, age, ethnic background, or having another psychiatric diagnosis.

Another limitation is that the Study 1 subjects were not asked the additional questions posed to the Study 2 subjects. Study 1 can be considered a pilot study (proof of concept). Once it was discovered that the intervention was effective, Study 2 was designed to replicate the effects and provide data about additional variables that describe the sample (e.g., a history of relatives with panic attacks or the use of psychotropic drugs, etc. (see **Table 1**).

The most serious limitation of both studies was the lack of a control group. This has implications for future research.

4.2. Implications

The results of this study support the fact that treatment of panic attacks can be successful in one session. Clinicians treating clients for multiple issues can help the client eradicate panic attacks quickly and then move on to other presenting problems. Mentioning this panic treatment to clients may prompt them to report a history of panic attacks when they come for treatment for other issues. Additionally, because this approach is a single session format, acute health care settings could refer to practitioners who use this model.

Given that one of the important characteristics of this study is that success is attained in a single session, the authors suggest that future research should continue to focus on that goal. A single session sets a standard of simplicity and elegance in research design that can counterbalance much current research which tends to involve costly mega studies with thousands of subjects and multiple locations, researchers and administrators.

Replicating the study described in this article with larger sample sizes and control groups would allow for greater generalization. Controlling for co-existing psychiatric disorders can contribute to understanding the application of this intervention. Including a pre- and post-test battery of psychological tests in future research could assist in assessing whether this approach affects the symptoms of other anxiety-based disorders.

5. Summary and Conclusion

In summary, the treatment approach described in this article demonstrated successful use of a powerful method to eliminate the occurrence of panic attacks. There were two major questions asked in this research project. The first was would the intervention result in a reduction in panic attack frequency? The second was whether a study with a new facilitator with differences in age, gender, and personality style would yield similar results in reducing panic attack frequency? The answer to both of these questions was yes. The affirmative answer to the second question seemed to indicate that the effect was created by the intervention itself and not by other variables such as the age, gender, or personality of the therapist. Suggestions for future research have been made and can contribute to further validation and extension of the use of the treatment protocol. The authors believe that utilizing this approach to treat panic attacks can be extremely beneficial to clients with those symptoms and encourage clinicians to try the method described in the article.

Within the constraints of publication space, an attempt has been made to give as full a presentation of the protocol as possible. Where questions remain unanswered, please email the first author, Ronald Robbins PhD, at rhythmicintegration@gmail.com and place "Panic project request" in the subject line to receive more information.

References

American Psychiatric Association (1994). *Diagnostic and Statistical Manual of Mental Disorders* (4th ed.). Washington, DC: Author.

Gloucester, A., Klotsche, J., Gerlach, A., Hamm, A., Strole, A., Gauggel, S., & Wittchen, H. (2014). Timing Matters: Change Depends on the Stage of Treatment in Cognitive Behavioral Treatment for Panic Disorder. *Journal of Consulting and Clinical Psychology, 82,* 141-153. http://dx.doi.org/10.1037/a0034555

Milrod, B., Leon, A., Busch, F., Rudden, M., Schwalberg, M., Clarkin, J., & Shear, K. (2007). A Randomized Controlled Clinical Trial of Psychoanalytic Psychotherapy for Panic Disorder. *The American Journal of Psychiatry, 164,* 265-272. http://dx.doi.org/10.1176/ajp.2007.164.2.265

Pagnini, F., Manzoni, G., Castelnuovo, G., & Molinari, E. (2009). The Efficacy of Relaxation Training in Treating Anxiety. *The International Journal of Behavioral Consultation and Therapy, 5,* 264-269.

Robbins, R. (1990). *Rhythmic Integration: Finding Wholeness in the Cycle of Change.* Barrytown, NY: Station Hill Press.

Stirman, S., Toder, K., & Crits-Cristoph, P. (2010). New Psychotherapies for Mood and Anxiety Disorders. *Canadian Journal of Psychiatry, 55,* 193-201.

Strohle, A., Feller, C., Onken, M., Godemann, F., Heinz, A., & Dimeo, F. (2005). The Acute Antipanic Activity of Aerobic Exercise. *American Journal of Psychiatry, 162,* 2376-2378. http://dx.doi.org/10.1176/appi.ajp.162.12.2376

Sweigard, L. (1974). *Human Movement Potential: Its Ideokinetic Facilitation.* New York, NY: Harper Row Publishing.

Teachman, B., Marker, C., & Clerkin, E. (2010). Catastrophic Misinterpretation as a Predictor of Symptom Change during Treatment for Panic Disorder. *Journal of Consulting Psychology, 78,* 964-973. http://dx.doi.org/10.1037/a0021067

Todd, M. E. (1937). *The Thinking Body: The Study of the Balancing Forces of Dynamic Man.* Brooklyn, NY: Dance Horizons.

White, K., Payne, L., Gorman, J., Shear, K., Woods, S., Saksa, J., & Barlow, D. (2012). Does Maintenance CBT Contribute to Long-Term Treatment Response of Panic Disorder with or without Agoraphobia? A Randomized Controlled Clinical Trial. *Journal of Consulting and Clinical Psychology, 81,* 47-57. http://dx.doi.org/10.1037/a0030666

Permissions

List of Contributors

Anna Vespa
Department of Neurology, INRCA-IRCCS Italian National Institute of Health and Science on Aging, Ancona, Italy

Maria Velia Giulietti
Unity of Neurology, INRCA-National Institute of Health and Science on Aging, Ancona, Italy

Marica Ottaviani, Olimpia Claudia Rossi, L. Paciaroni and Giuseppe Pelliccioni
Department of Neurology, INRCA-IRCCS National Institute of Health and Science on Aging, Ancona, Italy

R. Spatuzzi
U.O.C. Hospice/Palliative care Departments, A.O.R. San Carlo di Potenza, Italy

F. Merico
Hospice Casa di Betania Palliative Care Center, Lecce, Italy

Guido Gori
Director Day Alzheimer Center "Le Civette", ASL-Florence, Italy

Pietro Scendoni
Department of Rheumatology, INRCA-IRCCS National Institute of Health and Science on Aging, Fermo, Italy

Cristina Meloni
INRCA-IRCCS National Institute of Health and Science on Aging, Ancona, Italy

Wendy Boyd, Alan Foster and Jubilee Smith
School of Education, Southern Cross University, Lismore, Australia

William Edgar Boyd
School of Environment, Science & Engineering, Southern Cross University, Lismore, Australia

Aileen M. Pidgeon and Peta Stapleton
1PhD (Clin) Bond University, Gold Coast, Australia

Stephanie McGrath
Bond University, Gold Coast, Australia

Heidi B. Magya
ARNP, University of Florida, Gainesville, USA

Barbara C. Y. Lo
PhD University of Hong Kong, Hong Kong, China

SeoYoung Lee
GSI, Yonsei University, Seoul, Korea

Choon Khim Teh, Choon Wei Ngo, Rashidatul Aniyah binti Zulkifli, Rammiya Vellasamy and Kelvin Suresh
Melaka Manipal Medical College, Melaka, Malaysia

Murat Altin
Eli Lilly-Turkey, Istanbul, Turkey

Eiji Harada
Lilly Research Laboratories Japan, Eli Lilly Japan K.K., Kobe, Japan

Alexander Schacht and Lovisa Berggren
Eli Lilly and Company, Health Technology Appraisal Group, Bad Homburg, Germany

Daniel Walker
Lilly USA, LLC, Indianapolis, USA

Hector Dueñas
Eli Lilly de México, Mexico City, Mexico

Driss Boudhiba
High Institute of Sport and Physical Education, University of Sfax, Sfax, Tunisia

Najoua Moalla and Yassine Arfa
High Institute of Sport and Physical Education of Ksar Saïd, University of Manouba, Manouba, Tunisia

Noureddine Kridis
Faculty of Humanities and Social Sciences, University of Tunis, Tunis, Tunisia

Aileen M. Pidgeon, Alexandra C. Giufre
Bond University, Gold Coast, Australia

Timo Maljanen and Päivi Tillman
Social Insurance Institution, Helsinki, Finland

Tommi Härkänen, Esa Virtala and Olavi Lindfors
National Institute for Health and Welfare, Helsinki, Finland

Paul Knekt
National Institute for Health and Welfare, Helsinki, Finland

Biomedicum Helsinki, Helsinki, Finland

Borong Zhou, Shuangyan Xie, Jiajia Hu, Xiaofang Sun, Haitao Guan and Yanhua Deng
Department of Neurology, Key Laboratory of Reproduction and Genetics of Guangdong Higher Education Institutes, The Third Affiliated Hospital of Guangzhou Medical University, Guangzhou, China

Peyman Hashemian
Psychiatry and Behavioral Sciences Research Center, Faculty of Medicine, Mashhad University of Medical Sciences, Ibn-e-Sina Hospital, Mashhad, Iran

Amanda L. Schott and Betty Zimmerberg
Department of Psychology and Program in Neuroscience, Williams College, Williamstown, USA

Abdelgadir H. Osman
Department of Psychiatry, Faculty of Medicine University of Khartoum, Khartoum, Sudan

Taissier Y. Hagar and Abdelaziz A. Osman
Formerly Registrar in Sudan Medical Council, Currently Specialists in Saudi Arabia

Hussein Suliaman
Khartoum Neuropsychiatric Centre, Khartoum, Sudan

Teck Hwee Soh, Leslie Lim and Herng Nieng Chan
Department of Psychiatry, Singapore General Hospital, Singapore

Yiong Huak Chan
National University Health System, Singapore

Sei Ogawa, Risa Imai, Masaki Kondo and Tatsuo Akechi
Department of Psychiatry and Cognitive-Behavioral Medicine, Nagoya City University Graduate School of Medical Sciences, Nagoya, Japan

Toshi A. Furukawa
Department of Health Promotion and Human Behavior, Kyoto University Graduate School of Medicine/School of Public Health, Kyoto, Japan

Morteza Alibakhshi Kenari
Martyr Beheshti University of Medical Sciences and Health Services, Tehran, Iran

Mohammad Tajfard
Health Sciences Research Center, Department of Health and management, School of Health, Mashhad University of Medical Sciences, Mashhad, Iran
Department of Community Health, Faculty of Medicine and Health Sciences, Universiti Putra Malaysia, Serdang, Selangor, Malaysia

Latiffah A. Latiff and Rosliza A. Manaf
Department of Community Health, Faculty of Medicine and Health Sciences, Universiti Putra Malaysia, Serdang, Selangor, Malaysia

Majid Ghayour-Mobarhan
Cardiovascular Research Center, School of Medicine, Mashhad University of Medical Sciences, Mashhad, Iran

Hamid Reza Rahimi, Farzaneh Tajfiroozeh and Ramin Nazeminezhad
Student Research Committee, Department of Modern Sciences & Technologies, School of Medicine, Mashhad University of Medical Sciences, Mashhad, Iran

Mohsen Mouhebati and Homa Falsoleyman
Department of Cardiology, School of Medicine, Mashhad University of Medical Sciences, Mashhad, Iran

Habibollah Esmaeily and Ali Taghipour
Health Sciences Research Center, Department of Biostatistics, School of Health, Mashhad University of Medical Sciences, Mashhad, Iran

Gordon A. A. Ferns
Brighton & Sussex Medical School, Falmer, Brighton, UK

Nagmeh Mokhber
Departemet of Psychiatry, School of Medicine, Mashhad University of Medical Sciences, Mashhad, Iran

Ahmad Fazli Abdul Aziz
Department of Medicine, Faculty of Medicine and Health Sciences, University Putra Malaysia, Serdang, Selangor, Malaysia

Zahra Saghiri
Department of Biology-Biochemistry, Faculty of Science, Payame Noor University of Mashhad, Mashhad, Iran

Parichehr Hanachi
Faculty of Science, Biology Department, Biochemistry Unit, Alzahra University, Tehran, Iran

Sorin Saketi and Maryam Bananej
Biology Department, Faculty of Biological Sciences, Islamic Azad University, North Tehran Branch, Tehran, Iran

Mahsa Hadipour Jahromy
Medical Sciences Research Centre, Tehran Medical Sciences Branch, Islamic Azad University, Tehran, Iran

Isabel Serrano Pintado
Department Personalidad, Evaluación y Tratamiento Psicológico, Facultad de Psicología, Universidad de Salamanca, Salamanca, España

María del Camino Escolar Llamazares
Department Personalidad, Evaluación y Tratamiento Psicológico, Facultad de Humanidades y Educación, Universidad de Burgos, Burgos, España

Kaberi Majumder
Department of Orthodontics, SGT Dental College, Gurgaon, India

Shalender Sharma, Dayashankara Rao JK, Vijay Siwach, Varun Arya and Sunil Gulia
Department of Oral and Maxillofacial Surgery, SGT Dental College, Gurgaon, India

Valerie L. Alexander and B. Charles Tatum
Department of Psychology, National University, San Diego, USA

Pierluigi Diotaiuti, Filippo Petruccelli, Luigi Rea, Angelo Marco Zona and Valeria Verrastro
Department of Human, Social and Health Sciences, University of Cassino and South Latium, Cassino, Italy

Raziyeh Saeed Manesh, Azam Arabi and Mohamad Ali Sahami
1Yazd Health Network, Shahid Sadoughi University of Medical Sciences, Yazd, Iran

Sedigheh Fallahzadeh and Mohammad Sadegh Eshagh Panah
Abarkouh Health Network, Shahid Sadoughi University of Medical Sciences, Yazd, Iran

Naser Koochehbiuki
Afshar Hospitel, Shahid Sadoughi University of Medical Sciences, Yazd, Iran

Ron Robbins, Jan Parker and Charles Tatum
National University, San Diego, CA, USA